WITHDRAWN FROM STOCK

Adverse Drug Reactions

100540470

Adverse Drug Reactions

Second edition

Edited by

Anne Lee

MPhil, MRPharmS

Principal Pharmacist
National Services Scotland
Glasgow, UK

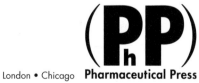

London • Chicago **Pharmaceutical Press**

100540 470
Rm
302.5
.L44

Published by the Pharmaceutical Press
Publications division of the Royal Pharmaceutical Society of Great Britain

1 Lambeth High Street, London SE1 7JN, UK
100 South Atkinson Road, Suite 200, Grayslake, IL 60030-7820, USA

© Pharmaceutical Press 2006

First edition published 2001
Second edition published 2006
Reprinted 2007

Typeset by Gray Publishing, Tunbridge Wells, Kent
Printed in Great Britain by TJ International, Padstow, Cornwall

ISBN   0 85369 601 2

All rights reserved. No part of this publication may be reproduced, stored in a retrieval system, or transmitted in any form or by any means, without the prior written permission of the copyright holder.

The publisher makes no representation, express or implied, with regard to the accuracy of the information contained in this book and cannot accept any legal responsibility or liability for any errors or omissions that may be made.

A catalogue record for this book is available from the British Library

For all my family

Contents

Preface

Adverse drug reactions continue to be an important public health issue, causing considerable patient harm and creating a burden on limited healthcare resources.

The safe use of medicines is a critical issue for all healthcare professionals, including prescribers, pharmacists and nurses, as well as regulatory authorities, the pharmaceutical industry and the public. There is a vast published literature on adverse reactions, and this book does not attempt to summarise it. Instead, it is intended as a resource for students and healthcare professionals who want to know more about the subject. There is a brief introduction, three new chapters (since the first edition) reviewing side effects and patients, pharmacogenetics and adverse reactions, and adverse reactions in pregnancy, followed by 12 revised chapters on reactions affecting particular organ systems. We have concentrated on the most common types of reaction, how to recognise them, and on the medicines most often implicated. Where possible we have tried to give practical guidance on the most appropriate management of suspected adverse drug reactions. We hope the book will be useful to healthcare professionals doing their best to ensure the safe use of medicines in their patients.

Anne Lee
September 2005

Acknowledgements

Thanks to all the contributors who have willingly given their time to write and update material for this edition. Time is precious, and no-one has much to spare for ventures such as this – I couldn't have done it without them. Thanks also to contributors from the first edition who have allowed their work to be updated. I am indebted to Paul Weller, Louise McIndoe and colleagues at Pharmaceutical Press for their continued support and encouragement.

About the editor

Anne Lee graduated in 1984 with a BSc in pharmacy from Heriot Watt University in Edinburgh, and went on to do her preregistration year at the Royal Infirmary of Edinburgh. In 1986 she took up a post at the Regional Drug Information Centre in the Wolfson Unit at the University of Newcastle upon Tyne, which is also a CSM Regional Monitoring Centre for adverse drug reactions. During her time there, working with Professor Sir Michael Rawlins, Dr Jim Smith, Dr Robin Ferner and Dr Nick Bateman, she became interested in adverse drug reactions. She researched aspects of causality assessment in adverse reactions for an MPhil, and was later involved in the Northern Region's successful pilot of hospital pharmacist reporting via the yellow card scheme. In 1996 Anne moved to a post in Medicines Information at Glasgow Royal Infirmary, where she maintained an interest in adverse drug reactions. She is currently a member of the CSM Scotland's advisory board. In 2005 she took up a post as Principal Pharmacist with National Services Scotland, working for the Scottish Medicines Consortium.

Contributors

Kwame N. Atuah
Research Pharmacist, Department of Pharmacology and Therapeutics, University of Liverpool, Liverpool

D Nicholas Bateman
Medical Director, CSM Scotland, Royal Infirmary of Edinburgh, Edinburgh

Keith Beard
Consultant Physician, Victoria Infirmary, South Glasgow University Hospitals, Glasgow

Karen Belton
Senior Manager, Global Safety, Amgen Ltd, Cambridge

Dianne Berry
Professor of Psychology and PVC for Research, University of Reading, Reading

Aileen Currie
Senior Pharmacist, Crosshouse Hospital, Kilmarnock, Ayrshire

Ewan Forrest
Consultant Gastroenterologist, Glasgow Royal Infirmary, North Glasgow University Hospitals, Glasgow

Karen Fraser
Principal Pharmacist – Mental Health, Pharmacy Department, Ailsa Hospital, Ayr

Donald G Grosset
Consultant Neurologist and Senior Lecturer, Institute of Neurological Sciences, South Glasgow University Hospitals, Glasgow

Sharon Hems
Formulary Pharmacist, Pharmacy Department, St Johns Hospital
at Howden, Livingston, West Lothian

Sheena Kerr
Principal Pharmacist, Medicines Information,
Royal Infirmary of Edinburgh, Edinburgh

Peter Knapp
Lecturer, School of Healthcare, University of Leeds, Leeds

Fiona MacLean
Principal Pharmacist, Cancer Care, Southern General Hospital,
South Glasgow University Hospitals, Glasgow

Patricia McElhatton
Consultant Teratologist, Head of NTIS, Lecturer in Reproductive
Toxicology, National Teratology Information Service, Wolfson
Unit, Newcastle upon Tyne

Moira McMurray
Senior Pharmacist, National Services Scotland, Glasgow

Fiona Needleman
Lead Pharmacist, Medicines Information, Southern General Hospital,
South Glasgow University Hospitals, Glasgow

Munir Pirmohamed
Professor of Clinical Pharmacology/Consultant Physician,
Department of Pharmacology and Therapeutics,
University of Liverpool, Liverpool

Christine Randall
Senior Pharmacist, North West Medicines Information Centre,
Liverpool

DK Theo Raynor
Professor of Pharmacy Practice, School of Healthcare,
University of Leeds, Leeds

John Thomson
Consultant Dermatologist, Drumbreck, Glasgow

W Stephen Waring
Consultant Physician and Senior Lecturer, Scottish Poisons
Information Bureau, Royal Infirmary of Edinburgh, Edinburgh

Janice Watt
Principal Pharmacist, Clinical Effectiveness, Glasgow Royal
Infirmary, North Glasgow University Hospitals, Glasgow

1

Introduction

Keith Beard and Anne Lee

Adverse drug reactions (ADRs) are important. They should be considered in the differential diagnosis of a wide range of conditions, as any bodily system can be affected and any disease process mimicked. An adverse drug reaction is an unwanted or harmful reaction experienced after the administration of a drug or combination of drugs under normal conditions of use and suspected to be related to the drug. Box 1.1 shows some commonly used adverse drug reaction terms and definitions. The safe use of medicines is a critical issue for doctors, pharmacists, nurses, regulatory authorities, the pharmaceutical industry and the public. Although prescribers aim to use medicines that help patients and do no harm, no drug is administered without risk. Healthcare professionals have a responsibility to their patients, who themselves are becoming more aware of problems associated with drug therapy. It is essential that all involved have some knowledge of the potential adverse effects of medicines. The main challenge is to prevent the occurrence of ADRs; to do this effectively requires an assessment of the balance between benefits and harms, taking into account the strength or quality of the evidence.[1] It is also important to be aware of the patient groups that are predisposed to drug toxicity. The key to appropriate management of ADRs is prompt recognition that the patient's new symptoms and signs may be drug related. This chapter provides an overview of the problem, focusing on the epidemiology, mechanisms, susceptible patient groups and the main systems used for detection.

ADRs have been known to cause significant morbidity and mortality for centuries.[2,3] In 400BC Hippocrates recommended that drugs should never be prescribed unless the patient had been thoroughly examined. In 1785, when William Withering described the benefits of digitalis, he also identified almost all its adverse effects and demonstrated how its toxicity could be minimised by careful dose titration.[4] With the development of new synthetic drugs in the early 20th century, governments became involved in some aspects of medicines control. In 1922, the Medical Research Council carried out a formal inquiry into jaundice following the use of arsenic to treat syphilis. In the United States, the

---

Box 1.1   Some adverse drug reaction terms and their definitions

Unexpected adverse reaction
An adverse reaction, the nature or severity of which is not consistent with domestic labelling or market authorisation, or expected from characteristics of the drug.

Serious adverse effect
Any untoward medical occurrence that at any dose results in death, requires hospital admission or prolongation of existing hospital stay, results in persistent or significant disability/incapacity, or is life-threatening.
* Cancers and congenital anomalies or birth defects should be regarded as serious.
* Medical events that would be regarded as serious if they had not responded to acute treatment should also be considered serious.
* The term 'severe' is often used to describe the intensity (severity) of a medical event, as in the grading 'mild', 'moderate', and 'severe'; thus a severe skin reaction need not be serious.

Adverse event/adverse experience
Any untoward occurrence that may present during treatment with a pharmaceutical product but which does not necessarily have a causal relationship to the treatment.

Signal
Reported information on a possible causal relationship between an adverse event and a drug, the relation being previously unknown or incompletely documented.
    Usually more than a single report is required to generate a signal, depending on the seriousness of the event and the quality of the information.

Source: Edwards IR, Aronson JK. Adverse drug reactions: definitions, diagnosis and management. *Lancet* 2000; 356: 1255–1259.

Food, Drug and Insecticide Administration (later the Food and Drug Administration) was established in 1927. It was the thalidomide disaster in the early 1960s, with the discovery of a large number of cases of phocomelia (a major congenital limb defect) in infants exposed *in utero*, that provided the catalyst for the development of drug safety legislation worldwide. In 1963, the UK Committee on Safety of Drugs was formed and the following year it established the world's first adverse drug reaction reporting system. In 1971 this became the Committee on Safety of Medicines (CSM). It has recently been announced that the CSM's functions will in future be undertaken by a new body, the Commission for Human Medicines.

Epidemiology

Many investigators have studied the incidence of ADRs in a variety of settings. The estimates of incidence in these studies vary widely, and this reflects differences in the methodologies used to detect suspected reactions, including differences in the definition of an ADR. Nevertheless, several key studies in the 1960s helped establish the epidemiological basis of drug-induced disease.[5–10] The Boston Collaborative Drug Surveillance Program (BCDSP) had a great impact in this field;[11] those investigators collected data on consecutive patients admitted to medical wards over a 10-year period. During that time, information was collected on over 50 000 patients, allowing much original research on the association between short-term drug exposures and acute ADRs to be carried out. In an interim analysis of 19 000 patients monitored, there were approximately 171 000 drug exposures and an adverse reaction rate of 30%.[12] Many ADRs were, however, minor, and the author concluded that drugs were 'remarkably non-toxic'. Detailed analysis of the data provided much information on patient characteristics predisposing to ADRs, and allowed some established adverse effects, such as excessive drowsiness or 'hangover' with flurazepam, to be quantified.[13,14]

The Harvard Medical Practice study showed that 3.7% of 30 195 patients admitted to acute hospitals in 1984 experienced adverse events.[15] Further data from this group suggested a 6% incidence of adverse drug events (ADEs) and a 5% incidence of potential ADEs among 4031 medical and surgical admissions over a 6-month period.[16] (Note that these investigators studied ADEs, a classification that included overdose and medication error). Of all events observed 1% were fatal, 12% life-threatening, 30% serious and 57% significant. Twenty-eight percent of observed ADEs, were considered preventable, with a greater proportion of the life-threatening and serious reactions in that category. The drug classes most frequently implicated were analgesics, antibiotics, sedatives, cytotoxics, cardiovascular drugs, anticoagulants, antipsychotics, antidiabetics and electrolytes. Another US study in hospital inpatients in 1992 found a similar frequency and type of adverse events to those observed in the Harvard study.[17] Data on nearly 15 000 patients discharged from 28 hospitals in two US states identified adverse events (not necessarily drug related) associated with 2.9% of hospitalisations. ADRs were the second most common type of adverse event, accounting for 19% of those identified. Antibiotics, cardiovascular agents, analgesics and anticoagulants were the drugs most commonly implicated. More than a third of these ADRs were considered avoidable, and nearly 1 in 10 caused irreversible harm. UK data from the mid 1990s suggested that 7% of over 20 000 medical inpatients experienced an ADR during their hospital stay.[18]

ADRs are responsible for a significant number of hospital admissions, with reported rates ranging from 0.3% to 11%.[19,20] Data from meta-analyses and systematic reviews suggest that the rate of admissions directly due to ADRs is 5%.[21–23] Recent work has suggested that many of these reactions are predictable and preventable.[24] Pirmohamed *et al.* undertook a prospective analysis of admissions caused by ADRs in two UK hospitals to define prevalence and outcome and to assess causality and preventability.[25] All adult patients admitted over a 6-month period were assessed to determine whether the admission had been caused by an ADR (according to the definition of Edwards and Aronson[22]). Patients were categorised as having an ADR if the cause of admission was consistent with the known adverse-effect profile of the drug; if there was a temporal relationship with the start of drug therapy; and if, after appropriate investigations, other causes were excluded. Causality assessment was carried out for all cases using two published methods. The avoidability of ADRs was assessed using the definitions developed by Hallas *et al.* (Box 1.2).[26] The main outcome measures were the prevalence of admissions due to an ADR, length of stay, avoidability and patient outcome.

There were 18 820 admissions over the 6-month period; 1225 of these were related to an ADR, giving a prevalence of 6.5% (95% confidence interval (CI) of 6.2–6.9%). Eighty percent of the ADRs were judged to have been directly responsible for the admission (termed causal),

---

Box 1.2 Avoidability of adverse drug reactions

Definitely avoidable – the ADR was due to a drug treatment procedure inconsistent with current knowledge of good medical practice.

Possibly avoidable – the ADR could have been avoided by an effort exceeding the obligatory demands of current knowledge of good medical practice.

Unavoidable – the ADR could not have been avoided by any reasonable means.

Source: Hallas J, Harvald B, Gram LF *et al*. Drug related hospital admissions: the role of definitions and intensity of data collection, and the possibility of prevention. *J Intern Med* 1990; 228: 83–90.

and 20% were identified through screening (termed coincidental). Patients admitted with ADRs (median age 76 years, interquartile range 65–83) were significantly older than those without ADRs (66 years, 46–79; 95% CI for difference 8 years to 10 years, $P < 0.0001$). Although most patients admitted with ADRs recovered, 28 (2.3%) died as a result of the ADR. The overall fatality rate was 0.15%. Only 340 (28%) of the 1225 ADR-related admissions were assessed as unavoidable, whereas 107 (9%) and 773 (63%) were classified as 'definitely avoidable' and 'possibly avoidable', respectively. Drug interactions accounted for 16.6% (15–19%) of ADRs. The most common reaction was gastrointestinal bleeding. The majority of the drugs commonly implicated as a cause of ADRs (non-steroidal anti-inflammatory drugs, diuretics, warfarin, digoxin, opioids) are consistent with the results of previous studies.[15,17] Aspirin was the suspect drug in 218 (18%) of 1225 patients, of whom 74% were taking a dose of 75 mg daily.

For ADRs occurring in the community, the reported incidence ranges from 2.6% to 41% of patients, but this is a much more difficult area to study and there are fewer well-designed studies.[12,27,28] Gandhi *et al.*[29] carried out a prospective cohort study in an ambulatory primary care setting in Boston, USA. Of 661 patients who responded to a telephone survey (response rate 55%), 162 described experiencing ADEs (25%; 95% CI 20–29%), with a total of 181 events. Twenty-four of the events (13%) were serious, 51 (28%) were ameliorable, and 20 (11%) were preventable. None was fatal or life-threatening. Of the 51 ameliorable events, 32 (63%) were attributed (by independent physicians) to the prescribing doctor's failure to respond to medication-related symptoms and 19 (37%) to the patient's failure to inform the prescriber of the symptoms. The most frequent types of ADE were central nervous system, gastrointestinal and cardiovascular disorders. The medications most frequently implicated were selective serotonin reuptake inhibitors (SSRIs) (10%), beta-blockers (9%), angiotensin-converting enzyme inhibitors (8%), and non-steroidal anti-inflammatory agents (8%). The authors concluded that ADEs in primary care are common and that many are preventable or ameliorable. Acting on early signs or symptoms and striving towards better communication were identified as important issues.

Gurwitz *et al.*[30] carried out a cohort study to assess the incidence and preventability of ADEs in elderly people in the ambulatory care setting in the USA. The study involved members of a New England health maintenance organisation aged 65 years and over (equivalent to 30 397 person-years of observation). Over a 1-year period possible drug-related incidents were studied using several methods, including discharge summaries, review of clinic and emergency department notes, and review of hospital discharge summaries. There were 1523 identified adverse events, of which 421 (27.6%) were considered preventable and 578 (38%) were categorised as serious, life-threatening or fatal. The classes of medication most frequently implicated were cardiovascular medicines, diuretics, non-opioid analgesics, antidiabetics and anticoagulants.

ADRs also have a significant impact on healthcare costs. Two US case–control studies have shown that the hospital stay was significantly longer in patients who experienced an ADR while in hospital.[31,32] Both studies estimated direct costs associated with ADRs and, not surprisingly, concluded that such costs may be substantial. Classen *et al.*[31] estimated that the occurrence of an ADR increased the cost of patient care by $2262 per patient. Bates *et al.*[32] estimated the cost of preventable ADRs in a 700-bed hospital to be $2.8 million per annum. In their recent UK study, Pirmohamed *et al.*[25] found that the median bed stay in patients with drug-related admissions was eight days, accounting for 4% of the hospital bed capacity. The authors estimated that, if these findings were extrapolated across the NHS in England, at any one time the equivalent of up to seven 800-bed hospitals would be occupied by patients admitted with ADRs. The projected annual cost of such admissions to the NHS was £466 m (€706 m, $847 m).

These recent studies from US primary care and UK hospitals demonstrate that ADRs remain a significant cause of patient harm. Recent studies have adopted more robust methodologies, so problems due to inconsistencies about the definition of an ADR the seriousness or avoidability of reactions are less of an issue than with earlier studies (although minor transatlantic differences in definitions persist). The burden of ADRs on healthcare is clearly high, accounting for considerable morbidity, mortality, and extra costs. The high proportion of ADRs classified as avoidable in recent studies suggests that inappropriate prescribing is common. It has been suggested that, if Pirmohamed's findings were extrapolated to the rest of England, drug-induced hospital admissions would be responsible for 5700 deaths every year (about twice the annual number of deaths from road traffic accidents).[25]

Measures need to be put into place to reduce the burden of ADRs and further improve the benefit–harm ratio of medicines. The imperative to reduce the number and severity of ADRs is a shared responsibility, presenting a considerable challenge to doctors, pharmacists and nurses.

Classification and mechanisms

ADRs have traditionally been classified into two broad categories.[33]

Type A ('augmented') reactions

Type A reactions include normal and augmented, but undesirable, responses to the drugs in question. They include an exaggerated therapeutic response at the target site (e.g. hypoglycaemia with a sulphonylurea), a desired pharmacological effect at another site (e.g. headache with GTN), and secondary pharmacological effects (e.g. orthostatic hypotension with a phenothiazine). Type A reactions are usually dose dependent and predictable, and are often recognised before a drug is marketed. However, some effects occur after a long latency, such as carcinogenesis or effects on reproduction. An example is vaginal adenocarcinoma in the daughters of women exposed to diethylstilbestrol during pregnancy. Many type A reactions have a pharmacokinetic basis, e.g. impaired hepatic metabolism (due to a genetic polymorphism or the effect of another concurrent medication), leading to increased plasma concentrations.

Type B reactions

Type B reactions are unrelated to the known pharmacological actions of the drugs in question. These reactions are often caused by immunological and pharmacogenetic mechanisms. Type B reactions are generally unrelated to dosage and, although comparatively rare, they are more likely to cause serious illness or death. Immunologic reactions such as anaphylaxis with penicillins fall into this category. Other examples include aplastic anaemia with chloramphenicol and malignant hyperthermia with anaesthetic agents. Because of their nature, type B reactions are more likely to result in withdrawal of marketing authorisation.

The main differences between type A and B reactions are shown in Table 1.1.

Although this classification is simple, some adverse reactions do not fit neatly into one type. Additional categories of ADR have subsequently been suggested,[22] to include type C (chronic), type D (delayed) and type E (end of use) reactions. Use of this extended classification does not mitigate all difficulties, however, and a new system has recently been proposed.[34] This takes into account properties of both the reaction and the affected individual, as well as those of the drug itself. The three-dimensional classification system, known as DoTS, is based on dose relatedness, time

Table 1.1 Characteristics of type A and type B reactions

Type A	Type B
Predictable	Unpredictable
Usually dose dependent	Rarely dose dependent
High morbidity	Low morbidity
Low mortality	High mortality
Responds to dose reduction	Responds to drug withdrawal

course and susceptibility. It may have some advantages over previous classifications.

The mechanisms of many ADRs are unknown. Known mechanisms are predominantly pharmacological or immunological.[35] Pharmacological ADRs can be an inevitable consequence of the therapeutic action of the drug (direct effects) or can occur when a drug exerts its action at a receptor or locus that is also present elsewhere ('collateral effects'). For example, the collateral effects of broad-spectrum antimicrobials can alter the bowel flora and increase the risk of *Clostridium difficile* overgrowth, culminating in pseudomembranous colitis. Many ADRs, including classic type 1 hypersensitivity reactions such as penicillin allergy, have an immunological basis. These reactions are generally classified into the four types of Coombs and Gell (see Chapter 5).

Susceptibility

The main factors that can influence the chance of patients experiencing an ADR are discussed below.

Age

The very old and the very young are more susceptible to ADRs. The elderly often have multiple and chronic diseases, and so generally consume large amounts of medicines. They are particularly vulnerable to adverse effects because of the physiological changes that accompany ageing. Most studies have shown a positive correlation between age and the number of ADRs, but this is a complex issue.[13,36–39] It is difficult to determine whether age alone renders these patients more susceptible to ADRs or whether this simply reflects increased drug exposure, multiple disease states and age-related pharmacokinetic changes. Not surprisingly, sick patients who have several diseases, receive many drugs and stay in hospital for longer, are more prone to ADRs. In such patients age has not been shown to be an independent predictor.[40] There is, however, evidence that age-related pharmacodynamic changes make the elderly more sensitive to the effects of some drugs.[41] Adverse reactions in elderly patients often present in a vague, non-specific fashion. Mental confusion, constipation, hypotension and falls may be the presenting features of illness, but may also suggest ADRs. Drugs that commonly cause problems in elderly patients include hypnotics, diuretics, non-steroidal anti-inflammatory drugs, antihypertensives, psychotropics and digoxin.[42–44] The list has remained remarkably constant.

All children, and particularly neonates, differ from adults in the way they handle and respond to drugs. In studies that have investigated the characteristics of ADRs specifically in children the reported incidence has varied considerably. This partly reflects the limited amount of high-quality research in the paediatric age group, but also the wide variations in study setting, patient group, and definition of adverse reaction used. A meta-analysis of observational studies on the incidence of ADRs in children in different healthcare settings has recently been published.[45] In hospitalised children the overall incidence of ADRs was 9.53%; severe reactions accounted for 12.29% of the total. The overall rate of paediatric hospital admissions due to ADRs was 2.09%; 39.3% of these were life-threatening. For outpatient children the overall incidence of ADRs was 1.46%.

These rates are broadly similar to the findings of systematic reviews and meta-analyses of studies focusing on adult patients (although the rate of drug-induced hospital admissions is somewhat lower than in adult studies).[20,21,23] However, the high proportion of severe ADRs in the hospital setting gives significant cause for concern (these are higher than the corresponding figures in studies in adults). Some studies reviewed suggested that the risk of ADRs associated with the use of unlicensed or off-label drug use may be greater than the corresponding risks for licensed medicines.[46] As in adults, polypharmacy was found to be a consistent risk factor for ADRs.

A review of all reports of suspected ADRs with a fatal outcome in children under 16 years received by the CSM from 1964 to 2000 showed that 331 deaths had been reported with 390 suspected medicines.[47] Limited conclusions can be drawn from a study based on data from a voluntary reporting scheme, but the study provides some insight into the drugs suspected of having caused deaths in children. The classes of medicine most frequently associated with fatalities were antiepileptics, cytotoxic agents, anaesthetic gases and antibiotics. The nature of the reported ADRs was diverse, with hepatic failure the most frequent.

Some medicines are particularly likely to cause problems in neonates but are generally well tolerated in older children, e.g. morphine. Others are associated with an increased risk of problems in children of any age, e.g. sodium valproate. Hazardous drugs for neonates include chloramphenicol, morphine and antiarrhythmics.[48] Specific examples of concern in children are Reye's syndrome with aspirin, and hepatotoxicity with sodium valproate.[49]

Gender

In general, women appear to be at greater risk of ADRs than men. Female patients appear to have a 1.5–1.7-fold greater risk of developing an ADR[50] than male patients. The reasons for this are not entirely clear, but include gender-related differences in pharmacokinetic, immunological and hormonal factors, as well as differences in the pattern of medicines use. Women are reputed to be more susceptible to blood dyscrasias with phenylbutazone and chloramphenicol,[51] to histaminoid reactions to neuromuscular blocking drugs,[52] and to drug-induced prolongation of the QT interval.[53]

Intercurrent disease

Drug handling may be altered in patients with renal, hepatic and cardiac disease, and this has implications for practical therapeutics. When faced with a possible ADR, one may have difficulty in attributing causality in view of other diseases and alternative explanations for the observed event. There are, however, specific disease states that may predispose to ADRs. HIV-positive patients suffer an increased rate of skin reactions with co-trimoxazole, antiretroviral drugs and other medicines.[54–56] Infectious mononucleosis (due to the Epstein–Barr virus) greatly increases the risk of rash in patients given amoxicillin. Immune deficiency is a complex clinical area with multiple drug exposures, multiple illness events, and consequent difficulty in interpreting drug toxicity data.

Abnormal metabolism and response to drugs

There is great variation in how the body handles and metabolises drugs. The dose required to produce a given pharmacological effect varies between individuals, as does the response to a defined dose. Patients with decreased hepatic or renal function may show considerable changes in drug disposition, leading to ADRs unless dose adjustments are made. Even in a normal population there may be great variation in drug metabolism because of genetic and environmental influences. Such variability may lead to subtherapeutic response or drug toxicity. Sound knowledge of a given drug's pharmacokinetics and the patient's individual characteristics may help prevent such ADRs.

Ethnic differences may affect drug handling and render some individuals more at risk of ADRs. Genetic factors are often responsible. For example, glucose-6-phosphate dehydrogenase (G6PD) deficiency renders affected individuals susceptible to drug-induced haemolysis. This enzyme is responsible for the oxidation of glucose-6-phosphate to the corresponding gluconolactone, generating reduced nicotinamide adenine dinucleotide phosphate (NADPH) in the process. NADPH protects red blood cells from oxidative damage, and in G6PD-deficient individuals drugs that are oxidising agents can cause haemolysis, which can be fatal. More than 200 genotypes of the enzyme have been described; the phenotype varies from a small increase in susceptibility to exquisite sensitivity to oxidising agents. G6PD deficiency is more prevalent in African, Middle Eastern and South East Asian populations.

Acute intermittent porphyria is an autosomal dominant disorder characterised by recurrent attacks of abdominal pain, neurological disturbance and excessive amounts of porphobilinogen in the urine. It is often provoked by drug therapy. The acute porphyrias are more prevalent in South African than in UK populations.

Individual predisposition to an ADR is, at least partly, genetically determined. Many ADRs that have a genetic basis have been identified (see Chapter 3).

Multiple drug therapy

The incidence of ADRs and interactions has been shown to increase with the number of medicines taken.[7,57] This suggests that the effects of multiple drug use are not simply additive. There is likely to be a synergistic effect, but the concept of confounding by multiple disease states must be borne in mind.

Drug allergy

Many ADRs have an immunological basis (see Chapter 5 for Coombs and Gell classification). True allergic reactions are immunologically mediated effects.

Allergic reactions vary from rash, serum sickness and angiooedema to life-threatening bronchospasm and hypotension associated with anaphylaxis. Many patients claim to be allergic to a drug, but close questioning reveals that they have experienced intolerance. For example, many patients who claim to be penicillin allergic have actually had vomiting or diarrhoea. A good history of drug allergy raises the possibility that the patient may be cross-reactive to other structurally similar drugs. This is perhaps most important with beta-lactam antibiotics, where cross-reactivity between penicillins and cephalosporins has been demonstrated.

Pharmaceutical factors

Predictable adverse reactions can occur because of the pharmaceutical aspects of a dosage form, because of alterations in the quantity of drug present or of its release characteristics. As a result of stringent requirements laid down by regulatory authorities, reactions due to variability in the quantity of drug present are now rare in developed countries. In 1983, a rate-controlled preparation of indometacin (Osmosin) was withdrawn after reports of localised intestinal bleeding and perforation that occurred as a consequence of the delayed-release mechanism. Pharmaceutical issues may also lead to type B reactions. These can arise from the presence of contaminants or degradation products, or because of the excipients used in formulation. The potentially fatal eosinophilia–myalgia syndrome associated with L-tryptophan was probably due to a contaminant.[58]

Detection and diagnosis

When an adverse event occurs during or after drug treatment, it may be a result of the drug, or the disease for which the drug was taken, or it may have another, unrelated cause. ADRs often mimic other diseases and may therefore go unrecognised. It is also known that healthy people who are not taking medicines often complain of symptoms typical of minor ADRs.[59] Placebos also cause side effects. When an adverse reaction is suspected, it is important to try to assess how likely it is that the symptom has occurred because of a drug. It is important to critically ascertain whether the signs and symptoms are in keeping with a drug-related problem. Knowledge of the adverse-effect profiles of all the medicines the patient is taking is important. This can be obtained from prescribing information, reference textbooks and/or medicines information centres. Inevitably, many patients are taking several medicines. In these cases, it can be difficult to decide which is most likely to be responsible. Following a few simple rules (remembered by the mnemonic TREND) may help in

---

Box 1.3   Steps to determine whether a drug is responsible for an adverse reaction (TREND)

Temporal relationship *What is the timing between the start of drug therapy and the reaction?*
Most reactions occur soon after commencing drug therapy: anaphylactic reactions can occur within hours, whereas hypersensitivity reactions typically take 2–6 weeks. Other reactions, such as bone density changes, may be delayed for years.

Rechallenge *What happens when the patient is rechallenged with the drug?*
Recurrence on rechallenge provides good evidence that the drug is responsible for the adverse effect. However, rechallenge is rarely possible, particularly for serious reactions, because of the danger to the patient. More rapid occurrence following re-exposure to the drug than on secondary exposure to the drug indicates an immune-mediated pathogenesis.

Exclusion *Have concomitant drugs and other non-drug causes been excluded?*
An adverse drug reaction is a diagnosis of exclusion, as no specific laboratory tests are available. It is important to exclude non-drug causes both clinically and by performing relevant investigations.

Novelty *Has the reaction been reported before?*
If the reaction is well recognised, it may be mentioned in the manufacturer's literature or have been reported in the medical literature. An opportunity should always be taken to search reference databases such as Medline systematically; this can provide valuable insight into the appropriate management of patients with what may be a relatively rare reaction. Drug information centres can also provide useful information.

Dechallenge *Does the reaction improve when the drug is withdrawn or the dose reduced?*
Most, but not all, reactions improve on drug withdrawal, although the recovery phase can be prolonged. In rare instances, an autoimmune phenomenon may be set up and thus the reaction will not improve on drug withdrawal.

---

the identification of the culprit drug (Box 1.3). Various decision tools have been developed specifically for causality assessment of ADRs, but these do not give consistent probability estimates of the likelihood that reactions are drug induced.[60,61]

Pharmacovigilance

By the time a medicine is granted a product licence, on average only about 1500 patients will have taken it and clinical trials will have detected only the most common adverse effects.[62] Type B reactions, particularly those with an incidence of 1 in 500 or less, are unlikely to have been identified. Exclusion criteria for most trials mean that patients with multiple disease states, children, the elderly and pregnant women are not well studied and the effect of long-term use is often unknown. The limitations of clinical trials in highlighting a drug's safety are shown in Box 1.4. Furthermore, analyses of safety reporting in the context of randomised controlled trials have demonstrated that the quality and quantity of safety reporting is variable and often inadequate.[63] The CONSORT statement (a checklist developed in an effort to standardise published reports of randomised controlled trials) has recently been extended in an attempt to improve the reporting of harms within such studies.[64]

Because of the limitations of premarketing studies described above, safety can only be regarded as provisional when a new medicine is first marketed and there is a need to collect more evidence arising from 'real world' usage. Postmarketing surveillance or 'pharmacovigilance' involves observational studies of patients who receive drugs in the course of clinical practice.

Box 1.4 Limitations of most clinical trials in highlighting a drug's safety

---

Homogeneous populations
Most trials assess relatively healthy patients with only one disease and mostly exclude specific groups such as pregnant women, children and elderly people.

Sample size
Small sample size (up to 1000 patients) reduces the chance of finding rare adverse effects.

Limited duration
Trials of short duration preclude the discovery of long-term consequences such as cancer.

Inability to predict the real world
Drug interactions can be substantial in a population as patients may take drugs concomitantly, a situation that can almost never be predicted from clinical trials.

Source: Stricker BHCh, Psaty BM. Detection, verification, and quantification of adverse drug reactions. *Br Med J* 2004; 329: 44–47.

Published case reports

Case reports have been vital in alerting healthcare professionals to serious ADRs, such as oculomucocutaneous syndrome with practolol, and *torsades de pointes* with cisapride. Such case reports are valuable in hypothesis generation and are complementary to spontaneous reporting systems and formal epidemiological studies.

Spontaneous reporting schemes

In the UK a system of spontaneous reporting of suspected adverse reactions to the CSM (the 'yellow card' scheme) has now been operating for more than 30 years. Its purposes are to provide early warnings or signals of possible ADRs and to enable study of factors associated with them. Spontaneous reporting schemes cannot provide estimates of risk because the true number of cases is invariably underestimated and the denominator (i.e. total number of patients exposed) unknown.[65,66] A complementary system of monitoring for postmarketing safety is Prescription Event Monitoring run by the Drug Safety Research Unit in Southampton. Information on events after exposure to certain drugs is sought by direct enquiry of patients' GPs.[67,68]

Formal studies

These may be either cohort or case–control in design, and are important epidemiological tools for establishing causation and quantification of the magnitude of any risk. They are often carried out using large multi-purpose databases linking drug exposure and illness events. The case–control method involves comparing drug exposure among cases of a particular condition, which may be drug induced, together with a control group. A significant excess of drug takers in the case group suggests that there may be an association with the drug. This is a useful retrospective method which can provide valuable information on a suspected link between a drug and a disease, especially if the condition is uncommon. However, these studies must be carefully designed to eliminate bias or confounding, and should be interpreted with caution. A cohort study is a longitudinal investigation of a group of patients exposed to a particular product. Comparison of event rates in exposed and non-exposed groups allows estimation of the risk of developing an ADR.

Healthcare professionals and adverse drug reactions

For every medicine a patient takes there is a balance between risk and benefit. Before giving any treatment the prescriber should consider this relationship. Wherever possible, the safest drug among those of similar efficacy should be chosen. The prescriber must explain to the patient the nature, purpose and risks associated with the treatment, and ensure that patient consent is based on an adequate understanding of the likely risks and benefits. Risk–benefit information is essential for prescribers, who must constantly make treatment choices. Prescribers must have access to good data and be able to interpret them and relate them to the patient. Some information is provided by textbooks, published literature and electronic databases. In the UK the *British National Formulary* is an essential and readily available tool for prescribers, giving much useful information. Medicines Information Centres, usually located in major teaching hospitals, are also useful sources of information and advice. All prescribers need to be aware of the importance of ADR reporting to public health.[69] They must be familiar with local or national guidance on which suspected reactions to report, and when to do so.

Patients, as the consumers of medicines, need more information about medicines and their side effects (see Chapter 2). Better communication between healthcare professionals and patients about the potential risks may help in the prevention and earlier detection of ADRs. Medication counselling should include alerting the patient to potential adverse effects, although there is a balance between giving important information and causing unnecessary alarm. The search for health-related information is one of the commonest uses of the World Wide Web. Information to be found there comes from many sources and varies significantly in quality and validity.[70] Moves to provide patients with valid up-to-date information on the risks and benefits of modern medicines must embrace this medium.

Some ways in which healthcare professionals can contribute to improving drug safety are summarised in Box 1.5.

The pharmacist's role

Ensuring that medicines are used safely is fundamental to the pharmacist's role. Several studies have demonstrated that pharmacists' involvement in patient care has resulted in the prevention and early detection of ADRs.[71,72] Based on knowledge of relevant patient and medication factors, pharmacists can ensure that prescribing is as safe as is reasonably

---

Box 1.5   Key points for prescribers and pharmacists on the safe use of medicines

- Consider whether drug therapy is really necessary. In all cases, consider the benefit of administering the medicine in relation to the risk involved.
- Always consider whether any new symptom(s) the patient is experiencing could indicate an adverse drug reaction (particularly important for rash, constipation, central nervous system effects).
- Be aware of 'at-risk' patient groups, particularly the elderly, children, patients with renal or liver impairment, and women who are pregnant, of childbearing age or breastfeeding.
- Take care with drugs known to produce predictable dose-related adverse effects; avoid their use where an equally effective and safer alternative exists.
- When possible use a familiar medicine. Consult an appropriate source of information before prescribing any medicine with which you are not thoroughly familiar. With a new medicine be particularly alert for ADRs or unexpected events.
- Check the patient's history of idiosyncratic reactions or drug allergy. Avoid the use of drugs known to cause problems.
- Ask if the patient is taking other medicines, including self-medication with over-the-counter medicines or complementary therapies.
- Ensure that patients are not exposed to risk through unnecessary drug use, disregard for warnings, special precautions or contraindications, or through drug interactions.
- Ensure that patients are informed about the risks/benefits of their medicines. Warn the patient if serious reactions are liable to occur.
- Identify patients who may have a compromised ability to take or use medicines. Ensure that the dosage form and treatment regimen are appropriate and that the patient is given clear instructions on how to take their medicines.
- Ensure that patients are counselled appropriately on the correct use of their medicines.
- Try to ensure that there is true concordance between prescriber and patient.
- Check whether there are any specific monitoring requirements (e.g. liver function tests, blood counts, therapeutic drug monitoring etc.) and ensure that they are carried out.
- Be vigilant for suspected ADRs. If appropriate, report them to the appropriate regulatory authority.

---

possible. The pharmacist also has a role in educating other healthcare professionals about the prevention, detection and reporting of ADRs.

Pharmacists, nurses and adverse drug reaction reporting

Several UK studies have explored the role of pharmacists in ADR monitoring and reporting.[73–75] The involvement of hospital and community pharmacists has been shown to increase the number of yellow cards submitted to the CSM without detracting from the quality of reporting.[76,77] Community pharmacists are well placed to assist in monitoring for problems with over-the-counter medicines, complementary therapies and new medicines (indicated with an inverted black triangle in prescribing information). All pharmacists and nurses in the UK are now encouraged to contribute to the yellow card scheme.[78] It seems likely that the role of pharmacists and nurses will become increasingly important as their roles as supplementary prescribers evolve.

References

1. Loke YK. Assessing the benefit–harm balance at the bedside. *Br Med J* 2004; 329: 7–8.
2. Lee A, Rawlins MD. Adverse drug reactions. In: Edwards C, Walker R, eds. *Clinical Pharmacy and Therapeutics*, 3rd edn. London: Churchill Livingstone, 2002.
3. Davies DM. 2000 years of adverse drug reactions. *Adv Drug Reaction Bull* 1999; 199: 759–762.
4. Rawlins MD. Pharmacovigilance: paradise lost, regained or postponed? *J Roy Coll Phys Lond* 1995; 29: 41–49.
5. Seidl LG, Friend D, Sadusk J. Meeting the problem. Panel discussion of experiences and problems involved in reporting adverse drug reactions. *JAMA* 1966; 196: 421–428.
6. Seidl LG, Thornton GF, Smith JW, *et al.* Studies on the epidemiology of adverse drug reactions, III. Reactions in patients on a general medical service. *Bull Johns Hopkins Med J* 1966; 119: 299–315.
7. Smith JW, Seidl LG, Cluff LE. Studies on the epidemiology of adverse drug reactions. *Ann Intern Med* 1966; 65: 629–634.
8. Ogilvie RJ, Reudy J. Adverse drug reactions during hospitalisation. *Can Med Assoc J* 1967; 97: 1450–1455.
9. Hurwitz N. Admissions to hospitals due to drugs. *Br Med J* 1969; i: 539–540.
10. Hurwitz N. Predisposing factors in adverse reactions to drugs. *Br Med J* 1969; i: 536–539.
11. Borda IT, Slone D, Jick H. Boston Collaborative Drug Surveillance Program. Assessment of adverse reactions within a drug surveillance program. *JAMA* 1968; 205: 645–647.
12. Jick H. Drugs – remarkably non-toxic. *N Engl J Med* 1974; 291: 824.
13. Greenblatt DJ, Allen MD, Shader RI. Toxicity of high-dose flurazepam in the elderly. *Clin Pharmacol Ther* 1977; 21: 355.
14. Jick H. The discovery of drug-induced illness. *N Engl J Med* 1977; 296: 481–485.
15. Brennan TA, Leape LL, Laird N, *et al.* The nature of adverse events in hospitalized patients. The results of the Harvard medical practice study II. *N Engl J Med* 1991; 324: 377–384.

16. Bates DW, Cullen DJ, Laird N, *et al.* Incidence of adverse drug events and potential adverse drug events. Implications for prevention. *JAMA* 1995; 274: 29–34.
17. Thomas EJ, Studdert DM, Burstin HR, *et al.* Incidence and types of adverse events and negligent care in Utah and Colorado. *Med Care* 2000; 38: 261–271.
18. Smith CC, Bennett PM, Pearce HM, *et al.* Adverse drug reactions in a hospital general medical unit meriting notification to the Committee on Safety of Medicines. *Br J Clin Pharmacol* 1996; 42: 423–429.
19. Beard K. Adverse reactions as a cause of hospital admission in the aged. *Drugs Aging* 1992; 2: 356–367.
20. Lazarou J, Pomeranz BH, Corey PN. Incidence of adverse drug reactions in hospitalised patients: a meta-analysis of prospective studies. *JAMA* 1998; 279: 1200–1205.
21. Wiffen P, Gill M, Edwards J, Moore A. Adverse drug reactions in hospital patients. A systematic review of the prospective and retrospective studies. *Bandolier Extra* 2002; June: 1–16.
22. Edwards IR, Aronson JK. Adverse drug reactions: definitions, diagnosis and management. *Lancet* 2000; 356: 1255–1259.
23. Einarson TR, Gutierrez LM, Rudis M. Drug-related hospital admissions. *Ann Pharmacother* 1993; 27: 832–840.
24. Green CF, Mottram DR, Rowe PH, *et al.* Adverse drug reactions as a cause of admission to an acute medical assessment unit: a pilot study. *J Clin Pharm Ther* 2000; 25: 355–361.
25. Pirmohamed M, James S, Meakin S, *et al.* Adverse drug reactions as cause of admission to hospital: prospective analysis of 18 820 patients. *Br Med J* 2004; 329: 15–19.
26. Hallas J, Harvald B, Gram LF, *et al.* Drug related hospital admissions: the role of definitions and intensity of data collection, and the possibility of prevention. *J Intern Med* 1990; 228: 83–90.
27. Mulroy R. Iatrogenic disease in general practice: its incidence and effects. *Br Med J* 1973; ii: 407–410.
28. Martys CR. Adverse reactions to drugs in general practice. *Br Med J* 1979; ii: 1194–1197.
29. Gandhi TK, Weingart SN, Borus J, *et al.* Adverse drug events in ambulatory care. *N Engl J Med* 2003; 348: 1556–1564.
30. Gurwitz JH, Filed TS, Harrold LR, *et al.* Incidence and preventability of adverse drug events among older persons in the ambulatory setting. *JAMA* 2003; 289: 1107–1116.
31. Classen DC, Pestotnik SL, Evans RS, *et al.* Adverse drug events in hospitalized patients: excess length of stay, extra costs, and attributable mortality. *JAMA* 1997; 277: 301–306.
32. Bates DW, Spell N, Cullen DJ, *et al.* The costs of adverse drug events in hospitalized patients. *JAMA* 1997; 277: 307–311.
33. Rawlins MD, Thompson JW. Mechanisms of adverse drug reactions. In: Davies DM, ed. *Textbook of Adverse Drug Reactions*, 4th edn. Oxford: Oxford Medical Publications, 1991: Chapter 3.
34. Aronson JK, Ferner RE. Joining the DoTS: new approach to classifying adverse drug reactions. *Br Med J* 2003; 327: 1222–1225.
35. Ferner RE. Adverse drug reactions. *Medicine* 2003; 31: 20–24.

36. Castleden CM, Pickles H. Suspected adverse drug reactions in elderly patients reported to the Committee on Safety of Medicines. *Br J Clin Pharmacol* 1988; 26: 347–353.

37. Hurwitz N, Wade OL. Intensive monitoring of adverse reactions to drugs. *Br Med J* 1969; i: 531–533.

38. Gurwitz JH, Avorn J. The ambiguous relation between aging and adverse drug reactions. *Ann Intern Med* 1991; 114: 956–966.

39. Thomas EJ, Brennan TA. Incidence and types of preventable adverse events in elderly patients: population based review of medical records. *Br Med J* 2000; 320: 741–744.

40. Carbonin P, Pahor M, Bernabei R, *et al.* Is age an independent risk factor of adverse drug reactions in hospitalized medical patients? *J Am Geriatr Soc* 1991; 39: 1093–1099.

41. Jacobs JR, Reves JG, Marty J, *et al.* Aging increases pharmacodynamic sensitivity to the hypnotic effects of midazolam. *Anesth Analg* 1995; 80: 143–148.

42. Lindley CM, Tully MP, Paramsothy V, *et al.* Inappropriate medication is a major cause of adverse drug reactions in elderly patients. *Age Ageing* 1992; 21: 294–300.

43. Cumming RG, Kineberg RJ. Psychotropics, thiazide diuretics and hip fractures. *Med J Aust* 1993; 158: 414–417.

44. Willcox SM, Himmelstein DU, Woolhandler S. Inappropriate drug prescribing for the community dwelling elderly. *JAMA* 1994; 272: 292–6.

45. Impicciatore P, Choonara I, Clarkson A, *et al.* Incidence of adverse drug reactions in paediatric in/out-patients: a systematic review and meta-analysis of prospective studies. *Br J Clin Pharmacol* 2001; 52: 77–83.

46. Turner S, Nunn AJ, Fielding K, *et al.* Adverse drug reactions to unlicensed and off-label drugs on paediatric wards: a prospective study. *Acta Paediatr* 1999; 88: 965–968.

47. Clarkson A, Choonara I. Surveillance for fatal suspected adverse drug reactions in the UK. *Arch Dis Child* 2002; 87: 462–467.

48. Knight M. Adverse drug reactions in neonates. *J Clin Pharmacol* 1994; 34: 128–135.

49. Choonara I, Gill A, Nunn A. Drug toxicity and surveillance in children. *Br J Clin Pharmacol* 1996; 42: 407–410.

50. Rademaker M. Do women have more adverse drug reactions? *Am J Clin Dermatol* 2001; 2: 349–351.

51. Lawson DH. Epidemiology. In: Davies DM, ed. *Textbook of Adverse Drug Reactions*, 4th edn. Oxford: Oxford Medical Publications, 1991: Chapter 2.

52. McKinnon RP, Wildsmith JAW. Histaminoid reactions in anaesthesia. *Br J Anaesth* 1995; 74: 217–228.

53. Drici M-D, Clement N. Is gender a risk factor for adverse drug reactions? The example of drug-induced long QT syndrome. *Drug Safety* 2001; 24: 575–585.

54. Ellis CJ, Leung D. Adverse drug reactions in patients with HIV infection. *Adv Drug React Bull* 1996; 178: 675–678.

55. Rotunda A, Hirsch R, Scheinfeld N, *et al.* Severe cutaneous reactions associated with the use of human immunodeficiency virus medications. *Acta Dermatol Venereol* 2003; 83: 1–9.

56. Heller HM. Adverse cutaneous drug reactions in patients with human immunodeficiency virus-1 infection. *Clin Dermatol* 2000; 18: 485–489.

57. Cadieux RJ. Drug interactions in the elderly. *Postgrad Med J* 1989; 86: 179–186.
58. Kilbourne EM, Philen RM, Kamb ML, Falk H. Tryptophan produced by Showa Denko and epidemic eosinophila-myalgia syndrome. *J Rheumatol* 1996: 23 (Suppl 46): 81–88.
59. Reidenberg MM, Lowenthal DT. Adverse non-drug reactions. *N Engl J Med* 1968; 279: 678.
60. Lanctot KL, Naranjo CA. Computer-assisted evaluation of adverse events using a Bayesian approach. *J Clin Pharmacol* 1994; 34: 142–147.
61. Frick PA, Cohen LG, Rovers JP. Algorithms used in adverse drug event reports: a comparative study. *Ann Pharmacother* 1997; 31: 164–167.
62. Stricker BHCh, Psaty BM. Detection, verification, and quantification of adverse drug reactions. *Br Med J* 2004; 329: 44–47.
63. Ioannidis JP, Lau J. Completeness of safety reporting in randomised trials: an evaluation of 7 medical areas. *JAMA* 2001; 285: 437–443.
64. Ioannidis JP, Evans SJ, Gotzsche PC, *et al.* Better reporting of harms in randomised trials: an extension of the CONSORT statement. *Ann Intern Med* 2004; 141: 781–788.
65. Waller PC. Measuring the frequency of adverse drug reactions. *Br J Clin Pharmacol* 1992; 33: 249–252.
66. Waller PC. Pharmacovigilance: evaluating and improving the safety of medicines. *Medicine* 1999; 27: 26–28.
67. Layton D, Riley J, Wilton LV, *et al.* Safety profile of rofecoxib as used in general practice in England: results of a prescription-event monitoring study. *Br J Clin Pharmacol* 2003; 55: 166–174.
68. Heeley E, Riley J, Layton D, *et al.* Prescription-event monitoring and reporting of adverse drug reactions. *Lancet* 2001; 358: 1872–1873.
69. Pirmohamed M, Breckenridge AM, Kitteringham NR, *et al.* Adverse drug reactions. *Br Med J* 1998; 316: 1295–1298.
70. Tatsioni A, Gerasi E, Charitidou E, *et al.* Important drug safety information on the internet: assessing its accuracy and reliability. *Drug Safety* 2003; 26: 519–527.
71. Lesar TS, Briceland L, Stein DS, *et al.* Factors related to errors in medication prescribing. *JAMA* 1997; 277: 312–317.
72. Leape LL, Cullen DJ, Clapp MD, *et al.* Pharmacist participation on physician rounds and adverse drug events in the intensive care unit. *JAMA* 1999; 282: 267–270.
73. Winstanley PA, Irvin LE, Smith JC, *et al.* Adverse drug reactions: a hospital pharmacy-based reporting scheme. *Br J Clin Pharmacol* 1989; 28: 113–116.
74. Wolfson DJ, Booth TG, Roberts PI. The community pharmacist and adverse drug reaction monitoring: (2) An examination of the potential role in the United Kingdom. *Pharm J* 1993; 251: 21–24.
75. Whittlesea C, Walker R, Houghton J, *et al.* Development of an adverse drug reaction reporting scheme for community pharmacists. *Pharm J* 1993; 251: 21–24.
76. Lee A, Bateman DN, Edwards C, Smith JM, Rawlins MD. Reporting of adverse drug reactions by hospital pharmacists: pilot scheme. *Br Med J* 1997; 315: 519.
77. Davis S, Coulson R. Community pharmacist reporting of suspected ADRs: The first year of the yellow card demonstration scheme. *Pharm J* 1999; 263: 786–788.
78. Morrison-Griffiths S, Walley TJ, Park BK, *et al.* Reporting of adverse drug reactions by nurses. *Lancet* 2003; 361: 1347–1348.

Further reading

Aronson JK, Ferner RE. Joining the DoTS: new approach to classifying adverse drug reactions. *Br Med J* 2003; 327: 1222–1225.

Edwards IR, Aronson JK. Adverse drug reactions: definitions, diagnosis and management. *Lancet* 2000; 356: 1255–1259.

Ferner RE. Adverse drug reactions. *Medicine* 2003; 31: 20–24.

Lee A, Rawlins MD. Adverse drug reactions. In: Edwards C, Walker R, eds. *Clinical Pharmacy and Therapeutics*, 3rd edn. London: Churchill Livingstone, 2002.

Pirmohamed M, James S, Meakin S, *et al.* Adverse drug reactions as cause of admission to hospital: prospective analysis of 18 820 patients. *Br Med J* 2004; 329: 15–19.

Stricker BH, Psaty BM. Detection, verification, and quantification of adverse drug reactions. *Br Med J* 2004; 329: 44–47.

2

Side effects and patients

Theo Raynor, Peter Knapp, Dianne Berry

Introduction

Any practical guide to adverse drug reactions (ADRs) and their management needs to pay particular attention to the relationship between patients and the side effects of their medicines. It is clearly important that healthcare professionals know about side effects and their frequency. However, the patient also needs to be informed about side effects, i.e.:

- What they are;
- How likely they are to happen;
- How to recognise them; and
- What to do if they happen.

Since the first edition of this book was written at the turn of the 21st century, there has been a marked change in the extent to which patients are expected to become involved in decisions about their medicines. In the UK, this is demonstrated in policy documents such as the National Plan for the NHS[1] and various National Service Frameworks. The origins of this change in context can be found in the consumer empowerment movement generally, but also specifically in the *concordance* or *partnership in medicine taking* initiative (Box 2.1).[2] This change in approach is exemplified in the recent decision by the UK Medicines and Healthcare products Regulatory Agency (MHRA) to take forward patient reporting of side effects – something that would have been unthinkable 5 years ago.

People taking medicines need to know about side effects for three reasons:

- It is their right to have understandable information about the harm that medicines might do to them.
- To make informed decisions about medicines, including their benefits and harms, people must be able to understand information about side effects and their frequency and apply it to their own circumstances.

> **Box 2.1** Definition of concordance
>
> Concordance is a new approach to the prescribing and taking of medicines. It is an agreement between a patient and a healthcare professional that respects the beliefs and wishes of the patient in determining whether, when and how medicines are to be taken. Although reciprocal, this is an alliance in which the professionals recognise the primacy of the patient's decisions about taking the recommended medications.
>
> From Britten N. Concordance and compliance. In: Jones R, Britten N, Culpepper L, et al., eds. *Oxford Textbook of Primary Medical Care*. Oxford: Oxford University Press, 2004.

- Minimising the impact of side effects depends crucially on the patient identifying a possible side effect early, and knowing what action to take.

The most likely source of information about side effects for patients is the patient information leaflet (PIL) now required by law to accompany every medicine pack.[3] Companies are required to include in the leaflet all side effects mentioned in the Summary of Product Characteristics (SPC), but in a form understandable to the patient. One of the practical issues with these leaflets is the amount of information to be included, e.g. the PIL for simvastatin lists over 20 side-effects. The European Union proposed that the likelihood of side effects occurring should be indicated in these leaflets by the use of verbal descriptors, such as *common* and *rare*.[4] As described later in the chapter, research into how patients interpret these words showed that they are grossly misunderstood, and this has led to an increased focus on finding the best method of describing the likelihood of side effects. There is an array of tools and aids to support healthcare professionals in informing people about the risks and benefits of treatment.[5] However, many people are not cognitively or emotionally equipped to understand, retain and use risk information, which is often complex and sometimes threatening.[6]

We have moved from a situation when in the 1970s people were not even given the name of their medicines, to 2004 where people are being empowered to report suspected side effects they experience to the regulatory authorities. The term side effect has passed into lay vocabulary, but people's understanding of the term and its implications is less clear.

In this chapter we will explore patients' new roles in terms of medicines and their side effects, how they perceive side effects, and the pitfalls associated with the various methods of describing the risk and frequency of side effects. It is an essential role of healthcare professionals to help patients understand the harms and benefits associated with their medicines, and this chapter will provide practical guidance.

Desire for information about side effects

There has been an increasing recognition of the need to provide people with information about their medicines. However, the extent to which people should be told about medication side effects has been a particular area of debate. This is despite several studies which show that people always rank side-effect information highly when asked about their medicine information needs.[7]

Berry and colleagues[7] investigated what people wanted to know about their medicines, and developed 16 categorisations of information type. They found that information about medication side effects was the most sought-after type of information, and that provision of this resulted in highly rated explanations (e.g. in terms of satisfaction). After side effects, people next wanted to know about what the medicine does, any lifestyle changes they would be required to make while taking it (such as whether they would have to stop drinking alcohol), and how it should be taken (details of dose, timing etc.). However, when they asked doctors, they found that there was almost no relationship between the patients' and the doctors' ratings of the priority of the information categories. The most noticeable difference was in terms of the patients' top two categories (namely, information about side effects and what the medicine actually does), where the doctors gave both of these categories low rankings (Table 2.1).[7]

Similar findings have been reported by Makoul and colleagues[8] and Mottram and Reed.[9] Makoul *et al.*, for example, examined a number of actual consultations between doctors and patients, and also asked doctors to rate the importance of providing particular types of information. They found that the doctors gave the highest ratings to providing full instructions for taking the medicine, and the lowest to explaining the side effects. Similarly, Mottram and Reed found that GPs rated the section on side effects in PILs as being least important.

There is also increasing evidence that patients want personalised or individualised information about their health and medicines, and that the provision of tailored information does have beneficial effects.[10] Following a review of the literature, Skinner *et al.*[11] suggested that tailored print communications are generally better read and remembered than generic

Table 2.1 Information categories wanted by people and what doctors thought[7]

Information category	Patients' ranking	Doctors' ranking
Possible side effects	1	10.5
What the medication does	2	10.5
Lifestyle changes	3	3
Detailed questions about taking medicine	4	2
What is it?	5	15
Interactions with medication	6	1
What to do if symptoms change	7	10.5
Probability medication will be effective	8	14
Any alternatives to medication	9	16
Is it known to be effective?	10	13
Does medication treat symptoms or cause?	11	6.5
What if I forget to take or take too much?	12	6.5
Interaction with non-prescription medicine	13	4
Risks of not taking the medicine	14	8
Interaction with currently prescribed medication	15	5
How will I know if medication is working?	16	10.5

communications, and that there is also evidence that they are more effective for influencing behaviour change. A key issue is how much tailoring is needed to produce a significant benefit. Interestingly, Berry and colleagues[12] reported beneficial effects from a simple personalisation of leaflets (e.g. using the words 'your medicine' rather than 'the medicine'). They found that such personalisation increased satisfaction with the information provided, reduced ratings of perceived risk to health, and increased the intention to take the medicine.

Berry[13] suggested that a potential compromise between the two extremes, of generic and fully individualised materials, might be to produce leaflets for particular subgroups of the population (e.g. elderly patients, or parents of young children). Kreuter et al.[14] similarly distinguished between targeted generic materials intended for a particular subgroup of the population and designed to take account of the specific needs and concerns of that subgroup, and fully tailored materials intended to reach a specific individual and derived from a specific assessment.

General perceptions

Later in this chapter we will give different examples of ways that patients can be informed about side effects, and their relative advantages. However, it is clear that a patient's understanding of side-effect information and their subsequent decision to take or not take the medicine are both influenced by additional factors. These might include information not from 'official' sources, which may potentially tell a conflicting story, as well as the patient's preconceptions of the medicine's riskiness, the values that they ascribe to the positive and negative outcomes of taking the medicine, and their emotional state.[6]

In order to determine the beliefs held by people about the risk of harm associated with taking a medicine, Knapp et al.[15] conducted a study in which participants were asked to imagine the scenario of being prescribed either ibuprofen (for a bad back) or penicillin (for a chest infection). They were then asked to estimate the likelihood of experiencing any side effect and the likelihood of each of two named side effects for the medicine. The results revealed an overestimation of the chance of experiencing any side effect (26.4% for penicillin compared with an incident rate of 18% established from several trials) and a larger overestimation of the chance of the individual side effects. For example, kidney damage was estimated at 14.9% in people taking ibuprofen compared with the incident rate in trials of 0.09%. What is equally striking is the variation in estimates given by the participants. For example, when asked to estimate the chance of any side effect for penicillin, the answers ranged from 1% to 90%.

The results of this single study confirm that the information that practitioners provide to patients may conflict with pre-existing beliefs. The variation noted in people's responses also mirrors work by Horne and Weinman.[16] They developed the 'Beliefs about Medicines Scale' to measure, among other things, people's estimates of the harmful effects of medicines generally and of specific medicines. The scale has been applied to medicines in many clinical areas, and the variation among participants is striking. Thus, any information provided about side effects should ideally take account of individual differences.

The increase in media reporting of health and healthcare means that patients are likely to read or hear more than a single account of the medicines they are taking. Increased access to the internet has had a similar effect. The result is that information provided by practitioners involved in their care is unlikely to be the only information the patient has access to. However, there are other important, more informal sources of information, including the patient's own experience of medicines and the experiences of people they know who have taken the medicine concerned. As a result, the patient may have to reconcile apparently conflicting pieces of information: a report from a practitioner of a very low side-effect incident rate and an account of a painful or inconvenient side effect from someone they know who took the medicine. Patients may not always make an objective, rational decision, and the epidemiological dataset may not always prevail.

The values a patient holds about the outcomes associated with a medicine (whether harmful or beneficial) are likely to be very influential in their interpretation of information about side effects. Because patients and practitioners may differ in their values, their decisions about taking the medicine may also vary. For example, Frankael et al.[17] report that many people with rheumatoid arthritis are unwilling to accept the chance of toxic effects of medicines that might be highly beneficial in treating the arthritis. Further, Berry et al.[7] noted that younger respondents in a scenario-based study were extremely concerned about the side effect of acne, whereas doctors in the study considered this a minor outcome.

Finally, interpretation of information and the decision to take or not take the medicine are likely also to be influenced by the patient's emotions. Information about the risk of side effects (and benefits) may be presented to the patient in a rational way, but it may be hard for them to make a decision entirely without emotion. Mayer[18] reports that a positive mood increases frequency estimates for positive outcome events, whereas negative mood increases estimates for negative outcomes. Lowenstein[19] argues that emotions will be dominant when the patient's emotions and their cognitions (thoughts) are in conflict. This may be particularly important when patients are considering treatments in highly emotive illnesses, such as in acute-onset conditions and those that are life-threatening.

Side effects and compliance

When considering providing side-effect information to patients, two possible implications are often raised. The first is the potential impact of the information on patient compliance, and the second is whether such information leads to spurious reporting of side effects by patients. We know that understandable and usable information about side effects can affect people's decisions about whether to take their medicine, and how much of it to take. Berry[20] showed in scenario-based research that the inclusion of negative information affected ratings of likely compliance. If we are to accept the concept of partnership in medicine taking, then we should aim for the situation where patients, when fully informed about the benefits and harm of their medicines, can decide appropriately not to take medicine.

Myers and Calvert[21] found that the rate of discontinuation was lower in patients given a leaflet that included information about transient side effects and encouraged the patient to keep taking the medicine. George and colleagues[22] found that leaflets about non-steroidal anti-inflammatory medicines and penicillin increased the awareness of side effects, but there was no evidence of increased reporting. However, when reported, side effects were significantly more likely to be attributed to the medicine. A further study from the same group showed some evidence of increased spurious reporting of side effects associated with a leaflet on benzodiazepines.[23] However, in general it seems that information on side effects has an attributing, rather than a suggesting, effect.

Mandatory patient information leaflets

Before the 1990s most patients received little or no information in written form about possible side effects of their medicines and their seriousness and frequency. However, in 1992 the European Union proposed a regulation requiring comprehensive written leaflets with every medicine as a package insert (for both prescribed and over-the-counter medicines).[3] This law was implemented in the UK in 1999 and resulted in a move from patients having little or no information about side effects to their having a list of all side effects included in the SPC (this is a legal requirement).

Subsequent to this legislation, the European Union produced a guideline on the readability of these leaflets, and proposed the use of verbal descriptors to describe the level of risk (see under Format).[24] The format of the patient information leaflet has significant drawbacks related to the nature of a folded package insert, its limited size and the consequent small print. As described later, individualisation of side-effect information is a goal, and this cannot be achieved with a standard package insert format. In practice, despite the recommendations of the guideline, most leaflets still give little or no information about the likelihood that the side effects listed will occur.

Format of side-effect data for patients

When it is desired to convey risk information to patients there are many different options to choose from. Essentially, there are three approaches: to use words, to use numbers or to use graphs. Of course, it may be possible, and indeed advisable in some cases, to use a combination of these approaches to increase the likelihood that the patient will understand the information. Some examples of each of the three approaches are given below. There is considerable variation in the extent to which these approaches have been evaluated, to see how well they actually convey the intended information. Furthermore, some of the examples have been shown not to be very effective, and so should be used with caution.

The EU's recommended scale of verbal descriptors of risk ranges from 'very common' (for incident rates of more than 1 in 10) to 'very rare' (for rates of less than 1 in 10 000) (Table 2.2). This mirrors the classification used by the Committee for the International Organisation of Medical Sciences (CIOMS)[25] for use by scientists working in pharmacovigilance. In a series of studies, Berry et al.[26] showed that the use of these verbal descriptors led to a gross overestimation of risk compared to their numerical equivalents. For example, in patients taking a statin the use of the term common to describe the risk of the side effect constipation resulted in a mean estimate of occurrence of 34%. Use of the terms also resulted in increased estimates of the severity of the side effect and, importantly, a reduction in the number of participants who said they would take the medicine.

Calman's[27] proposed risk scale pre-dates the EU scale and uses seven points (rather than the EU's five) ranging from high (for rates of more than 1 in 100) to negligible (for rates of less than 1 in 1 million). Like the EU, Calman appeared not to have tested his scale before publication, and Berry et al.[4] showed that the scale led to overestimation of risk to a similar extent to the EU scale. Both scales produce estimates of risk that show great variation, as described earlier, and, perhaps most worryingly, produce the greatest overestimation in the lower frequency bands. These bands are likely to be used mostly for infrequent but severe side effects.

Table 2.2 Verbal descriptors

EC Guideline descriptor	Mean (SD) estimate (%) from study participants	Frequency assigned by EU (%)
Very common	65 (24.3)	>10
Common	45 (22.2)	1–10
Uncommon	18 (13.0)	0.1–1
Rare	8 (7.5)	0.01–0.1
Very rare	4 (6.7)	<0.01

If numbers are to be used, then many different methods can be chosen. Using percentages may seem the most obvious approach, so that the risk of a side effect might be given as 1%, for example. However, care needs to be taken because percentages are misunderstood by many people. Gigerenzer[28] showed that interpretations of '40%' were often inaccurate, with some respondents in a research study thinking it meant 1 in 4 or 1 in 40 persons. Gigerenzer advocates the use of 'natural frequencies', that is whole numbers related to individuals receiving a treatment, and he has shown that presenting natural frequencies, e.g. '1 person out of every 10 taking the medicine', is more likely to be understood than the percentage equivalent.

However, even the use of the expression '1 in x' is not simple. When giving data on two side effects with different rates, is it better to keep the top row (the numerator) or the bottom row (the denominator) constant? For example, will '1 in 60' and '3 in 60' be better understood than '1 in 60' and '1 in 20'? There is no firm research evidence to suggest which is the best option here.

Providing information on the difference in risk between two treatments can present further problems. The effects of relative and absolute risk reduction presentations are detailed below, but an alternative approach is to use the expression 'number needed to harm' (NNH). This format has been used more often in recent years,[29] and one study suggests that it is better understood by patients than conventional ways of expressing risk reduction.[30] The NNH is the inverse of the absolute increase in harm when comparing two treatments. For example, if headache occurs in 2% of patients with treatment A and 6% with treatment B, the NNH is 1/0.04 = 25. That is, 25 patients will have to use treatment A rather than B for one fewer patient to experience headache. Further research is needed to determine whether the population generally would find NNH acceptable and understandable.

Data on side effects are not often displayed in the form of a graph and this format has been little evaluated, but if space allows, graphical presentation may help the patient's understanding. One of the most common approaches is to use a bar chart, in which the rates of different outcomes are displayed in separate bars. If used, care should be taken to ensure that the vertical scale does not mislead the patient. Pie charts can be useful, but should probably be avoided unless colour printing is available. Other less common but interesting presentations include the 'faces' grid, in which 100 faces (i.e. patients) are shown in different colours according to outcome, to show an incident rate. Linear graphs may also be used, particularly to show two or more incident rates on one scale.

A useful summary of graphical approaches can be found in an article by Paling.[31]

It is hard to recommend a single best approach to describe side-effect data, as there has been little research comparing alternatives. A combination of methods may help the patient best, as they may complement each other. The choice of approach may depend on the amount and complexity of the data to convey, as well as on the paper size and the available colours.

Key effects to consider when presenting side-effect data

A number of key effects must be borne in mind when considering the issue of presenting side-effect data. They include the concept of heuristics (mental shortcuts), relative versus absolute data, framing and context.

Use of heuristics

We noted at the start of this chapter that many people are not cognitively equipped to interpret risk information effectively. Connected to this is the fact that responses to risk are not simple quantitative analyses, but people often use simplified rules, or 'heuristics'. One reason is that we are all subject to various cognitive biases and heuristics (shortcuts, or rules of thumb). The use of heuristics when making probability judgements often leads to the correct answer but can be associated with systematic errors or biases. An example of such a heuristic is 'availability'. This is called into play when people are asked to judge the frequencies of events. Rather than employing standard normative methods, people using the availability heuristic make the estimate on the basis of how easy or difficult it is to bring particular instances to mind. Tversky and Kahneman,[32] for example, asked people to consider words in the English language of three letters or more and to judge whether it is more likely that such words start with the letter 'r', or have 'r' as the third letter. They found that the majority of participants believed that a word starting with 'r' was more likely, whereas in reality the reverse is the case. According to Tversky and Kahneman, people respond incorrectly because words beginning with the letter 'r' can be more easily retrieved from memory (i.e. are more available).

Studies have also shown that availability judgements can be based on actual frequency of occurrence, in that we tend to recall those things that have been encountered most frequently in the past. However, such judgements are often influenced by the relative salience of instances. A classic experiment by Lichtenstein et al.[33] showed that, contrary to the true state of affairs, causes of death that attract more publicity (e.g. murder) are judged more likely to occur than those that attract less (e.g. suicide, certain types of cancer).

Relative and absolute forms of presenting risk information

People's judgements of risk information are also influenced in other ways, particularly by how the information is presented. One example of this is whether absolute or relative forms of presentation are used to convey risk reductions (and increases). A relative risk reduction, for example, indicates a *ratio* and compares a risk level for one group with that for another group, whereas an absolute risk reduction indicates a *difference* between two risk levels. Thus, a risk reduction from 4% to 2% can be expressed as 'reduced by 50%' (relative risk reduction) or as an absolute risk reduction of 2%. To date, relative risk reductions have been much more commonly used than absolute risk reductions. Moynihan *et al.*,[34] for example, investigated the different ways in which the benefits and risks of three medications were presented in 207 media reports, and found that 83% of reports presented benefits, such as risk reductions, only in relative terms, 2% communicated only absolute benefits, and 15% communicated both relative and absolute benefits.

The predominance of relative risk reductions in risk communications is hardly surprising, given that over the past 10 years a number of studies have shown what are reported to be 'significant advantages' of conveying information about treatment benefits in terms of relative risk reductions. It has been found, for example, that physicians are more likely to prescribe, and patients are more willing to choose, medical treatments if the risk reductions are communicated in relative formats.[35]

However, in recent years people have become increasingly aware of the potential biasing effects of using relative forms of presentation. This has arisen partly as a result of highly publicised health scares, such as the 1995 oral contraceptive 'pill scare' and the more recent controversy over hormone replacement therapy. The pill scare, for example, was provoked by warnings of an almost doubled risk of venous thrombosis for women taking oral contraceptives containing third-generation progestogens. This led many women to stop taking the pill, which resulted in a sharp rise in unwanted pregnancies and terminations. What was not made sufficiently clear was that the absolute level of risk involved was very low. Use of the third-generation pill increased the risk of venous thrombosis from around 15 cases per 100 000 pill users to around 25 cases.[36] A crucial point, however, is that the risk of venous thrombosis associated with pregnancy is actually four to five times higher. So, telling women about the doubled risk of thrombosis from taking these pills led to many pregnancies, thereby actually incurring a greater risk of thrombosis for these women.

Framing

Another way in which risk judgements are influenced is in terms of whether the information is framed in a positive or a negative way. It is now well established that people are more likely to opt for a particular treatment if told that there is a 95% chance of survival (i.e. using a positive frame) rather than if they are told that there is a 5% risk of dying (i.e. using a negative frame). Gurm and Litaker,[37] for example, presented patients with one of two videos describing angioplasty and its associated risks. They found that the patients were more likely to opt for treatment when the video framed the procedure as 99% safe rather than there being a 1 in 100 likelihood of complications. Such effects are not limited to lay people. McNeil *et al.*[38] found that framing information in terms of risk of dying significantly reduced the likelihood that doctors would recommend radiation therapy over surgery.

Whereas positive framing has generally been found to be more influential than negative framing, other studies have shown that framing information in terms of losses can be more influential than framing the same information in terms of gains. Thus, when encouraging people to undergo some form of health screening, it has been found that telling them about the risks of not being screened (loss framing) leads to a greater uptake than telling them about the benefits of being screened (gain framing). The findings are not entirely consistent in this area, however. Rothman and Salovey[39] suggested that the differences in effectiveness might result from whether the behaviour being promoted is a detection or a prevention behaviour. After reviewing a number of studies, they argued that loss framing is generally more effective in relation to detection behaviours, such as undergoing screening, whereas gain framing is generally more effective in relation to prevention behaviours, such as being vaccinated.

Context

Evidence has consistently shown that people's interpretations of risk information are influenced by the particular context in which the judgement is made. As noted by Parducci as early as 1968,[40] a student may think that if her contraceptive failed on 5% of occasions this would be 'often', whereas if she were absent from 5% of her classes this would be 'almost never'. Parducci's claims have been backed up by findings from a number of empirical studies. Weber and Hilton,[41] for example, reported that probability judgements were influenced by severity of outcome, with lower estimates being given in relation to 'likely' number of murders than to 'likely' number of injuries. Similarly, in a medical context, Merz et al.[42] reviewed over 450 informed consent decisions and found that verbal expressions of probability were influenced by the severity of the consequences. Studies in our own research group have shown that people vary in their interpretation of European Commission-recommended verbal descriptors, such as 'common', depending on whether they are used to describe mild or severe side effects,[43] and whether the medicine in question is being prescribed for an adult or a 1-year-old child.[13]

Interestingly, several investigators have shown that interpretations of numeric probability expressions are not immune to context effects. Windschitl and Weber,[44] for example, found that when people were told that a woman had a 30% chance of contracting malaria on a forthcoming trip, their degree of certainty as to whether or not she would develop the disease varied according to whether the trip was to India or to Hawaii.

Uncertainty

A significant issue to consider when preparing information about ADRs is the confidence you have in the available data. Assessing causality at individual patient level is fraught with difficulty, and there are limitations in the various methods currently used to support pharmacovigilance (see Chapter 1). Confidence in the data will depend on its source. Randomised clinical trials (RCTs), for example, allow the capture of safety information under a controlled setting that minimises biases in the comparison of different therapeutic options. Nevertheless, evidence suggests that the reporting of safety information in clinical trials is often neglected and receives less attention than do efficacy outcomes. In an analysis of 192 RCTs, Ioannidis and Lau[45] found that reasons for withdrawal owing to side effects were specified in only 46% of the trial reports, and that adequate reporting of adverse effects and laboratory-determined toxicity occurred in only 39 and 29% of the trials, respectively. The authors concluded that safety data from RCTs need to be collected and analysed in a systematic fashion using standard categorisations of ADR severity in order to improve the safety data gained.

In a further study Papanikolaou and Ioannidis found that reporting of adverse effects could also be improved in systematic reviews.[46] They searched the Cochrane Database of Systematic Reviews for reviews containing quantitative data on specific, well-defined harms for at least 4000 randomised subjects (the minimum sample required for adequate power to detect an adverse event due to an intervention in 1% of subjects). Of 138 reviews that included evidence on 4000 or more subjects, only 25 (18%) had eligible data on adverse events, 77 had no harms data, and 36 had data on harms that were non-specific or pertained to fewer than 4000 subjects.

Data derived from postmarketing surveillance techniques (including spontaneous reporting schemes) will give an indication of a medicine's side-effect profile, but establishing rates is extremely difficult (see Chapter 1), mainly because there is so much uncertainty about the denominator, i.e. the number of people taking the medicine. For example, if four patients experience gastrointestinal (GI) bleeding after taking a medicine but it is unclear whether the number of patients taking it in a given population is 20 000 or 40 000, then there is potentially a twofold difference in estimated incidence rate. This may be less of an issue in relation to a side effect with a very low frequency, as in this example, as regardless of which is the true rate, you can say that the risk of GI bleeding is unlikely to be more than 1 in 5000.

The difficulty in establishing definitive incidence rates is corroborated by how often estimates of ADR incidence in this book are given as a range. In practice we simply do not know how often each side effect occurs. It is often difficult to convey this uncertainty to patients: knowledge gaps are not something people necessarily understand or accept.

The 'truth' or validity concerning the incidence rate of side effects is also influenced by the changing evidence base. As incidence rates are initially based on relatively limited patient exposure data they may need significant revision with the publication of new evidence, whether in the form of a large trial or a systematic review. Although it would be unreasonable to expect practitioners to be aware of all new evidence, patients may well be aware of new research, particularly if a trial outcome (whether beneficial or harmful) is widely publicised. As with new treatments, practitioners will need to respond to patients' enquiries about the possible side effects of medicines, and so need to be aware of sources that may be helpful in accessing the relevant information, such as medicines information centres.

Patient reporting of ADRs

The road to patient reporting of suspected ADRs in the UK has been long. From the introduction of the yellow card scheme in 1964, doctors, dentists and coroners were eligible to report. All pharmacists have been eligible to report since 1999, and all nurses since 2002. A recent review of the yellow card system recommended the establishment of pilot schemes to explore the most effective way for patients to report side effects directly.

The potential benefits of patient reporting include earlier signal generation, reporting of a greater spectrum of adverse events, and more complete accounts of the suspected adverse events, medications taken and possible risk factors. Concerns about patient reporting relate mainly to the quality of reports. These include whether patients can distinguish between possible ADRs and other complaints (if not, these reports would generate 'noise' rather than true signals), and the completeness of the information that will be documented by patients. Another concern is whether patient reporting might leave the scheme open to misuse by individuals or groups through the submission of fraudulent reports.

It is known that patients with HIV infection were first to raise the possible association between protease inhibitors and lipodystrophy. However, few formal studies have investigated the potential contribution of patient reports on possible ADRs. Solovitz et al. reported that users of medicines are capable of distinguishing between adverse effects and other complaints or symptoms.[47–49] In a retrospective study Egberts et al. assessed data gathered from a Dutch telephone service that enabled patients to consult a pharmacist for medicines information, focusing on questions asked about side effects of paroxetine.[50] The time at which the first report of a previously unrecognised reaction was identified from the information service data was compared with the time of receipt for the first health-professional report to the regulatory authority database of the same reaction. They found that for each of the new ADRs reported by both patients and healthcare professionals, the reactions were reported first by patients, with the first professional report received on average 273 days later. Also focusing on patients' concerns about ADRs with paroxetine, an analysis of patient reports in the UK showed that spontaneous reports from healthcare professionals and patients are complementary.[51] Other recent studies have shown that patients are willing and able to report suspected ADRs if asked to do so.[52,53]

Regulatory authorities in several countries (e.g. Canada, US, Denmark and Australia) currently accept ADR reports directly from patients.[54]

The report on the Independent Review of Access to the UK Yellow Card scheme[55] (published in 2004) recommended that the MHRA should accept ADR reports from patients. The MHRA are currently developing proposals to pilot different arrangements for patient reporting to gauge effectiveness. There will be much interest in whether patient reporting will ultimately lead to more timely detection of signals of possible ADRs.

The way forward

We should remember that, if the patient cannot play their part in the identification and management of side effects, much of the content of this book is of limited value. Patients need the facts about the risk of harm from a medicine they may take, so that they can make a reasoned decision on whether the medicine is right for them. Informing patients effectively can help minimise the impact of side effects, both from the perspective of the individual as well as in the wider public health context.

Improving the utility of side-effect information that many patients say they want involves consideration of both the content and the presentation of the material. This chapter has shown that there are some techniques that we can apply to help improve patients' understanding. These include:

- Using frequency (1 in 100) rather then percentage data (1%);
- Using absolute risk data (and not relative risk data alone);
- Taking care when framing data – be even-handed where possible;
- Balancing benefit and harm (in similar terms) when the information is available.

We have also described other approaches that have face validity but which need further research and so should be used with care. These include the use of graphical representations. You can argue that healthcare professionals need a range of formats so that they can use the most appropriate one to aid discussions with individual patients. However, at present some healthcare professionals may regard these approaches as gold standard, and we are still a long way from using them as part of routine practice. In addition, as a practical issue, PILs in current use are too small to incorporate some of the methods for indicating risk described in this chapter.

Risk perception is complex and influenced by many factors, and we have seen that the ways in which people make choices may not always be rational. However, individuals' existing values, beliefs and attitudes must be respected. Finally, we should put the risk of harm from medicines into context. With almost all medicines, the journey to and from the pharmacy (whether by driving, walking or cycling) is likely to be far riskier than taking the medicine itself.

References

1. The NHS Plan. A plan for investment. A plan for reform. London: Stationery Office, 2000.
2. Royal Pharmaceutical Society of Great Britain. From compliance to concordance. Achieving shared goals in medicine taking. London: RPSGB, 1997.
3. European Commission. European Commission Council Directive 92/27/EEC (OJ NoL 113 of 30.4.1992, p.8) m1992.
4. Berry DC, Knapp P, Raynor DK. Provision of information about drug side effects to patients. *Lancet* 2002; 359: 853–854.
5. Cranney A. Decision aids in clinical practice. *Br Med J* 2004; 329: 39–40.
6. Berry D. Risk, communication and health psychology. Maidenhead: Open University Press, 2004.
7. Berry DC, Michas IC, Gillie T, *et al*. What do patients want to know about their medicines and what do doctors want to tell them? A comparative study. *Psychol Health* 1997; 12: 467–480.
8. Makoul G, Arntson P, Schofield T. Health promotion in primary care: Physician-patient communication and decision making about prescription medications. *Soc Sci Med* 1995; 41: 1241–1254.
9. Mottram DR, Reed C. Comparative evaluation of patient information leaflets by pharmacists, doctors and the general public. *J Clin Pharmacol Ther* 1997; 22: 127–134.
10. Straus SE. Individualizing treatment decisions: the likelihood of being helped or harmed. *Evaluation & The Health Professions* 2002; 25: 210–224.
11. Skinner CS, Campbell MK, Rimer BK, Curry S, Prochaska JO. How effective is tailored print communication? *Ann Behav Med* 1999; 21: 290–298.
12. Berry DC, Michas IC, Bersellini E. Communicating information about medicine: the benefits of making it personal. *Psychol Health* 2003; 18: 127–139.
13. Berry DC. Interpreting information about medication side effects: differences in risk perception and intention to comply when medicines are prescribed for adults or young children. *Psychol Health Med* 2004; 9: 227–234.
14. Kreuter MW, Strecher VJ, Glassman B. One size does not fit all: the case for tailoring print materials. *Ann Behav Med* 1999; 21: 276–283.
15. Knapp PK, Coppack Z, Raynor DK. What do people think is the likelihood of harm and benefit from two common medicines? HSRPP conference 2004 http://www.hsrpp.org.uk/abstracts/2004_46.shtml
16. Horne R, Weinman J. Patients' beliefs about prescribed medicines and their role in adherence to treatment in chronic physical illness. *J Psychosom Res* 1999; 47: 555–567.
17. Frankael L, Bogardus S, Concato J, Felson D. Risk communication in rheumatoid arthritis. *J Rheumatol* 2003; 30: 443–448.
18. Mayer JD, Gaschke YN, Braverman DL, Evans TW. Mood congruent judgement is a general effect. *J Personality Soc Psychol* 1992; 63: 119–152.

19. Lowenstein GF, Weber EU, Hsee CK, Welch N. Risk as feelings. *Psychol Bull* 2001: 127: 267–286.
20. Berry DC, Michas IC, DeRosis F. Evaluating explanations about drug prescriptions: Effects of varying the nature of information about side effects and its relative position in explanations. *Psychol Health* 1998; 13: 767–784.
21. Myers ED, Calvert EJ. Information, compliance and side-effects. *Br J Clin Pharmacol* 1984; 17: 21–25.
22. George LF, Waters WE, Nicholas JA. Prescription information leaflets, a pilot study in general practice. *Br Med J* 1983; 287: 1193–1196.
23. Gibbs S, Waters WE, George CF. The benefits of prescriptions information leaflets. *Br J Clin Pharmacol* 1989; 28: 345–351.
24. European Commission. A guideline on the readability of the label and package leaflet of medicinal products for human use. EC Pharmaceutical Committee, 1998.
25. Guidelines for Preparing Core Clinical-Safety Information on Drugs, 2nd edn. (Report of CIOMS Working Group III & V) 1998. ISBN 92 9036 070 4.
26. Berry DC, Raynor DK, Knapp P, Bersellini E. Patients' understanding of risk associated with medication use. *Drug Safety* 2003; 26: 1–11.
27. Calman KC. Cancer, science and society and the communication of risk. *Br Med J* 1996; 313: 799–802.
28. Gigerenzer G. *Reckoning with risk*. London: Penguin, 2002.
29. http://www.jr2.ox.ac.uk/bandolier/band59/NNT1.html
30. Misselbrook D, Armstrong D. Patients' responses to risk information about the benefits of treating hypertension. *Br J Gen Pract* 2001; 51: 276–279.
31. Paling J. Strategies to help patients understand risks. *Br Med J* 2003; 327: 745–748.
32. Tversky A, Kahneman D. Judgement under uncertainty: heuristics and biases. *Science* 1974; 185:1124–1131.
33. Lichtenstein S, Slovic P, Fischoff B, Layman M, Combs B. Judged frequency of lethal events. *J Exp Psychol* 1978; 4: 551–578.
34. Moynihan R, Bero L, Ross-Degnon D, *et al.* Coverage by the news media of the benefits and risks of medication. *N Engl J Med* 2000; 342: 1645–1650.
35. Lacy C, Barone J, Suh D, *et al.* Impact of presentation of research results on likelihood of prescribing medications in patients with left ventricular presentations. *Am J Cardiol* 2001; 87: 203–207.
36. Berry DC, Raynor DK, Knapp P, Bersellini E. Official warnings on thromboembolism risk with oral contraceptives fail to inform users adequately. *Contraception* 2002; 66: 305–307.
37. Gurm HS, Litaker DG. Framing procedural risks to patients: is 99% safe the same risk as a risk of 1 in 100? *Acad Med* 2000; 75: 840–842.
38. McNeil BJ, Pauker SG, Sox HC, Tversky A. On the elicitation of preferences for alternative therapies. *N Engl J Med* 1982; 306: 1259–1262.
39. Rothman AJ, Salovey P. Shaping perceptions of vulnerability: personal relevance and use of experiential information in health judgements. *Personality Soc Psychol Bull* 1997; 121: 3–19.
40. Parducci A. Often is often. *Am Psych* 1968; 24: 828.
41. Weber EU, Hilton DJ. Contextual effects in the interpretations of probability words. *J Exp Psychol* 1990; 16: 781–789.
42. Merz JF, Druzdel MJ, Mazur DJ. Verbal expressions of probability in informed consent litigation. *J Med Decision Making* 1991; 1: 273–281.

43. Berry DC, Raynor DK, Knapp P. Communicating risk of medication side effects: an empirical evaluation of EU recommended terminology. *Psychol Health Med* 2003; 8: 251–263.
44. Windschitl PD, Weber EU. The interpretation of 'likely' depends on the context, but 70% is 70% right? *J Exp Psychol* 1999; 25: 1514–1533.
45. Ioannidis JP, Lau J. Improving safety reporting from randomised trials. *Drug Safety* 2002; 25: 77–84.
46. Papanikolaou PN, Ioannidis JP. Availability of large-scale evidence on specific harms from systematic reviews of randomized trials. *Am J Med* 2004; 117: 582–589.
47. Solovitch BL, Fisher S, Bryand SG, *et al.* How well can patients discriminate drug-related side effects from extraneous new symptoms? *Psychopharmacol Bull* 1987; 23: 189–192.
48. Mitchell AS, Henry DA, Sanson-Fischer R, *et al.* Patients as a direct source of information on adverse drug reactions. *Br Med J* 1988; 297: 891–893.
49. Fisher S, Bryant SG. Postmarketing surveillance: accuracy of patient drug attribution judgements. *Clin Pharmacol Ther* 1990; 48: 102–107.
50. Egberts TC, Smulders M, de Koning FH, *et al.* Can adverse drug reactions be detected earlier? A comparison of reports by patients and professionals. *Br Med J* 1996; 313: 530–531.
51. Anon. Adverse effects: direct reporting by patients is beneficial. *Prescrire Int* 2004; 13: 234–235.
52. van der Bemt PM, Egberts AC, Lendering AW, *et al.* Adverse drug events in hospitalized patients: a comparison of doctors, nurses and patients as sources of reports. *Eur J Clin Pharmacol* 1999; 55: 155–158.
53. Jarernsiripornkul N, Krska J, Capps PA, *et al.* Patient reporting of potential adverse drug reactions: a methodological study. *Br J Clin Pharmacol* 2002; 53: 318–325.
54. van Grootheest K, de Graaf L, de Jong-van den Berg LT. Consumer adverse drug reaction reporting. *Drug Safety* 2003; 26: 211–217.
55. Independent Steering Committee. Report of an Independent Review of Access to the Yellow Card Scheme. The Stationery Office, May 2004 (accessed online http://medicines.mhra.gov.uk/ourwork/monitorsafequalmed/yellowcard/yellowcardreport.pdf)

Further reading

Berry DC, Raynor DK, Knapp P, Bersellini E. Patients' understanding of risk associated with medication use. *Drug Safety* 2003; 26: 1–11.
Edwards A. Communicating risks. *Br Med J* 2003; 327: 691–692.
Gigerenzer G. *Reckoning with Risk*. London: Penguin, 2002.
Misselbrook D, Armstrong D. Patients' responses to risk information about the benefits of treating hypertension. *Br J Gen Pract* 2001; 51: 276–279.
Number needed to treat (NNT): Bandolier http://www.jr2.ox.ac.uk/bandolier/band59/NNT1.html
Paling J. Strategies to help patients understand risks. *Br Med J* 2003; 327: 745–748.

3

Pharmacogenetics and adverse drug reactions

Munir Pirmohamed and Kwame N. Atuah

Introduction

It is widely known that people respond differently to medicines, and this is an important clinical problem. Why does one patient suffer an adverse reaction and another not? Why does a particular medicine work well for one patient, yet have little or no effect on someone else? It is now clear that much individuality in drug response is inherited. This genetically determined variability defines the research area known as pharmacogenetics. This chapter provides an overview of pharmacogenetics in the context of adverse drug reactions (ADRs). Note that definitions of some specific terms with which you may not be familiar are included in the glossary at the end of the chapter.

The Human Genome Project has revealed that there are approximately 50 000 genes in the human genome.[1,2] It has also revealed a high frequency of nucleotide variants in gene sequence. Generally, when present in the general population at a frequency of 1% or more these variants are called genetic polymorphisms, and at lower frequencies are known as mutations. The most frequently encountered form of genetic polymorphism is a single nucleotide polymorphism (SNP), which is estimated to occur about once every 185 nucleotides.

The presence of a genetic polymorphism or mutation may lead to an amino acid substitution in the protein the gene codes for. This alteration may render the protein non-functional. For example, in sickle cell disease a single nucleotide substitution of thymine (T) with the normal adenine (A) in the haemoglobin gene results in the amino acid valine replacing glutamate in the haemoglobin polypeptide. The hydrophobic nature of valine causes polymerisation of the haemoglobin molecules, resulting in red blood cell membrane rigidity, with the formation of crescent-shaped red blood cells known as sickle cells and the well-known clinical sequelae such as local tissue hypoxia and anaemia.

The frequency of SNPs in the human genome suggests that any individual may possess a unique set of polymorphisms, which may correspond to individual variations in protein structure and function. These genetic alterations may affect proteins involved in the action of a drug (e.g. metabolising enzymes) and cause variations in drug response. Pharmacogenetics (PG) can thus be defined as the study and elucidation of the genetic basis of individual variations in drug response.

Adverse drug reactions

Adverse drug reactions are commonly classified into two types, A and B[3] (see Chapter 1). Type A reactions feature an augmentation of the known pharmacological actions of the drug and usually show a good relationship with the dose. Type B reactions, which are often referred to as idiosyncratic, are not usually predictable from the known pharmacological actions of the drug. There is no simple relationship with dose, but clearly some degree of dose dependency exists, as the reaction does not develop unless the patient is administered the drug. Examples of type B reactions include agranulocytosis with clozapine, and toxic epidermal necrolysis (TEN) with sulfonamides. Other types of reaction, such as delayed-onset reactions, can be considered to be subclasses or hybrids of type A and B ADRs.[4] An alternative classification system, which considers the relationship with dose, timing and patient susceptibility, has also been proposed.[5]

Drug action

The clinical action of a drug is determined primarily by its pharmacokinetic and pharmacodynamic properties. Pharmacokinetics (PK) describes the serum or blood concentrations of the drug with time; the main processes involved are absorption, distribution, metabolism and excretion. The proteins involved in each of these processes may have a direct effect on the drug's pharmacokinetics. For example, energy-dependent transmembrane transporter proteins that mediate the passage of xenobiotics into and out of cells may affect the absorption of drugs from the gut lumen. Hence, genetic polymorphisms that alter the function of these transporter proteins may effect changes in the rate of drug absorption. This can result in drug toxicity if the individual has an overactive transporter phenotype, or drug ineffectiveness in the case of inactivity. Thus, polymorphisms in the genes coding for pharmacokinetic proteins affect drug plasma levels, and may cause increases (toxicity) or decreases (lack of drug action) in drug levels, both of which can result in an adverse outcome.

Pharmacodynamics (PD) describes the relationship between concentration of the drug at its site of action and the magnitude of its biological effect. Specific molecular interactions between the drug and its target protein (an ion channel or receptor, for example) are the main determinants of the pharmacodynamic properties of a drug. Genetic polymorphisms also affect the function of drug target proteins. An important example is the variation in the efficacy of the beta$_2$-agonist salbutamol owing to the polymorphic nature of the gene that codes for beta$_2$-adrenergic receptors.

It follows, then, that proteins that mediate the pharmacokinetic and pharmacodynamic properties of a drug, and thereby drug action, are determinants of both safety and efficacy. In this chapter, the different mechanisms by which polymorphisms may cause ADRs are described, and the associations of certain genetic variations with ADRs discussed.

Genetics revisited

A genotype describes the genetic make-up of an individual; the phenotype is the observable trait of the genotype, for example eye colour or enzyme activity. Every gene in a diploid cell (containing 46 chromosomes, including the two sex chromosomes, X and Y) exists as an allelic pair. The dominant allele may be expressed as the phenotype, or an intermediate phenotype may be observed, as in tall (dominant), short (recessive) or medium height (codominant or intermediate). Likewise, the activity of an enzyme may be extremely high, non-existent or intermediate. Some genes are closely associated or linked, and the set of alleles of these linked genes, or haplotype, are usually inherited together. Polymorphisms or sequence variants on the same chromosomal region that are associated more often than would be expected by chance are said to be in linkage disequilibrium.

Throughout this chapter, the name of a gene will always be italicised, whereas that of the corresponding protein will be in normal typeface. Thus *MDR1* refers to the gene that codes for the MDR1 protein. It is convention for different variants of a gene to be represented by a sequence of numbers preceded by an asterisk (*) after the name of the gene. For example, *CYP2C9*3* is one of the identified genetic variants of *CYP2C9*; other variants include *CYP2C9*2* and *CYP2C9*4*.

Genetic polymorphism and drug transporters

Absorption

Efflux proteins: multiple drug resistance transporter (MDR1)

The rate and magnitude of the oral absorption of a drug are key determinants of its bioavailability. Transporter proteins within the cells of the gut wall pump xenobiotics (including drugs) out of the intracellular space. This cellular efflux action is energy dependent and acts against a concentration gradient. The best-studied of these transport proteins is a glycoprotein named P-glycoprotein (P-gp).[6] In more recent nomenclature, P-gp is known as MDR1 or ABCB1.[7] This is one of a group of transporter proteins that belong to the adenosine triphosphate (ATP) binding cassette (ABC) superfamily (consisting of *ABCA* to *ABCG* families, and the associated subfamilies).[8] Overexpression of MDR1 in tumour cells confers resistance to a range of anticancer drugs. MDR1 is expressed in cells of various organs, including the intestines, liver, blood–brain barrier (BBB) and kidney. In the intestines, it is found in the brush border membranes of enterocytes. The protein limits the absorption of drugs by actively pumping the molecules back into the intestinal lumen. Therefore, the absorption of drugs that are MDR1 substrates may be affected by genetic polymorphisms that influence the intestinal activity of MDR1.

Digoxin absorption and toxicity

The cardiac glycoside digoxin is an MDR1 substrate. Induction of the MDR1 protein by rifampicin directly affects the bioavailability of digoxin. Coadministration of rifampicin with digoxin reduces the oral bioavailability of digoxin by 30% owing to the induction of intestinal MDR1.[9] Thus, MDR1 activity in the gut affects the plasma concentration of any drug that may be a transporter substrate. It therefore follows that a genetic polymorphism that increases the amount of MDR1 in the gut will also reduce drug plasma levels through decreased absorption.

A correlation between polymorphic variants in the *MDR1* gene, expression of the protein and oral bioavailability was first demonstrated in 2000.[10] Fifteen SNPs were identified in *MDR1*. One of them (a cytosine (C) to thymine (T) substitution at position 3435 on exon 26 of the *MDR1* gene) correlated with duodenal levels of MDR1 protein. Individuals who were homozygous for the thymine allele (TT) displayed more than twofold lower expression of MDR1, compared with those who were homozygous for the cytosine allele (CC). Heterozygote individuals displayed an intermediate phenotype. More importantly, TT individuals had higher digoxin plasma levels than those with the C-allele homozygous genotype. This trend has been observed in other studies.[11,12] However, a similar study showed the opposite trend, i.e. individuals with the TT genotype had the lowest digoxin bioavailability after a single dose.[13] MDR1 is expressed not only in the intestine, but also on the surfaces of hepatocytes and renal proximal tubular cells,[14] i.e. the transporter is also involved in renal and biliary excretion. The association between higher plasma levels of digoxin and the TT individuals (homozygous for the weaker form of the MDR1) may be explained by a reduced excretion of the drug.[13] A subsequent study reported a correlation between the digoxin plasma concentration and *MDR1* haplotypes, and agreed that analysis of single SNPs and drug plasma concentrations may not always give consistent trends.[15] Clearly, further studies are required to establish the effect of polymorphisms in the *MDR1* gene on digoxin plasma levels. It is likely that the variations in digoxin, and indeed other drug plasma levels, are mediated not by individual SNPs, but by particular combinations (haplotypes). In addition, the effect of other transporters cannot be discounted. It is also important to note that variations in plasma levels of an MDR1 substrate, as a result of polymorphisms in the gene, will be of greatest significance when the drug has a narrow therapeutic index and is present in low concentrations in the intestine. At low doses, or for drugs with low dissolution rates (e.g. ciclosporin), the transporter will not be saturated, and hence genetically determined variations in transporter activity can affect the absorption of the drug.[16]

Distribution

Drug transporters are important in the distribution of drugs across organ and tissue membranes, such as the BBB and placenta. In this regard, evidence for the role of MDR1 in drug disposition is derived mainly from animal models. A transgenic mouse strain that lacks one of the *MDR1* genes (*mdr1a −/−*) showed increased neurotoxic effects of ivermectin, an MDR1 substrate.[17] Further, accumulation of the drug in the brain was 80 times higher in these mice than in the strain with normal *MDR1* expression. Similarly, loperamide, a peripherally acting opioid derivative and MDR1 substrate, shows few central nervous system (CNS) side effects. This has been ascribed to MDR1-mediated efflux at the BBB. In support of this, pronounced CNS side effects were observed in *MDR1* knockout mice (*mdr1a −/−*) administered loperamide.[18] In humans, inhibition of the MDR1 transporter by quinidine resulted in marked CNS toxicity (respiratory depression), with no corresponding increase in loperamide plasma concentrations.[19] However, no correlation was found between the *MDR1* variant genotypes (SNPs and haplotypes) and respiratory depression in humans.[20] It is possible that other transporters that are as yet unidentified or not studied in this context, may have genetic variants that are in linkage disequilibrium with the MDR1 polymorphisms. Continuing research may well reveal specific gene–gene interactions that will explain the mechanisms behind these contrasting and sometimes confusing observations.

Excretion

Uptake systems: the organic anion transporter proteins

Several groups of uptake carrier systems have been characterised. These include the dipeptide transporters (PEPTs), concentrative nucleoside transporters (CNTs), organic cation transporters (OCTs) and organic anion transporters (OATPs). Genetic polymorphisms have been reported in the genes coding for many of these transport proteins, although their functional and clinical relevance has not been defined. However, such studies are now beginning to be performed. For instance, OATPs are expressed in various organs, including the liver. Drug substrates of this transporter include enalapril, fexofenadine and pravastatin. OATP-C, an isoform of the OATP family of carrier systems, is expressed in the basolateral membrane of hepatocytes. There are at least 17 polymorphisms of this isoform, including *OATP-C*1b*, *OATP-C*5*, and *OATP-C*15*. The pharmacokinetics of pravastatin have recently been studied in relation to the OATP-C polymorphisms.[21] Pravastatin undergoes excretion via the biliary tract, and its use has been associated with raised liver enzymes. The bioavailability of the drug has been shown to be elevated in individuals expressing the *OATP-C*15* allele. The highest AUC (area under the curve) and lowest non-renal clearance values were found in individuals homozygous for the *OATP-C*15* polymorphism. However, large intergenotypic variation was observed in heterozygous carriers, and it was noted that other as yet unknown factors might also contribute to the overall pharmacokinetics of the drug. Larger studies are required to confirm the association and establish the clinical consequence of OATP-C (and other transporter protein) polymorphisms. Some examples of drugs that are substrates for transporters with identified polymorphisms are listed in Table 3.1.

Table 3.1 Examples of drugs that are known substrates of transporter proteins with genetic polymorphisms[7,10,21,22]

Transporter	Gene	Substrate drugs
ATP-binding cassette (ABC)	ABCB1 (MDR1)	Digoxin Nelfinavir Ciclosporin Fexofenadine Loperamide Erythromycin
ATP-binding cassette (ABC)	ABCC2 (MRP2)	Cisplatin Methotrexate Vincristine
ATP-binding cassette (ABC)	ABCA4 (ABCR)[a]	Chloroquine Hydroxychloroquine
Breast-cancer-related protein	ABCG2 (BCRP)	Mitoxantrone, daunorubicin, doxorubicin, topotecan
Organic anion transporters	OATP	Pravastatin, fexofenadine, enalapril

[a]Genetic variants associated with retinopathy.[22]

Metabolism

Phase I metabolism involves oxidation, reduction or hydrolysis of drugs. Oxidation is usually undertaken by the cytochrome P450 (CYP) enzymes. This is a family of haem-containing mono-oxygenases that represent a powerful and versatile group of *in vivo* oxidising agents.[23,24] Phase II metabolism results in the conjugation of the phase I product with a polar molecule, which renders it more water soluble and allows it to be eliminated by the kidney or bile.

Many drugs that cause ADRs are metabolised by CYP enzymes, and the relationship between CYPs and predisposition to ADRs has been extensively reviewed.[25] A complete treatise of all the potential ADRs associated with all known CYP polymorphisms is beyond the scope of a single chapter. As such, we shall discuss the underlying principles and highlight these with a few examples.

The *CYP* gene superfamily codes for many CYP enzymes. In humans, CYP2C9, CYP2D6 and CYP3A4 account for 60–70% of all phase I drug metabolism.[26] Because the biological effect of a drug is related to its plasma concentration, differences in the rates of metabolism will be expected to predispose to certain adverse effects. Table 3.2 shows

Table 3.2 Metabolising enzyme polymorphisms ADRs, adapted from ref. 27

Metabolising enzyme	Gene	Substrate drugs	ADR	Ref
CYP1A2	CYP1A2	Typical antipsychotics	Tardive dyskinesia	28
		Theophylline	Tachycardia, convulsions	29
CYP2C9	CYP2C9	Warfarin	Haemorrhage,	30
		Phenytoin	Phenytoin toxicity	27
CYP2C19	CYP2C19	Mephenytoin	Neurotoxicity	27
		Diazepam	Prolonged sedation	27
CYP2D6	CYP2D6	Antiarrhythmics	Arryhthmias	31
		Beta-blockers	Bradycardia	27
		Opioids	Dependence	27
		Perhexilene	Hepatotoxicity	32
CYP3A4	CYP3A4	Etoposide Teniposide	Treatment-related leukaemia	33
Thiopurine S-methyl transferase	TPMT	6-Mercaptopurine, azathioprine	Haemotoxicity, myelotoxicity	34–37
N-acetyl transferase 2	NAT2	Sulfasalazine	Infectious mononucleosis-like syndrome	38
		Sulfamethoxazole	Sulfamethoxazole hypersensitivity	39,40
Uridine diphosphate-glucuronosyl-transferases	UGT1A1	Irinotecan	Neutropenia	41,42
Dihydropyrimidine dehydrogenase	DPYD	5-Fluorouracil	Myelotoxicity	43
Plasma butyrylcholinesterase	BCHE	Suxamethonium	Prolonged apnoea	44
NAD(P)H dehydrogenase	NQO2	Clozapine	Agranulocytosis	45

For many of these associations conflicting data have been reported, or the associations have not undergone replication studies in different populations. An example is the association between CYP3A4 gene polymorphisms and treatment-related leukaemia, which was not reported in another study.[46]

examples of CYP polymorphisms and their associated potential ADRs. An updated list of CYP polymorphisms may be found at the website of the Human Cytochrome P450 Allele Nomenclature Committee [http://www.imm.ki.se/cypalleles].

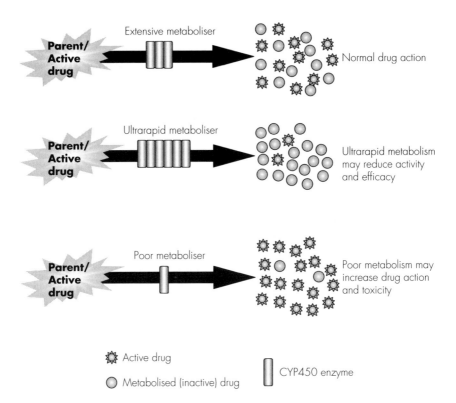

Figure 3.1 A simplified diagrammatic representation showing the effects cytochrome P450 (CYP) metaboliser status on drug action. The quantitative presence of the CYP enzymes determines the ratio of active and inactive drug in the blood serum. Thus, a poor metaboliser of a drug (active parent drug) will have a higher active:inactive drug ratio, increasing their susceptibility to drug toxicity.

Polymorphism in genes coding for CYP enzymes may lead to:[25]

- Abolished activity: the gene may be deleted, or altered in such a way as to render the resulting CYP protein non-functional.
- Reduced activity or altered activity: a change in the shape of the CYP protein affects the active site, so that substrate specificity is affected.
- Increased activity: two or more copies of the same genes may be present, resulting in multiple copies of the same CYP enzyme. This increases the metabolic capacity of the enzyme.

The clinical effects of CYP polymorphisms can be categorised into different metabolic capacities, which have been termed poor metabolisers (PM), extensive metabolisers (EM) and ultrarapid metabolisers (UM). Figure 3.1 is a diagrammatic explanation of the potential consequences of CYP activity.

As is the case with transporter proteins, the presence of a genetic polymorphism expressed as a phenotypic variant may not necessarily lead to a significant clinical effect *per se*. An important aspect to consider is the route of metabolism of the drug. If the drug is metabolised exclusively by one CYP enzyme, the effect of a polymorphism that reduces the enzyme activity will usually lead to a large increase in the plasma level. Alternatively, if a drug is metabolised by a range of CYP enzymes, a polymorphism in one of the CYP isoforms may have little clinical impact.

Cytochrome P450 2D6 (CYP2D6)

In the 1970s it was noted that the metabolism of debrisoquine and sparteine showed interindividual variation.[47,48] The enzyme responsible for the metabolism of both drugs was later shown to be CYP2D6. CYP2D6 is involved in the metabolism of a wide range of drugs, including beta-blockers (e.g. alprenolol and propranolol), antipsychotics (e.g. haloperidol and risperidone) and antidepressants (e.g. paroxetine and venlafaxine).[25,49] As with most other genetic polymorphisms, there are interethnic differences in the frequencies of the polymorphisms. For example, the prevalence of CYP2D6 poor metabolisers (PM) is about 6–8% in Swedish Caucasians, and 7–10% in other European countries,[50,51] but much lower in Chinese,[52] Japanese[53] and Koreans.[54] Ultra-rapid metabolisers have also been characterised, with one study reporting a Swedish family possessing 12 extra copies of a functional CYP2D6*2 gene.[55] The prevalence of the UM phenotype in Swedish Caucasians is about 1–2%, increasing to 3–6% in Germany, 10% in Italy, and 30% in Ethiopia.[50]

Clinical implications of the CYP2D6 polymorphism

The antianginal agent perhexiline is metabolised by CYP2D6. Its therapeutic use is associated with peripheral neuropathy and hepatotoxicity. The high lipophilicity of the molecule necessitates hepatic hydroxylation and conjugation for subsequent renal elimination.[56] Genetically determined impairment of CYP2D6 activity results in an increase in the plasma levels of the parent drug, with associated adverse effects. In order to establish a link between CYP2D6 metaboliser status and perhexiline-induced neuropathy, Shah *et al.*[57] compared the rate of hydroxylation of debrisoquine (a phenotypic marker of CYP2D6 activity) in neuropathic and non-neuropathic patients on perhexiline therapy. The investigators noted a clear association between the occurrence of perhexiline-induced neuropathy and diminished debrisoquine hydroxylation (poor CYP2D6 metaboliser status); the median debrisoquine metabolic ratio (unchanged debrisoquine/hydroxylated debrisoquine) in the neuropathic group was 14.4, compared with 0.65 in the non-neuropathic group.[57] A later study in healthy volunteers identified poor and extensive metabolisers in whom 0.014% and 1.4% (respectively) of the administered dose was excreted in the urine as monohydroxyperhexiline, 12–24 hours after ingestion. Higher parent drug plasma concentrations were also detected concomitantly in poor metabolisers.[56] Likewise, patients phenotyped as CYP2D6 PM treated with propafenone displayed more than a fourfold reduction in oral clearance, increased elimination half-life and higher plasma drug concentrations, which was associated with a higher incidence of CNS side effects.[31]

Genetic research techniques such as polymerase chain reaction (PCR) and restriction fragment length polymorphism (RFLP) analysis allow a phenotype to be rapidly linked to the corresponding gene sequence (genotype). Using these techniques, the effect of the specific allelic variants on the phenotype can be established, and any association with the clinical effect investigated. For example, the allelic variants CYP2D6*3, *4, *5 and *6 were identified in schizophrenic patients being treated with a range of CYP2D6-metabolised antipsychotics (including haloperidol, fluphenazine and zuclopenthixol). Patients with the *4/*4 or *4/*5 genotype were characterised as being poor metabolisers. All of these patients suffered extrapyramidal adverse effects (such as tardive dykinesia and parkinsonism).[58] However, because of the small numbers in the study, only a tentative conclusion of a correlation between the presence of defective CYP2D6 alleles and the incidence of EPS (extrapyramidal syndrome) was made. A similar trend was also reported by an earlier study,[59] although again the numbers studied were small, but the trend has since been confirmed in two other studies.[60,61] The following case study (p. 54) illustrates the problems that can occur.

Despite these trends and observations, there are contradictory data in the literature. For instance, a recent study of 125 patients randomised to either fluoxetine or nortriptyline outpatient treatment failed to show an association between antidepressant-induced adverse effects and the CYP2D6 PM genotype.[63] At present, no firm recommendations can be given with regard to genotyping for CYP2D6 prior to the commencement of psychotropic treatment – there is an urgent need to conduct large prospective studies which take into account not only genetic factors but also environmental factors, such as compliance and the placebo effect.

CASE STUDY 3.1

A 69-year-old patient on nortriptyline 25 mg three times daily suffered dizziness, tiredness, vertigo and confusion. Analysis of the blood plasma showed that the drug level was more than twice the recommended upper limit (1300 nM; recommended range 200–600 nM). Reduction of the dose to 25 mg once daily reduced the drug plasma level to 742 nM after 12 days. Further reduction to 20 mg once daily resulted in complete recovery from the adverse effects. The patient was later confirmed to be a poor metaboliser for CYP2D6.[62]

CYP2C9 polymorphism

The CYP2C subfamily accounts for around 18% of the CYP protein content in human hepatocytes. The *CYP2C9* gene is located on chromosome 10, and is more than 55 kb in length.[64] Currently about 12 allelic variants have been identified at this gene locus (*CYP2C9*1* to *CYP2C9*12*) [http://www.imm.ki.se/cypalleles]. The frequency of the CYP2C9 allelic variants is variable in different populations. Approximately two-thirds of Caucasian and Turkish individuals express the *1/*1 genotype, but less than 2.5% express the variant *2/*2, *2/*3 and *3/*3 genotypes. These variants appear to be rare in African-American, Japanese, Chinese and Korean populations.[64] One of the important drugs metabolised by CYP2C9 is warfarin, which has been the subject of numerous pharmacogenetic studies.

Warfarin and CYP2C9 polymorphism

Warfarin is a coumarin anticoagulant used for the prevention and treatment of thrombotic events, such as venous thromboembolism and systemic arterial embolism in patients with atrial fibrillation. It is administered clinically as a racemic mixture of the R and S enantiomers. The S form is about three to five times more potent than the R enantiomer. The drug has a narrow therapeutic index, and serum concentrations above or below the therapeutic range may cause haemorrhagic events or thrombosis, respectively. Thus, maintaining a steady plasma level of warfarin, which is clinically assessed by the International Normalised Ratio (INR), is a routine aspect of warfarin therapy, necessitating frequent clinic visits.

However, despite the frequent monitoring, many patients fail to consistently achieve an INR within the therapeutic range, and the dose range required can vary from 0.5 to 15 mg/day.

The more active S enantiomer of warfarin is metabolised by CYP2C9. Allelic variation at the *CYP2C9* gene locus can alter the metabolic clearance of warfarin; this has been most extensively studied with the *CYP2C9*2* and *CYP2C9*3* variants, which are known to reduce enzyme activity to between 5 and 12% of wildtype activity.[65] Thus, in relation to warfarin, individuals homozygous for the *1* allele (*CYP2C9*1/*1*) have 'normal' warfarin metabolic rates, whereas the *CYP2C9*3/*3* genotype is associated with the lowest metabolic clearance rate.[66]

The most important adverse effect associated with warfarin therapy is serious haemorrhage; the major risk factors for this include age, diet and concomitant medication. In a retrospective cohort study, it was found that patients who carry the *CYP2C9*2* and *3* variant alleles required a longer time to achieve stable warfarin dosing, and also required lower doses of warfarin to maintain a therapeutic INR;[30] the mean daily maintenance dose of warfarin in the *1/*1* genotype group was 5.63 mg, whereas in the *2/*2* and *3/*3* genotypes the mean doses were 4.07 and 1.60 mg, respectively. It was also noted that patients with variant *CYP2C9* genotypes were more likely to have INRs above the therapeutic range, and correspondingly, the rate of serious and life-threatening bleeding events was higher in the variant genotypic patients (10.92 and 1.56 per 100 patient-years, respectively) than in the wildtype genotypes (4.89 and 0.7 per 100 patient-years, respectively).[30] These observations were consistent with those of a previous study, in which significantly higher numbers of serious haemorrhagic episodes occurred in individuals requiring low-dose warfarin.[65] However, Taube et al.[67] reported no increase in the risk of overanticoagulation, but did demonstrate the relationship between the CYP2C9 genotype and warfarin dose. Thus, genotyping may identify a subpopulation of individuals who may require extra attention and monitoring during the initiation phase of warfarin therapy. However, the predictive value of CYP2C9 genotyping for the individual is low, and cannot at present be used to indicate the final maintenance dose. It is also important to note that all studies to date have been retrospective and small, and have not consistently taken account of environmental factors determining warfarin dose requirement, nor the interaction between genetic and environmental factors. Large prospective studies evaluating the role of genetic factors in determining the response to warfarin, and the utility of genotyping, are being undertaken, and will provide us with valuable answers as to whether we can improve the benefit–risk ratio of warfarin therapy.

Other metabolising enzymes: thiopurine S-methyl transferase

Thiopurine S-methyl transferase (TPMT) is responsible for the inactivation of 6-mercaptopurine (6-MP) and azathioprine, a prodrug of 6-MP. It mediates this action by methylation of the drug and its active metabolites.[68] 6-MP has been used largely in children with acute lymphoblastic leukaemia, whereas azathioprine is used as an immunosuppressant for the treatment of inflammatory bowel disease, rheumatoid arthritis and other autoimmune conditions. The sequential conversion of 6-MP results in the formation of 6-thioguanine nucleotides, which are incorporated into chromosomal DNA and arrest cell replication; cellular accumulation of active thioguanine further suppresses proliferation.[34]

TPMT gene polymorphisms were first identified in man in the 1980s[69] and are now well characterised.[35] *TPMT* genetic polymorphisms have been identified in Caucasians, Asians and Africans. There are about 19 alleles associated with low TPMT activity, the most common being *3A, *3C and *2,[34,35,68] which comprise about 95% of *TPMT* mutant alleles in Caucasians, African-Americans and Asians.[70] These polymorphisms result in proteins that are rapidly degraded after translation, rendering the homozygous individual phenotypically deficient.[35] This can result in fatal toxicity.[70] In a prospective cohort study of patients prescribed azathioprine for rheumatic disease, all compliant patients with the *TPMT*3A* allele suffered from leukopenia and discontinued therapy within 1 month of initiation.[37] A larger study undertaken to characterise 6-MP metabolism and tolerance in patients with ALL (acute lymphoblastic leukaemia) showed that cellular accumulation of TGN (thioguanine) metabolites caused significant haematotoxicity in heterozygous patients. This can therefore be considered a high-risk group that requires dose reduction and closer monitoring of therapy.[36] Another study of patients on thiopurines (azathioprine and 6-MP) showed more than a sixfold overrepresentation of TPMT deficiency (homozygous *3A/*3A) or heterozygosity in patients who developed dose-limiting toxicity.[70] The median concentration of thioguanine nucleotides in the erythrocytes of homozygous *3A/*3A variants was $200 \, pmol/8 \times 10^8$ red blood cells (RBC), compared with 89.5 and 87 in heterozygotes and homozygous wildtypes, respectively. A median dose reduction of 90.8% in the homozygous-deficient and 66.7% in the heterozygotes allowed continuation of therapy. The example of TPMT genetics therefore provides a very good paradigm of how pharmacogenetics may be successfully used to continue therapy by altering dose and thereby preventing toxicity.

Genetically determined pharmacodynamic variations

Interindividual variation in drug response (efficacy and toxicity) is reproducibly large and may be more pronounced than pharmacokinetic variability by itself.[71,72] Therefore, pharmacodynamic factors accounting for variability also have to be considered, and may in fact contribute to variability to a greater extent than do pharmacokinetic factors. Specific molecular interactions between the drug molecule and the target agent such as receptors, ion channels and enzymes are key determinants of the pharmacodynamic properties of a drug. Table 3.3 lists a few examples.

Genetic variations in drug targets

Beta2-adrenergic receptor

A classic example of a polymorphically expressed drug receptor is the beta2-adrenergic receptor ($\beta_2 AR$). Beta2-agonists such as salbutamol activate receptors on airway smooth muscle cells via a G-protein-coupled mechanism to effect a relaxation of smooth muscle tone. Long-term exposure to beta2-agonists is known to induce receptor desensitisation and down-regulation.[80] The two most common polymorphisms of the $\beta_2 AR$

Table 3.3 Examples of drug targets with identified genetic polymorphisms associated with ADRs

Drug target	Gene	Drug	Potential ADR	Ref
Dopamine D3 receptors	DRD3	Antipsychotics (dopamine antagonists)	Drug-induced tardive dyskinesia	73
Delta opioid receptor	OPRM1	Methadone, heroin, fentanyl	Addiction	73
Potassium channel	KCNH2 (HERG)	Cisapride, quinidine	Drug-induced LQT/TdP	74
Potassium channel	KCNQ1	Terfenadine, disopyramide mefloquine	Drug-induced LQT	75
	KCNE2	Clarithromycin	Drug-induced arrhythmia	76
Ryanodine receptor	RYR1	Halothane, suxamethonium	Malignant hyperthermia	77
Beta2-adrenergic receptor	$\beta_2 AR$	Salbutamol	Lack of efficacy	78, 79

LQT, long QT. TdP, *torsades de pointes*.

gene result in amino acid substitutions at positions 16 (Arg→Gly16) and 27 (Gln→Glu27). The Gly16 variant had been shown to undergo enhanced agonist-promoted down-regulation compared to the wildtype, whereas the Glu27 variant appears to attenuate down-regulation.[79,80] Asthmatic patients with the Gly16 genotype are more likely to suffer from nocturnal symptoms, and have a higher degree of airway reactivity to histamine.[81] A clinical investigation showed that 80% of patients with nocturnal asthma (defined as a 20% reduction in peak expiratory flow rate, PEFR) possessed the genotype for Gly16, compared to 52% of the control group (patients with non-nocturnal asthma).[79] Additionally, 74% of patients with a history of nocturnal worsening of asthma symptoms (i.e. not classed according to PEFR) were homozygous for the Gly16 genotype, compared to 7% of the control group.[79] A more recent study investigated the association between beta$_2$ haplotypes and beta$_2$-agonist effects in asthmatic patients. In keeping with the observed attenuated beta$_2$-receptor down-regulation of the Arg16 variant, there was a greater reduction in serum K^+ and diastolic blood pressure in the Arg16-Gln27 haplotypes than in the Gly16-Glu27 haplotype.[78] This suggests that increased responsiveness of patients with the Arg16-Gln27 haplotype may lead to an increased risk of beta$_2$-adrenoceptor-mediated systemic adverse effects from high-dose salbutamol. By contrast, investigators retrospectively examined asthma control during long-term treatment with salbutamol and salmeterol in a double-blind three-way crossover study. It was found that the major exacerbation rate during treatment with salbutamol was five times greater for homozygous Arg16 than for homozygous Gly16 patients.[82] These observations probably reflect the multifactorial aetiology of asthma. Further studies in this area are warranted and should perhaps be prospective in design, taking into account both environmental and multiple genetic factors.

Dopamine receptors and tardive dykinesia

Tardive dyskinesia (TD) is a motor disorder that occurs as a result of chronic neuroleptic drug treatment (see Chapter 15). It occurs in about 20–30% of schizophrenic patients.[83] A postulated mechanism of the adverse reaction is the up-regulation of dopamine receptors in the nigrostriatal pathway[84] as a result of long-term blockade by dopamine antagonists. In fact, the severity of TD is increased by dopamine agonists and reduced by antagonists. The dopamine D3 receptor, coded by the *DRD3* gene, has a polymorphism characterised by a serine to glycine substitution in the D3 receptor protein (ser9Gly). Several studies, including a meta-analysis, have now shown an association between the ser9Gly variant and the incidence and severity of TD.[85–88]

Cardiac potassium-channel polymorphisms

The interval between the action potential and repolarisation of the ventricular fibres is measured as the QT interval on the surface ECG (electrocardiograph). An outward current of potassium ions (the potassium rectifier current, I_{Kr}) mediates ventricular depolarisation via specific K^+ ion channels. A reduction in I_{Kr} delays repolarisation and lengthens the QT interval. This condition may be congenital or drug-induced, and may lead to *torsades de pointes* (TdP) or ventricular fibrillation. Variations in the gene coding for the K^+ ion channel have been postulated to increase the sensitivity of the channel to specific drugs. This may increase the risk of LQTS (long QT syndrome) in association with certain drugs. For example, a patient with clarithomycin-induced TdP was found to have a mutation in the *KCNE2* gene. This mutation resulted in the K^+ channel being three times more sensitive to drug inhibition than the non-mutated channel.[89] However, to date, no large-scale studies have been performed to corroborate these results, and so the implications of these observations remain tentative. A difficulty in this area is the lack of careful definition of the phenotype and the uncertain relationship between the degree of QT-interval prolongation and the risk of TdP.

Human leukocyte antigens and adverse drug reactions

The human leukocyte antigen (HLA) system

The short arm of human chromosome 6 contains a region known as the major histocompatibility complex (MHC). Approximately 60% of the genes in this region code for proteins that regulate the immune response. The HLA system, which resides within the MHC, encodes proteins whose function is to bind peptides and present them as antigens on the surface of antigen-presenting cells for interaction with T-cell receptors. There are two forms of antigen, in terms of protein structure and function, namely HLA class I and class II. This is a vital system that governs our ability to fight off infections and other harmful substances within the environment. Given the need to recognise a large array of infecting organisms, this system has adapted through the course of evolution to be the most polymorphic system in the human genome. This huge degree of variability unfortunately also leads to the development of aberrant immune responses in certain individuals, leading to autoimmune diseases, and in the case of drugs, to allergic reactions.

HLA class I antigens consist of HLA-A, HLA-B, and HLA-C sub-families, whereas the class II antigens comprise the HLA-DP, HLA-DQ and HLA-DR subfamilies. A good account of the HLA system and associated polymorphisms can be found elsewhere[90,91] and on the website of the Australasian and South East Asian Tissue Typing Association [http://www.aseatta.org.au/]. As stated above, by virtue of the polymorphic nature of the HLA antigens some individuals may develop immune-mediated ADRs, some of which are listed in Table 3.4.

Clozapine-induced agranulocytosis

The antipsychotic drug clozapine causes agranulocytosis in about 1% of patients (see Chapter 12). Several studies have investigated the association between HLA alleles and haplotypes and clozapine-induced agranulocytosis (CA) in order to identify genetic risk factors.[45,8–100,104,105] Initial studies indicated that patients of Jewish ancestry with CA displayed an increased frequency of *HLA-B38*, *HLA-DR4* and *HLA-DQ3*.[98] The frequency of this haplotype in the general population in the

Table 3.4 Examples of HLA alleles and haplotypes associated with ADRs[92]

Allele or haplotype	Drug	ADR associated with HLA	Ref
HLA-B*1502	Carbamazepine	Stevens–Johnson syndrome	93
HLA-DRB1*1501, *HLA-DQB1*0602,* *HLA-DRB5*0101*	Amoxicillin– clavulanic acid	Hepatitis	94,95
HLA-DQ7	Pyrazolones	Pyrazolone hypersensitivity	96
HLA-A29, HLA-B12, *HLA-DR7*	Sulfonamides	Toxic epidermal necrolysis	97
HLA-B38, HLA-DR4, *HLA-DQ3, HLA-Cw*7,* *HLA-DQB*0502,* *HLA-DRB*0101,* *HLA-DRB3*0202*	Clozapine	Agranulocytosis	98–100
HLA-B*5701, *HLA-DR7, HLA-DQ3*	Abacavir	Abacavir hypersensitivity reaction	101–103
HLA-DR4	Hydralazine	Systemic lupus erythematosus	92

northeastern USA is about 0.4–0.8%, but was estimated to be 10–12% in the American (USA) and Israeli Jewish populations.[105] These observations were largely corroborated in a larger study involving Jewish and non-Jewish patients with CA.[99] The study also showed an association between a different haplotype (*HLA-DR*02, HLA-DQB1*0502, HLA-DQA1* 0102*) and CA in non-Jewish patients. Hence different haplotypes were associated with CA in different races.[99] Whether these genes are causal variants or are linked to other genes on the same region of the genome in predisposing to CA is not known. Positive associations with polymorphisms in the heat shock proteins (HSP) and tumour necrosis factor-alpha (TNF-alpha) loci suggests that other genes and protein products may be involved in the pathogenesis of CA.[99,104] For instance, HSPs are a group of proteins involved in the conservation of protein structure and cellular function. TNF-alpha is an important cytokine that induces apoptosis in human polymorphonucleocytes (PMNs).[106] Clozapine or its metabolites may interact with HSP-70 and result in apoptosis of bone marrow granulocyte precursors, or inhibit the protective role of HSP in variant individuals.[105] Further studies are needed to determine the mechanisms of CA.

Abacavir hypersensitivity and HLA

Abacavir is a nucleoside reverse-transcriptase inhibitor used in HIV treatment regimens. Its use is associated with a hypersensitivity reaction in about 5% of patients.[102,107] Several studies have now shown that certain haplotypes in Caucasians are predictive of abacavir hypersensitivity.[101–103] The alleles on the MHC define the presence of an ancestral haplotype, 57.1. A combination of *HLA-B*5701* and *HSP-Hom M4937*, both of which are located on the ancestral haplotype, has recently been reported to increase the discrimination between hypersensitive individuals and controls in Australia, compared to *HLA-B*5701* alone.[102] Whether this is true in all populations awaits further study, and the precise mechanism by which this haplotype predisposes to abacavir hypersensitivity is unknown.

Utility of pharmacogenetics in the clinical setting

The ultimate aim of pharmacogenetics is to individualise drug therapy, where the choice of medicine is determined by the genetic status of the patient. In this scenario, genetically determined variations in drug response will be identified prior to prescription, and the potential for reduced efficacy and/or increased toxicity reduced. Some commentators have suggested that there may well come a time when it will be considered unethical to prescribe a medicine without elucidating the genetic profile beforehand. However, in reality this is a long way off, and the case for routine pharmacogenetic testing prior to drug administration is yet to be made.

Current limitations

Genomic research technology permits the rapid acquisition of large amounts of data. New genetic polymorphisms are being discovered at an increasing rate. However, not all genetically determined protein variants have pharmacokinetic or pharmacodynamic consequences. If a polymorphism is shown to affect either the pharmacokinetics or the pharmacodynamics of a drug, this will need to be related to clinical effects, which may be either lack of efficacy or increased toxicity. This relation between drug pharmacology and a clinical effect may be unclear, and the situation might be further compounded by discordant results in the literature. In this typical scenario, the clinical applicability of a particular polymorphism is difficult to evaluate. Other factors that may affect the clinical utility of pharmacogenetics include the predictive power and technical accuracy of pharmacogenetic tests, and associated ethical and social implications.[108] Regarding the prediction of adverse reactions, cost savings may be made not only through the preventing the adverse effect, but also by avoiding the prescription of an (ultimately) ineffective therapy.[109]

Furthermore, for many drugs therapeutic drug monitoring (TDM) allows the dose to be titrated against efficacy and adverse effects, especially when patients are taking multiple (and interacting) medicines. Thus, pharmacogenetics, if and when introduced, will have to further increase the utility of current drug therapy (see Table 3.5). Nevertheless, the value and potential usefulness of this technology is not trivial.

Potential advantages of pharmacogenetic technology

An evaluation of the role of pharmacogenomics in reducing the incidence of ADRs showed that 59% of drugs known to cause ADRs are metabolised by at least one enzyme with a variant allele known to reduce metabolism.[111] Interestingly, CYP1A2 was involved in the metabolism of 75% of the drugs implicated in causing ADRs, but in only 5% of all prescribed drugs. The study indicates that prior knowledge of a patient's pharmacogenetic profile may prevent some ADRs. Indeed, determination of

Table 3.5 Some considerations of the use of pharmacogenetic testing[110]

Is the drug subject to polymorphism-determined variations in pharmacokinetics
  (PK) or pharmacodynamics (PD)?
Is the variation in the PK or PD clinically significant?
Does the available information regarding the clinical effect of the genetic variation
  apply to the patient (e.g. ethnic background)?
Is there an alternative drug that is not subject to pharmacogenetic variation?
Is the patient on other medication that will negate the effects of
  pharmacogenetically determined dose adjustments?
Can ADRs be avoided by normal therapeutic drug monitoring?

the genotype may reduce the adverse effects of warfarin[112] and azathioprine[36] in patients lacking the enzymes responsible for metabolism of
these drugs. This concept may be extended to the early stages of drug
development. Individuals with genotypes associated with ADRs may be
identified earlier in the development process, so that the drug will be
avoided or used with caution in these individuals, when the drug is
licensed and used in the wider population. This targeted approach has
been successfully applied in terms of efficacy for the anticancer agent
trastuzumab. The drug is a monoclonal antibody directed against the
human epidermal growth factor receptor (HER) 2 protein. The drug
shows good efficacy in tumours that overexpress this protein, and is
therefore licensed for the treatment of cancer only in this patient population.[113] Likewise, it can be envisaged that patients who have a genetic
risk factor strongly associated with an ADR may be excluded (if
causative) from receiving that drug. In this way, it may be possible to
further improve the harm–benefit ratio of a drug.

Cost-effectiveness of pharmacogenetic testing

Another factor precluding routine pharmacogenetic testing of patients is
proof of clinical utility and the cost-effectiveness of the technology.
Numerous reports have outlined the rationale for clinical genotyping
and advocate its use in preventing or reducing ADRs.[110,111,114] What is
required is proof of the clinical reliability and cost-effectiveness. Pharmacogenetic testing may be viable if the economic benefits of treating fewer
patients and preventing adverse effects exceed the costs of testing.[115]
Using a decision analysis model, a study was conducted to evaluate the
effectiveness of testing for TPMT polymorphisms before initiating azathioprine therapy, compared to initiation without testing.[116] Adoption

of the prescreening strategy resulted in modest cost reductions, with about half of all serious haematological toxicities being avoided. The main determinants of the savings included the costs of PCR, which is time-consuming and requires technical expertise. A more recent similar study showed that genotyping for *HLA B*5701* prior to the initiation of abacavir therapy may be a cost-effective strategy.[117] Other issues to be considered include the potential reduction in drug sales as a consequence of genetic stratification of patients. The effect of this may be an increase in the price, or even withdrawal of the drug on the grounds of lack of economical viability. However, there is a potential for cost savings to be made during the clinical development of the drug by using a smaller pharmacogenetically relevant patient group.

In summary, progress in genetic research will continue to provide new insights into individual genotypic variations in the general population. One of the important challenges facing pharmacogenetics is a robust testimony of the cost and clinical effectiveness of the technology, particularly in relation to the prevention or management of ADRs. Much work needs to be done before this becomes a clinical reality and is accepted into clinical practice.

References

1. Lander ES, Linton LM, Birren B, *et al*. Initial sequencing and analysis of the human genome. *Nature* 2001; 409: 860–921.
2. Venter JC, Adams MD, Myers EW, *et al*. The sequence of the human genome. *Science* 2001; 291: 1304–1351.
3. Rawlins MD. Clinical pharmacology. Adverse reactions to drugs. *Br Med J* (Clin Res Ed) 1981; 282: 974–976.
4. Edwards IR, Aronson JK. Adverse drug reactions: definitions, diagnosis, and management. *Lancet* 2000; 356: 1255–1259.
5. Aronson JK, Ferner RE. Joining the DoTS: new approach to classifying adverse drug reactions. *Br Med J* 2003; 327: 1222–1225.
6. Juliano RL, Ling V. A surface glycoprotein modulating drug permeability in Chinese hamster ovary cell mutants. *Biochim Biophys Acta* 1976; 455: 152–162.
7. Sakaeda T, Nakamura T, Okumura K. MDR1 genotype-related pharmacokinetics and pharmacodynamics. *Biol Pharm Bull* 2002; 25: 1391–1400.
8. Hyde SC, Emsley P, Hartshorn MJ, *et al*. Structural model of ATP-binding proteins associated with cystic fibrosis, multidrug resistance and bacterial transport. *Nature* 1990; 346: 362–365.
9. Greiner B, Eichelbaum M, Fritz P, *et al*. The role of intestinal P-glycoprotein in the interaction of digoxin and rifampin. *J Clin Invest* 1999; 104: 147–153.
10. Hoffmeyer S, Burk O, von Richter O, *et al*. Functional polymorphisms of the human multidrug-resistance gene: multiple sequence variations and correlation

of one allele with P-glycoprotein expression and activity in vivo. *Proc Natl Acad Sci USA* 2000; 97: 3473–3478.

11. Verstuyft C, Schwab M, Schaeffeler E, *et al*. Digoxin pharmacokinetics and MDR1 genetic polymorphisms. *Eur J Clin Pharmacol* 2003; 58: 809–812.

12. Morita Y, Sakaeda T, Horinouchi M, *et al*. MDR1 genotype-related duodenal absorption rate of digoxin in healthy Japanese subjects. *Pharm Res* 2003; 20: 552–556.

13. Sakaeda T, Nakamura T, Horinouchi M, *et al*. MDR1 genotype-related pharmacokinetics of digoxin after single oral administration in healthy Japanese subjects. *Pharm Res* 2001; 18: 1400–1404.

14. Marzolini C, Paus E, Buclin T, *et al*. Polymorphisms in human MDR1 (P-glycoprotein): recent advances and clinical relevance. *Clin Pharmacol Ther* 2004; 75: 13–33.

15. Johne A, Kopke K, Gerloff T, *et al*. Modulation of steady-state kinetics of digoxin by haplotypes of the P-glycoprotein MDR1 gene. *Clin Pharmacol Ther* 2002; 72: 584–594.

16. Lin JH, Yamazaki M. Role of P-glycoprotein in pharmacokinetics: clinical implications. *Clin Pharmacokinet* 2003; 42: 59–98.

17. Lankas GR, Cartwright ME, Umbenhauer D. P-glycoprotein deficiency in a subpopulation of CF-1 mice enhances ivermectin-induced neurotoxicity. *Toxicol Appl Pharmacol* 1997; 143: 357–365.

18. Ayrton A, Morgan P. Role of transport proteins in drug absorption, distribution and excretion. *Xenobiotica* 2001; 31: 469–497.

19. Sadeque AJ, Wandel C, He H, *et al*. Increased drug delivery to the brain by P-glycoprotein inhibition. *Clin Pharmacol Ther* 2000; 68: 231–237.

20. Pauli-Magnus C, Feiner J, Brett C, *et al*. No effect of MDR1 C3435T variant on loperamide disposition and central nervous system effects. *Clin Pharmacol Ther* 2003; 74: 487–498.

21. Nishizato Y, Ieiri I, Suzuki H, *et al*. Polymorphisms of OATP-C (SLC21A6) and OAT3 (SLC22A8) genes: consequences for pravastatin pharmacokinetics. *Clin Pharmacol Ther* 2003; 73: 554–565.

22. Shroyer NF, Lewis RA, Lupski JR. Analysis of the ABCR (ABCA4) gene in 4-aminoquinoline retinopathy: is retinal toxicity by chloroquine and hydroxychloroquine related to Stargardt disease? *Am J Ophthalmol* 2001; 131: 761–766.

23. Nebert DW, Russell DW. Clinical importance of the cytochromes P450. *Lancet* 2002; 360: 1155–1162.

24. Danielson PB. The cytochrome P450 superfamily: biochemistry, evolution and drug metabolism in humans. *Curr Drug Metab* 2002; 3: 561–597.

25. Pirmohamed M, Park BK. Cytochrome P450 enzyme polymorphisms and adverse drug reactions. *Toxicology* 2003; 192: 23–32.

26. Ingelman-Sundberg M, Oscarson M, McLellan RA. Polymorphic human cytochrome P450 enzymes: an opportunity for individualized drug treatment. *Trends Pharmacol Sci* 1999; 20: 342–349.

27. Pirmohamed M, Park BK. Genetic susceptibility to adverse drug reactions. *Trends Pharmacol Sci* 2001; 22: 298–305.

28. Basile VS, Ozdemir V, Masellis M, *et al*. A functional polymorphism of the cytochrome P450 1A2 (CYP1A2) gene: association with tardive dyskinesia in schizophrenia. *Mol Psychiatry* 2000; 5: 410–417.

29. Obase Y, Shimoda T, Kawano T, *et al.* Polymorphisms in the CYP1A2 gene and theophylline metabolism in patients with asthma. *Clin Pharmacol Ther* 2003; 73: 468–474.

30. Higashi MK, Veenstra DL, Kondo LM, *et al.* Association between CYP2C9 genetic variants and anticoagulation-related outcomes during warfarin therapy. *JAMA* 2002; 287: 1690–1698.

31. Siddoway LA, Thompson KA, McAllister CB, *et al.* Polymorphism of propafenone metabolism and disposition in man: clinical and pharmacokinetic consequences. *Circulation* 1987; 75: 785–791.

32. Meyer UA. Pharmacogenetics and adverse drug reactions. *Lancet* 2000; 356: 1667–1671.

33. Felix CA, Walker AH, Lange BJ, *et al.* Association of CYP3A4 genotype with treatment-related leukemia. *Proc Natl Acad Sci USA* 1998; 95: 13176–13181.

34. Evans WE. Pharmacogenetics of thiopurine S-methyltransferase and thiopurine therapy. *Ther Drug Monit* 2004; 26: 186–191.

35. Krynetski EY, Evans WE. Pharmacogenetics as a molecular basis for individualized drug therapy: the thiopurine S-methyltransferase paradigm. *Pharm Res* 1999; 16: 342–349.

36. Relling MV, Hancock ML, Rivera GK, *et al.* Mercaptopurine therapy intolerance and heterozygosity at the thiopurine S-methyltransferase gene locus. *J Natl Cancer Inst* 1999; 91: 2001–2008.

37. Black AJ, McLeod HL, Capell HA, *et al.* Thiopurine methyltransferase genotype predicts therapy-limiting severe toxicity from azathioprine. *Ann Intern Med* 1998; 129: 716–718.

38. Ohtani T, Hiroi A, Sakurane M, *et al.* Slow acetylator genotypes as a possible risk factor for infectious mononucleosis-like syndrome induced by salazosulfapyridine. *Br J Dermatol* 2003; 148: 1035–1039.

39. Alfirevic A, Stalford AC, Vilar FJ, *et al.* Slow acetylator phenotype and genotype in HIV-positive patients with sulphamethoxazole hypersensitivity. *Br J Clin Pharmacol* 2003; 55: 158–165.

40. Zielinska E, Niewiarowski W, Bodalski J. The arylamine N-acetyltransferase (NAT2) polymorphism and the risk of adverse reactions to co-trimoxazole in children. *Eur J Clin Pharmacol* 1998; 54: 779–785.

41. Innocenti F, Iyer L, Ratain MJ. Pharmacogenetics of anticancer agents: lessons from amonafide and irinotecan. *Drug Metab Dispos* 2001; 29: 596–600.

42. Innocenti F, Undevia SD, Iyer L, *et al.* Genetic variants in the UDP-glucuronosyltransferase 1A1 gene predict the risk of severe neutropenia of irinotecan. *J Clin Oncol* 2004; 22: 1382–1388.

43. van Kuilenburg AB, Muller EW, Haasjes J, *et al.* Lethal outcome of a patient with a complete dihydropyrimidine dehydrogenase (DPD) deficiency after administration of 5-fluorouracil: frequency of the common IVS14 + 1G > A mutation causing DPD deficiency. *Clin Cancer Res* 2001; 7: 1149–1153.

44. Barta C, Sasvari-Szekely M, Devai A, *et al.* Analysis of mutations in the plasma cholinesterase gene of patients with a history of prolonged neuromuscular block during anesthesia. *Mol Genet Metab* 2001; 74: 484–488.

45. Ostrousky O, Meged S, Loewenthal R, *et al.* NQO2 gene is associated with clozapine-induced agranulocytosis. *Tissue Antigens* 2003; 62: 483–491.

46. Blanco JG, Edick MJ, Hancock ML, *et al.* Genetic polymorphisms in CYP3A5, CYP3A4 and NQO1 in children who developed therapy-related myeloid malignancies. *Pharmacogenetics* 2002; 12: 605–611.
47. Mahgoub A, Idle JR, Dring LG, *et al.* Polymorphic hydroxylation of debrisoquine in man. *Lancet* 1977; 2: 584–586.
48. Eichelbaum M, Spannbrucker N, Steincke B, *et al.* Defective N-oxidation of sparteine in man: a new pharmacogenetic defect. *Eur J Clin Pharmacol* 1979; 16: 183–187.
49. Cascorbi I. Pharmacogenetics of cytochrome p4502D6: genetic background and clinical implication. *Eur J Clin Invest* 2003; 33(Suppl 2): 17–22.
50. Bertilsson L, Dahl ML, Dalen P, *et al.* Molecular genetics of CYP2D6: clinical relevance with focus on psychotropic drugs. *Br J Clin Pharmacol* 2002; 53: 111–122.
51. Alvan G, Bechtel P, Iselius L, *et al.* Hydroxylation polymorphisms of debrisoquine and mephenytoin in European populations. *Eur J Clin Pharmacol* 1990; 39: 533–537.
52. Bertilsson L, Lou YQ, Du YL, *et al.* Pronounced differences between native Chinese and Swedish populations in the polymorphic hydroxylations of debrisoquin and S-mephenytoin. *Clin Pharmacol Ther* 1992; 51: 388–397.
53. Nakamura K, Goto F, Ray WA, *et al.* Interethnic differences in genetic polymorphism of debrisoquin and mephenytoin hydroxylation between Japanese and Caucasian populations. *Clin Pharmacol Ther* 1985; 38: 402–408.
54. Sohn DR, Shin SG, Park CW, *et al.* Metoprolol oxidation polymorphism in a Korean population: comparison with native Japanese and Chinese populations. *Br J Clin Pharmacol* 1991; 32: 504–507.
55. Johansson I, Lundqvist E, Bertilsson L, *et al.* Inherited amplification of an active gene in the cytochrome P450 CYP2D locus as a cause of ultrarapid metabolism of debrisoquine. *Proc Natl Acad Sci USA* 1993; 90: 11825–11829.
56. Cooper RG, Evans DA, Whibley EJ. Polymorphic hydroxylation of perhexiline maleate in man. *J Med Genet* 1984; 21: 27–33.
57. Shah RR, Oates NS, Idle JR, *et al.* Impaired oxidation of debrisoquine in patients with perhexiline neuropathy. *Br Med J* (Clin Res Ed) 1982; 284: 295–299.
58. Scordo MG, Spina E, Romeo P, *et al.* CYP2D6 genotype and antipsychotic-induced extrapyramidal side effects in schizophrenic patients. *Eur J Clin Pharmacol* 2000; 56: 679–683.
59. Vandel P, Haffen E, Vandel S, *et al.* Drug extrapyramidal side effects. CYP2D6 genotypes and phenotypes. *Eur J Clin Pharmacol* 1999; 55: 659–665.
60. Mihara K, Kondo T, Yasui-Furukori N, *et al.* Effects of various CYP2D6 genotypes on the steady-state plasma concentrations of risperidone and its active metabolite, 9–hydroxyrisperidone, in Japanese patients with schizophrenia. *Ther Drug Monit* 2003; 25: 287–293.
61. Charlier C, Broly F, Lhermitte M, *et al.* Polymorphisms in the CYP2D6 gene: association with plasma concentrations of fluoxetine and paroxetine. *Ther Drug Monit* 2003; 25: 738–742.
62. Bertilsson L, Mellstrom B, Sjokvist F, *et al.* Slow hydroxylation of nortriptyline and concomitant poor debrisoquine hydroxylation: clinical implications. *Lancet* 1981; 1: 560–561.

63. Roberts RL, Mulder RT, Joyce PR, *et al*. No evidence of increased adverse drug reactions in cytochrome P450 CYP2D6 poor metabolizers treated with fluoxetine or nortriptyline. *Hum Psychopharmacol* 2004; 19: 17–23.
64. Lee CR, Goldstein JA, Pieper JA. Cytochrome P450 2C9 polymorphisms: a comprehensive review of the in-vitro and human data. *Pharmacogenetics* 2002; 12: 251–263.
65. Aithal GP, Day CP, Kesteven PJ, *et al*. Association of polymorphisms in the cytochrome P450 CYP2C9 with warfarin dose requirement and risk of bleeding complications. *Lancet* 1999; 353: 717–719.
66. Schwarz UI. Clinical relevance of genetic polymorphisms in the human CYP2C9 gene. *Eur J Clin Invest* 2003; 33(Suppl 2): 23–30.
67. Taube J, Halsall D, Baglin T. Influence of cytochrome P-450 CYP2C9 polymorphisms on warfarin sensitivity and risk of over-anticoagulation in patients on long-term treatment. *Blood* 2000; 96: 1816–1819.
68. Baker DE. Pharmacogenomics of azathioprine and 6-mercaptopurine in gastroenterologic therapy. *Rev Gastroenterol Disord* 2003; 3: 150–157.
69. Weinshilboum RM, Sladek SL. Mercaptopurine pharmacogenetics: monogenic inheritance of erythrocyte thiopurine methyltransferase activity. *Am J Hum Genet* 1980; 32: 651–662.
70. Evans WE, Hon YY, Bomgaars L, *et al*. Preponderance of thiopurine S-methyltransferase deficiency and heterozygosity among patients intolerant to mercaptopurine or azathioprine. *J Clin Oncol* 2001; 19: 2293–2301.
71. Levy G. Predicting effective drug concentrations for individual patients. Determinants of pharmacodynamic variability. *Clin Pharmacokinet* 1998; 34: 323–333.
72. Lapka R, Sechser T, Rejholec V, *et al*. Pharmacokinetics and pharmacodynamics of conventional and controlled-release formulations of metipranolol in man. *Eur J Clin Pharmacol* 1990; 38: 243–247.
73. Shi J, Hui L, Xu Y, *et al*. Sequence variations in the mu-opioid receptor gene (OPRM1) associated with human addiction to heroin. *Hum Mutat* 2002; 19: 459–460.
74. Moss AJ, Zareba W, Kaufman ES, *et al*. Increased risk of arrhythmic events in long-QT syndrome with mutations in the pore region of the human ether-a-go-go-related gene potassium channel. *Circulation* 2002; 105: 794–799.
75. Kubota T, Horie M, Takano M, *et al*. Evidence for a single nucleotide polymorphism in the KCNQ1 potassium channel that underlies susceptibility to life-threatening arrhythmias. *J Cardiovasc Electrophysiol* 2001; 12: 1223–1229.
76. Abbott GW, Sesti F, Splawski I, *et al*. MiRP1 forms IKr potassium channels with HERG and is associated with cardiac arrhythmia. *Cell* 1999; 97: 175–187.
77. Girard T, Urwyler A, Censier K, *et al*. Genotype–phenotype comparison of the Swiss malignant hyperthermia population. *Hum Mutat* 2001; 18: 357–358.
78. Lee DK, Bates CE, Lipworth BJ. Acute systemic effects of inhaled salbutamol in asthmatic subjects expressing common homozygous beta2-adrenoceptor haplotypes at positions 16 and 27. *Br J Clin Pharmacol* 2004; 57: 100–104.
79. Liggett SB. Beta(2)-adrenergic receptor pharmacogenetics. *Am J Respir Crit Care Med* 2000; 161: S197–S201.
80. Fenech A, Hall IP. Pharmacogenetics of asthma. *Br J Clin Pharmacol* 2002; 53: 3–15.
81. Xu J, Levitt RC, Panhuysen CI, *et al*. Evidence for two unlinked loci regulating total serum IgE levels. *Am J Hum Genet* 1995; 57: 425–430.

82. Taylor DR, Drazen JM, Herbison GP, *et al.* Asthma exacerbations during long term beta agonist use: influence of beta(2) adrenoceptor polymorphism. *Thorax* 2000; 55: 762–767.

83. Casey DE. Neuroleptic drug-induced extrapyramidal syndromes and tardive dyskinesia. *Schizophrenia Res* 1991; 4: 109–120.

84. Gordon JH, Fields JZ. A permanent dopamine receptor up-regulation in the ovariectomized rat. *Pharmacol Biochem Behav* 1989; 33: 123–125.

85. Segman R, Neeman T, Heresco-Levy U, *et al.* Genotypic association between the dopamine D3 receptor and tardive dyskinesia in chronic schizophrenia. *Mol Psychiatry* 1999; 4: 247–253.

86. Lerer B, Segman RH, Fangerau H, *et al.* Pharmacogenetics of tardive dyskinesia: combined analysis of 780 patients supports association with dopamine D3 receptor gene Ser9Gly polymorphism. *Neuropsychopharmacology* 2002; 27: 105–119.

87. Steen VM, Lovlie R, MacEwan T, *et al.* Dopamine D3-receptor gene variant and susceptibility to tardive dyskinesia in schizophrenic patients. *Mol Psychiatry* 1997; 2: 139–145.

88. Basile VS, Masellis M, Badri F, *et al.* Association of the MscI polymorphism of the dopamine D3 receptor gene with tardive dyskinesia in schizophrenia. *Neuropsychopharmacology* 1999; 21: 17–27.

89. Sesti F, Abbott GW, Wei J, *et al.* A common polymorphism associated with antibiotic-induced cardiac arrhythmia. *Proc Natl Acad Sci USA* 2000; 97: 10613–10618.

90. Tomlinson IP, Bodmer WF. The HLA system and the analysis of multifactorial genetic disease. *Trends Genet* 1995; 11: 493–498.

91. Williams TM. Human leukocyte antigen gene polymorphism and the histocompatibility laboratory. *J Mol Diagn* 2001; 3: 98–104.

92. Park BK, Pirmohamed M, Kitteringham NR. Idiosyncratic drug reactions: a mechanistic evaluation of risk factors. *Br J Clin Pharmacol* 1992; 34: 377–395.

93. Chung WH, Hung SI, Hong HS, *et al.* Medical genetics: a marker for Stevens–Johnson syndrome. *Nature* 2004; 428: 486.

94. O'Donohue J, Oien KA, Donaldson P, *et al.* Co-amoxiclav jaundice: clinical and histological features and HLA class II association. *Gut* 2000; 47: 717–720.

95. Hautekeete ML, Horsmans Y, Van Waeyenberge C, *et al.* HLA association of amoxicillin–clavulanate–induced hepatitis. *Gastroenterology* 1999; 117: 1181–1186.

96. Kowalski ML, Woszczek G, Bienkiewicz B, *et al.* Association of pyrazolone drug hypersensitivity with HLA-DQ and DR antigens. *Clin Exp Allergy* 1998; 28: 1153–1158.

97. Roujeau JC, Huynh TN, Bracq C, *et al.* Genetic susceptibility to toxic epidermal necrolysis. *Arch Dermatol* 1987; 123: 1171–1173.

98. Lieberman JA, Yunis J, Egea E, *et al.* HLA-B38, DR4, DQw3 and clozapine-induced agranulocytosis in Jewish patients with schizophrenia. *Arch Gen Psychiatry* 1990; 47: 945–948.

99. Yunis JJ, Corzo D, Salazar M, *et al.* HLA associations in clozapine-induced agranulocytosis. *Blood* 1995; 86: 1177–1183.

100. Dettling M, Schaub RT, Mueller-Oerlinghausen B, *et al.* Further evidence of human leukocyte antigen-encoded susceptibility to clozapine-induced agranulocytosis independent of ancestry. *Pharmacogenetics* 2001; 11: 135–141.

101. Hetherington S, Hughes AR, Mosteller M, *et al*. Genetic variations in HLA-B region and hypersensitivity reactions to abacavir. *Lancet* 2002; 359: 1121–1122.
102. Mallal S, Nolan D, Witt C, *et al*. Association between presence of HLA-B*5701, HLA-DR7, and HLA-DQ3 and hypersensitivity to HIV-1 reverse-transcriptase inhibitor abacavir. *Lancet* 2002; 359: 727–732.
103. Martin AM, Nolan D, Gaudieri S, *et al*. Predisposition to abacavir hypersensitivity conferred by HLA-B*5701 and a haplotypic Hsp70-Hom variant. *Proc Natl Acad Sci USA* 2004; 101: 4180–4185.
104. Turbay D, Lieberman J, Alper CA, *et al*. Tumor necrosis factor constellation polymorphism and clozapine-induced agranulocytosis in two different ethnic groups. *Blood* 1997; 89: 4167–4174.
105. Corzo D, Yunis JJ, Salazar M, *et al*. The major histocompatibility complex region marked by HSP70-1 and HSP70-2 variants is associated with clozapine-induced agranulocytosis in two different ethnic groups. *Blood* 1995; 86: 3835–3840.
106. Salamone G, Giordano M, Trevani AS, *et al*. Promotion of neutrophil apoptosis by TNF-alpha. *J Immunol* 2001; 166: 3476–3483.
107. Clay PG. The abacavir hypersensitivity reaction: a review. *Clin Ther* 2002; 24: 1502–1514.
108. Shah J. Criteria influencing the clinical uptake of pharmacogenomic strategies. *Br Med J* 2004; 328: 1482–1486.
109. Nuffield Pharmacogenetics Working Party Report, September 2003; Pharmacogenetics: ethical issues. Nuffield Council on Bioethics, London. Available online at [www.nuffieldbioethics.org/pharmacogenetics]
110. Fishbain DA, Fishbain D, Lewis J, *et al*. Genetic testing for enzymes of drug metabolism: does it have clinical utility for pain medicine at the present time? A structured review. *Pain Med* 2004; 5: 81–93.
111. Phillips KA, Veenstra DL, Oren E, *et al*. Potential role of pharmacogenomics in reducing adverse drug reactions: a systematic review. *JAMA* 2001; 286: 2270–2279.
112. Ablin J, Cabili S, Eldor A, *et al*. Warfarin therapy is feasible in CYP2C9*3 homozygous patients. *Eur J Intern Med* 2004; 15: 22–27.
113. Miles DW. Update on HER-2 as a target for cancer therapy: herceptin in the clinical setting. *Breast Cancer Res* 2001; 3: 380–384.
114. Kirchheiner J, Brosen K, Dahl ML, *et al*. CYP2D6 and CYP2C19 genotype-based dose recommendations for antidepressants: a first step towards subpopulation-specific dosages. *Acta Psychiatr Scand* 2001; 104: 173–192.
115. Danzon P, Towse A. The economics of gene therapy and of pharmacogenetics. *Value Health* 2002; 5: 5–13.
116. Marra CA, Esdaile JM, Anis AH. Practical pharmacogenetics: the cost effectiveness of screening for thiopurine s-methyltransferase polymorphisms in patients with rheumatological conditions treated with azathioprine. *J Rheumatol* 2002; 29: 2507–2512.
117. Hughes D, Vilar J, Ward C, *et al*. Cost-effectiveness of HLAB*5701 genotyping in preventing abacavir hypersensitivity. *Pharmacogenetics* 2004; 14: 335–342.

Further reading

Ensom MH, Chang TK, Patel P. Pharmacogenetics: the therapeutic drug monitoring of the future? *Clin Pharmacokinet* 2001; 40: 783–802.

Evans WE, Relling MV. Pharmacogenomics: translating functional genomics into rational therapeutics. *Science* 1999; 286: 487–491.

Fishbain DA, Fishbain D, Lewis J, *et al.* Genetic testing for enzymes of drug metabolism: does it have clinical utility for pain medicine at the present time? A structured review. *Pain Med* 2004; 5: 81–93.

Ingelman-Sundberg M. Pharmacogenetics: an opportunity for a safer and more efficient pharmacotherapy. *J Intern Med* 2001; 250: 186–200.

Lin JH, Yamazaki M. Role of P-glycoprotein in pharmacokinetics: clinical implications. *Clin Pharmacokinet* 2003; 42: 59–98.

Marzolini C, Paus E, Buclin T, *et al.* Polymorphisms in human MDR1 (P-glycoprotein): recent advances and clinical relevance. *Clin Pharmacol Ther* 2004; 75: 13–33.

Meyer UA. Pharmacogenetics and adverse drug reactions. *Lancet* 2000; 356: 1667–1671.

Ozdemir V, Shear NH, Kalow W. What will be the role of pharmacogenetics in evaluating drug safety and minimising adverse effects? *Drug Safety* 2001; 24: 75–85.

Park BK, Pirmohamed M, Kitteringham NR. Idiosyncratic drug reactions: a mechanistic evaluation of risk factors. *Br J Clin Pharmacol* 1992; 34: 377–395.

Pirmohamed M, Park BK. Genetic susceptibility to advese drug reactions. *Trends Pharmacol Sci* 2001; 22: 298–305.

Vandebriel RJ. Gene polymorphisms within the immune system that may underlie drug allergy. *Naunyn Schmiedebergs Arch Pharmacol* 2004; 369: 125–132.

Glossary

Allele   One of the variant forms of a gene at a particular locus, or location, on a chromosome. Different alleles produce variations in inherited characteristics, such as hair colour or blood type. In an individual, one form of the allele (the dominant one) may be expressed more than another form (the recessive one).

Amino acid   A building block of proteins. There are 20 different kinds of naturally occurring amino acid.

Base pair   Two bases which form a 'rung of the DNA ladder'. A DNA nucleotide is made of a molecule of sugar, a molecule of phosphoric acid, and a molecule called a base. The bases are the 'letters' that spell out the genetic code.

Candidate gene   A gene located in a chromosome region suspected of being involved in a disease.

Carrier   An individual who possesses one copy of a mutant allele that causes disease only when two copies are present. Although carriers not affected by the disease, two carriers can produce a child who has the disease.

Chromosome   A structure found in the cell nucleus that contains the genes; chromosomes are composed of DNA and proteins. Each parent contributes one chromosome to each pair, so children get half of their chromosomes from their mother and half from their father.

Cloning   Using specialised DNA technology to produce multiple exact copies of a single gene or other segment of DNA to obtain enough material for further study.

Deoxyribonucleic acid (DNA)   The substance of heredity; a large molecule that carries the genetic information necessary for all cellular functions, including the building of proteins. DNA is composed of the sugar deoxyribose, phosphate, and the bases adenine, thymine, guanine and cytosine.

Dominant   A gene that almost always results in a specific physical characteristic even though the patient's genome possesses only one copy. With a dominant gene, the chance of passing on that gene, which may cause a condition or disease, to children is 50/50 in each pregnancy.

Double helix   The structural arrangement of DNA, which looks something like an immensely long ladder twisted into a helix, or coil. The sides of the 'ladder' are formed by a backbone of sugar and phosphate molecules, and the 'rungs' consist of nucleotide bases joined weakly in the middle by hydrogen bonds.

Gene   The functional and physical unit of heredity passed from parent to offspring. Genes are pieces of DNA, and most genes contain the information for making a specific protein.

Genetic code (ATGC)   The language in which DNA's instructions are written. It consists of triplets of nucleotides, with each triplet corresponding to one amino acid in a protein's structure or to a signal to start or stop protein production.

Genome   All the DNA contained in an organism or a cell, which includes both the chromosomes within the nucleus and the DNA in mitochondria.

Genotype   The genetic identity of an individual that does not show as outward characteristics.

Haplotype   A set or combination of alleles or linked genetic markers found on a single chromosome, which tend to be inherited together in a given individual.

Heterozygous   Possessing two different forms of a particular gene, one inherited from each parent.

Homozygous   Possessing two identical forms of a particular gene, one inherited from each parent.

Human Genome Project   An international research project to map each human gene and to completely sequence human DNA.

Inherited   Transmitted through genes from parents to offspring.

Knockout   Inactivation of specific genes. Knockouts are often created in laboratory organisms such as yeast or mice, so that scientists can study the knockout organism as a model for a particular disease.

Linkage disequilibrium   The occurrence, on the same chromosome, of some combinations of alleles of closely linked genes more often than would be predicted by chance.

Mutation   A permanent structural alteration in DNA. In most cases DNA changes either have no effect or cause harm, but occasionally a mutation can improve an organism's chance of surviving and passing the beneficial change on to its descendants.

Nucleotide   One of the structural components, or building blocks, of DNA and RNA. A nucleotide consists of a base (one of four chemicals: adenine, thymine, guanine, and cytosine) plus a molecule of sugar and one of phosphoric acid.

Oncogene   A gene that is capable of causing the transformation of normal cells into cancer cells.

Pharmacogenetics   The study of how people respond differently to medicines due to their genetic inheritance. The term is made up of the words pharmacology and genetics. An ultimate goal of pharmacogenetics is to understand how someone's genetic make-up determines how well a medicine works in the body, as well as what side effects are likely to occur. In the future, advances gleaned from pharmacogenetics research will provide information to guide prescribers in individualising drug therapy.

Phenotype   The observable traits or characteristics of an organism, for example hair colour, weight, or the presence or absence of a disease.

Polymerase chain reaction (PCR)   A method of rapidly synthesising many copies of a specific segment of DNA.

Polymorphism   A common variation in the sequence of DNA among individuals.

Recessive   A genetic condition that appears only in individuals who have received two copies of a mutant gene, one from each parent.

Restriction fragment length polymorphism (RFLP)   A common variation in DNA sequence which manifests itself in the variation in length of one or more restriction fragments.

Ribonucleic acid (RNA)   A single-stranded molecule that carries genetic information. RNA is composed of the sugar ribose, phosphate, and the bases adenine, uracil, guanine and cytosine.

Sex chromosome   One of the two chromosomes that specify an organism's genetic sex. Humans have two kinds of sex chromosome, one called X and the other Y.

Single nucleotide polymorphism (SNP)   Common but minute variations that occur in human DNA at a frequency of one every 1000 bases (see **Base pair**). These variations can be used to track inheritance in families. SNP is pronounced 'snip'.

4

Adverse drug reactions in pregnancy

Patricia McElhatton

Introduction

Some medicines when taken during pregnancy can harm the developing baby (i.e. act as teratogens). The warning labels on medicines and information leaflets concerning possible adverse effects of medicines during pregnancy are often outdated, misleading, and contain little information that is of practical help to the healthcare professional. Furthermore, such warnings are often unheeded by the patient prior to use of the medication but read only after it has been taken. This is a source of concern for both the patient and the prescriber.

The care of the pregnant woman is one of the paradoxes of modern medicine. Risk perception among pregnant women (and many healthcare professionals) is often poor. Most pregnant women expect to have a healthy pregnancy resulting in the birth of a healthy child. They are often unaware of the background incidence of congenital malformations (2–3%) or miscarriages (10–20% – often associated with fetal malformation incompatible with extrauterine life) in clinically confirmed pregnancies. Many women do have uneventful pregnancies and require little if any medical intervention. Some, however, for a variety of reasons, may incur a high risk of damage to their own health or that of their unborn child without appropriate intervention, often involving drug treatment. Although there has been much emphasis on the adverse effects of medication on the fetus, less attention has been paid to the potential adverse effects from maternal illness, which may be exacerbated during pregnancy, particularly if the illness is left untreated or treated inappropriately.

It is estimated that about 80% women still take between three and eight medicines, either prescribed or over-the-counter (OTC), during pregnancy, often before they realise that they are pregnant.[1] Analgesics are taken by about 12% of pregnant women and a further 9% take medicines for chronic diseases such as hypertension or asthma. Few data are available on complementary remedies or on the effects of paternal exposure to medicines on fetal development.

Effective risk communication is one of the major challenges facing healthcare professionals caring for pregnant women (see section on Risk Assessment). There are two main areas of risk communication that require different approaches: risk communication before a therapeutic choice is made or pregnancy initiated, and communicating risks after drug exposure in pregnancy has occurred. In the latter case, questions as to whether or not fetal development will be adversely affected may have to be addressed. This may involve discussions on whether additional invasive diagnostic procedures or termination of pregnancy should be considered.

Teratogens

An agent is a teratogen if its administration to a pregnant woman directly or indirectly causes structural or functional abnormalities in the fetus, or in the child after birth, which may not be apparent until later life.[2–4] Thus fetal toxicity can occur at any stage of pregnancy, not just in the first trimester. The range of teratogenic effects is shown in Table 4.1. Note that definitions of some specific terms are included in the glossary at the end of the chapter.

Table 4.1 Effects induced by teratogens

Chromosomal abnormalities
Impairment of implantation of the conceptus
Resorption or abortion of the early embryo
Structural malformations
Intrauterine growth retardation
Fetal death
Functional impairment in the neonate, e.g. deafness
Behavioural abnormalities
Central nervous system (CNS) dysfunction, e.g. mental retardation
Transplacental carcinogenesis

Physiological and pharmacological changes during pregnancy

There is no specific placental barrier to the passage of drugs, so the fetus is inevitably exposed, and although an agent can be either beneficial or harmless to the mother, it can none the less be harmful, even lethal, to the embryo or fetus.

The metabolism and kinetics of some drugs change during pregnancy. Overall, the effective drug concentration is influenced by four main factors: 1) the uptake, distribution, metabolism and excretion by the mother; 2) the passage and metabolism of the substance via the yolk sac and placenta; 3) the distribution, metabolism and excretion by the fetus;

and 4) reabsorption and swallowing of the substance by the fetus from the amniotic fluid. The main physiological changes that influence drug and chemical metabolism are summarised in Table 4.2.

Teratogenic effects are usually dose dependent; agents can act synergistically, and the time of administration after conception is critically important in determining the possible effects on the fetus. Risk can differ among individuals, as a result of genetic variation in drug metabolism or other factors.

Table 4.2 Changes in drug pharmacokinetics during pregnancy

Resorption	
Gastrointestinal motility	⇓
Lung function	⇑
Skin blood circulation	⇑
Distribution	
Plasma volume	⇑
Body water	⇑
Plasma protein	⇓
Fat deposit	⇑
Metabolism	
Liver activity	⇑⇓
Excretion	
Glomerular filtration	⇑

Adapted from ref. 5.

Risk assessment in pregnancy

Little is known about specific teratogenic mechanisms.[3,6] Most medicines given in pregnancy are for treatment of the mother, but in most instances this means that the fetus is also exposed. Therefore, it is important to balance the risk to the fetus from the drug-related effects against the risks to both the mother and the fetus from failing to treat the maternal illness. Unfortunately, the effects of a drug in pregnancy are often unknown, and the majority of drugs either carry a warning against use in pregnancy unless the potential benefits outweigh the risks (usually undefined), or are contraindicated.

Timing of exposure

Drugs and other chemicals can cause adverse effects at any stage of pregnancy. Consequently, limiting cautionary advice statements to the first trimester is an underestimation of the risks involved to the embryo/fetus. Also, when a woman first learns she is pregnant organogenesis may have already begun, e.g. neural tube closure may already be in progress, or be completed (up to 28 days post conception). Therefore, in many instances the embryo is inadvertently exposed to maternal drug therapy in the very early stages of development.

Detecting teratogenic effects

In Europe, the incidence of spontaneous malformations in newborn babies is approximately 2–3% (1 in 40 live births). This makes it difficult to detect any change in incidence due to maternal drug therapy. For example, to be reasonably sure that a drug doubles the incidence of a malformation such as cleft palate (<1:1000 expected in the general population), a study of 23 000 pregnancies would be needed.[7] Even when a very rare, severe defect (amelia/phocomelia) occurred, it took approximately 10 years and several hundred malformed babies to establish a causal relationship with a newly marketed drug, thalidomide.

Evaluation of studies

For most drugs and chemicals data on human exposure are scarce, as these are not routinely tested in women of childbearing age, but the need to include women in clinical trials is increasingly recognised. Although the evaluation of data from the limited number of epidemiological studies and human case reports of drug use in pregnancy provides useful information, often the only information available on reproductive toxicology is from preclinical studies in animals or from *in vitro* tests. It is very difficult to extrapolate the data from such studies to human pregnancy.[1–3]

Prescribing in pregnancy

Making decisions on whether or not to prescribe or to take medicines, during pregnancy, and the choice of drug to recommend for a particular condition, is difficult and a frequent source of anxiety for both the prescriber and the patient. It is particularly difficult in situations where the preferred drug for an illness is also a known teratogen, for example the use of sodium valproate in the treatment of epilepsy or bipolar disorder. Current knowledge of the effects of drugs on the developing infant can be classified into three main categories: 1) drugs for which there is consistent

Table 4.3 Drugs known to cause fetotoxic effects when taken in the first trimester of pregnancy

Drug taken by the mother	Possible effect on the infant
ACE inhibitors and angiotensin-II receptor antagonists	Lung and kidney hypoplasia, hypocalvaria[8]
Antiepileptics	Cardiac, facial and limb defects, mental retardation, neural tube defects[1,4]
Cytotoxic drugs	Multiple defects,[9] abortion[10]
Drugs of abuse	Multiple defects[11,12]
Ethanol	Fetal alcohol syndrome (FAS)[13,14]
Hormones – androgens	Virilisation of female fetus[1,4]
Diethylstilbestrol	Genital anomalies in female and male infants, transplacental carcinogen[4,6]
Other oestrogens	Feminisation of male fetus[4,6]
Lithium	Cardiovascular and other defects[15]
Misoprostol – as an abortifacient	Moebius sequence[16]
Retinoids	Ear, cardiovascular, skeletal defects CNS dysfunction[17,18]
Thalidomide	Limb reduction and other defects[1,4,6]
Warfarin	Nasal hypoplasia, chondrodysplasia punctata[19]

NB. Absence of a drug from this table does not imply safety.
ACE, angiotensin-converting enzyme. CNS, central nervous system.

evidence of teratogenic effects (Tables 4.3 and 4.4); 2) drugs where there is a high index of suspicion of adverse fetal effects but fewer data about causality (Table 4.5); and 3) drugs about which the effects in pregnancy are not known. Category (3) is the largest group, comprising the majority of drugs on the market.

Knowledge of the general principles of teratogenesis may guide healthcare professionals towards effective and safe prescribing for pregnant women. It should not be necessary to state that drug treatment should only be given if it is clearly needed. Conversely, it should not be withheld in situations where the wellbeing of the mother and the fetus would be at risk if medication were discontinued, e.g. in epilepsy, diabetes, hypertension and psychosis. Because the fetus is most at risk of structural malformations, e.g. spina bifida or cleft palate, during the first trimester, treatment should, wherever possible, be withheld until later in pregnancy. However, if treatment is needed, then the lowest effective dose of a single agent should be used, and treatment should stop as soon as possible. New medicines are best avoided, because information on them is necessarily

Table 4.4 Drugs known to cause fetotoxic effects when taken in the second and third trimesters of pregnancy

Drug taken by the mother	Possible effect on the infant
ACE inhibitors and angiotensin-II receptor antagonists	Oligohydramnios, growth retardation, lung and kidney hypoplasia, hypocalvaria, neonatal convulsions, hypotension, anuria[8,20]
Aminoglycosides	Deafness, vestibular damage[21]
Antidepressants	Neonatal withdrawal symptoms[119]
Antiepileptics	Mental retardation, ?autism/Asperger syndrome[83]
Benzodiazepines	Floppy infant syndrome, neonatal respiratory depression, withdrawal symptoms[4]
Beta-adrenoceptor antagonists	?Intrauterine growth retardation, neonatal bradycardia, hypoglycaemia[22]
Cytotoxic drugs	Intrauterine growth retardation, stillbirth[9,10]
Diethylstilbestrol	Vaginal adenocarcinoma – transplacental carcinogen[1,4,6]
Drugs of abuse	CNS dysfunction, intrauterine growth retardation[4,107]
Non-steroidal anti-inflammatory drugs (NSAIDs)	?Prolongation of gestation and labour, premature closure of ductus arteriosus, neonatal pulmonary hypertension[4,67,68]
Opioids	Neonatal respiratory depression, withdrawal symptoms[4]
Phenothiazines	Neonatal withdrawal symptoms, impaired thermoregulation, extrapyramidal effects[4,17]
Retinoids	CNS dysfunction[17]
Salicylates	Fetal/neonatal haemorrhage[4,67,68]
Sex hormones	Virilisation of female fetus/feminisation of male fetus[4,6]
Sulfonamides	Hyperbilirubinaemia, kernicterus[4]
Tetracyclines	Staining of deciduous teeth, impairs bone growth[4,21]
Warfarin/coumarins	Fetal haemorrhage, CNS abnormalities[23]

NB. Absence of a drug from this table does not imply safety.

sparse. It is best, if possible, to avoid using known teratogens (Tables 4.3 and 4.4) in women of childbearing age. Where the nature of potential abnormalities is known, then ultrasound scanning at approximately 20 weeks of pregnancy and subsequently can give accurate information on gestational age and may detect some major anomalies while therapeutic

Table 4.5 Drugs for which there is a high index of suspicion of fetal and long-term postnatal developmental toxicity

Drug taken by the mother	Possible effect on the infant
Bisphosphonates	Skeletal defects in animals,[24] accumulates in bone, very long half life
Ecstasy (methylenedioxymethamfetamine)	Multiple defects, mainly CVS and musculoskeletal[25,26]
Leflunomide	CNS and skeletal defects in animals at drug concentration lower than those associated with therapy in humans[27,28]
Methotrexate (maternal exposure)	Multiple, diverse malformations – dose dependent?[9,65]
Methotrexate (paternal exposure)	Chromosomal abnormalities?[9,29]
Quinolones	Animal data – damage to the cartilage of immature animals and the fetus resulting in joint arthropathies[21,48,149]
Statins (few data)	Multiple, diverse malformations – several CNS malformations[30,31]

NB. Absence of a drug from this table does not imply safety.
CVS, cardiovascular system.

abortion is still possible (normally up to 24 weeks). It is important to remember that prenatal diagnostic scans are tools to aid assessment of the magnitude of the teratogenic risk, but the limits of detection of the technique do not permit all malformations to be detected or excluded.

There is growing concern about the potential pre- and postnatal effects of drugs that are taken during pregnancy for the long-term treatment of chronic illness, e.g. depression, psychosis, epilepsy. There is evidence from experimental studies that drugs such as antipsychotics, antidepressants and antiepileptics may cause CNS dysfunction and adverse effects on postnatal behaviour. Some of these effects may not be manifest until the child is several years old, and causality is difficult to prove. At present, there are no prenatal diagnostic tests to detect such functional abnormalities.

Specific agents

The drugs for which there are consistent data concerning fetal toxicity are shown in Tables 4.3 and 4.4. In the following sections, selected drugs cited in Tables 4.3–4.5, which are commonly referred for risk assessment to the UK National Teratology Information Service, will be discussed in more detail.

Drugs used to treat selected cardiovascular system disorders

In this section the adverse effects of drugs used in the treatment of hypertension, hypercholesterolaemia/hyperlipidaemia and anticoagulation will be described.

Antihypertensive therapy

Although hypertensive disorders complicate about 10–16% of pregnancies and are a leading cause of maternal, fetal and neonatal morbidity and mortality worldwide, the choice of treatment remains controversial.[22,32–37]

Diuretics

Diuretics reduce placental perfusion and may cause a decrease in plasma volume expansion, oligohydramnios and electrolyte disturbances. They are generally contraindicated in pregnancy, and should only be used in rare circumstances such as heart failure or pulmonary oedema.[38] The best-studied are the thiazides, in particular hydrochlorothiazide. In a study of 567 women treated in the first 3 months of pregnancy there was no increase in the overall malformation rate or in any specific malformation.[39] In situations where a diuretic is clinically indicated, hydrochlorothiazide is recommended and maternal electrolytes, haematocrit and amniotic fluid volume should be monitored.[38] If used long term during pregnancy, neonatal hypoglycaemia should be excluded.

Methyldopa

Results of a 7.5-year follow-up study of children born to hypertensive women treated with methyldopa during pregnancy were inconclusive.[40] However, there is no clear evidence of an increased risk of malformations directly attributable to the drug.[41–43] Methyldopa is one of the preferred drugs for the treatment of hypertension in pregnancy.

Beta-adrenoceptor antagonists

Beta-adrenoceptor antagonists are not known teratogens.[44–46] Atenolol significantly retarded growth compared to acebutolol, pindolol and labetalol, but not by comparison with a control group.[47–50] There is a theoretical risk of neonatal beta-adrenoceptor blockade causing neonatal bradycardia, hypotension and hypoglycaemia.[22] Neonatal breathing difficulties and apnoea have been reported following *in utero* exposure to propranolol, but such adverse effects are rare.[39] Labetalol, propranolol and metoprolol have been in long-term use and are among the drugs of choice for treating hypertension in pregnancy. Timolol eye drops may be used to treat glaucoma throughout pregnancy.[51]

Calcium channel blockers

Nifedipine and verapamil are the best-studied calcium antagonists in human pregnancy.[52] Although embryogenesis is a highly calcium-dependent process, there are no substantial data to indicate that calcium channel blockers disrupt this process or cause a significant increase in fetotoxicity in humans.[53–55] In the first trimester, calcium antagonists are considered to be second-line therapy. Nifedipine capsules that act rapidly should not be used because they can cause a precipitous fall in blood pressure. The long-acting nifedipine preparations given once daily are preferred. Profound hypotension could also be a problem when parenteral magnesium sulphate is used in addition to nifedipine for either prophylaxis or treatment of eclampsia, because of the effects of magnesium ions on calcium channel function.

Angiotensin-converting enzyme (ACE) inhibitors

ACE inhibitors such as captopril and lisinopril are contraindicated in pregnancy except in cases where the illness is severe and there is no other effective treatment. They can cause oligohydramnios, renal tubular dysgenesis, neonatal anuria, hypocalvaria, pulmonary hypoplasia, persistent patent ductus arteriosus, intrauterine growth retardation, and fetal or neonatal death. A direct action of ACE inhibitors on the fetal renin–angiotensin system, and ischaemia due to maternal hypertension and subsequent reduction in fetoplacental blood flow, have been implicated.[8] Although the major adverse effects associated with ACE inhibitors have been reported after second- and third-trimester exposure (Tables 4.3, 4.4), experimental evidence is accumulating to indicate that these effects are initiated in the first trimester owing to the profound hypotensive effects of ACE inhibitors on the developing fetal cardiovascular system.

Angiotensin-II receptor antagonists

Angiotensin-II receptor antagonists such as losartan and valsartan are thought to have a similar action to ACE inhibitors on fetal kidney metabolism, and are suspected to cause similar fetal lesions.[20,56–59] As their role in the management of hypertension has yet to be established, the use of angiotensin-II receptor antagonists in pregnancy is contraindicated unless all other treatment regimens have been ineffective.

Inadvertent exposure to either an ACE inhibitor or an angiotensin-II receptor antagonist in the first trimester is not sufficient grounds to recommend termination. However, in cases involving long-term prenatal therapy the fetus should be monitored for the potential development of oligohydramnios, and fetal growth and development should be assessed with detailed ultrasound scans.

Statins

Statins are competitive inhibitors of 3-hydroxy-3-methylglutaryl coenzyme A (HMG-CoA) reductase, the rate-limiting step in *de novo* cholesterol biosynthesis. They are used orally to treat hyperlipidaemia and hypercholesterolaemia. In the UK, statins are now available without a prescription and health promotion campaigns encourage their use.

One of the normal physiological changes that occurs during pregnancy is a steady increase in serum lipids and cholesterol. By the third trimester triglyceride levels are 300–400 times higher and cholesterol levels are 25–90% higher than in the prepregnancy state, and do not return to normal until about 8 weeks after delivery. The pregnancy-induced hypertriglyceridaemia is usually moderate except in women with diabetes or familial hypercholesterolaemia.[60] Because of the safety profile of the statins they are not generally recommended for use in pregnancy, but inadvertent exposure has been reported.

As cholesterol is required for the synthesis of steroid hormones, there are concerns that HMG-CoA reductase inhibition may impair adrenal and gonadal endocrine function and synthesis of steroid hormones.[61,62] Cholesterol-binding to a protein known as Sonic Hedgehog protein is required for it to play a signalling role in embryo development. A collection of spontaneous uncontrolled reports of human malformations possibly linked to abnormal Sonic Hedgehog signalling after exposure to HMG-CoA reductase inhibitors, including lovastatin, simvastatin and atorvastatin, has been published.[63]

No epidemiological studies of pregnancy outcome in infants born to women treated with statins during pregnancy have been reported. However, there are several conflicting reports of adverse pregnancy outcomes following such exposures, and it is not always clear how many individual babies with congenital malformations are involved.[30,31,64–66]

The current estimate from the literature is 16–20 babies with congenital malformations out of about 520 live births (3–4%), including neural tube defects (NTD), limb reduction defects (LRD), holoprosencephaly, and the VACTERL syndrome (Vertebral, Anal, Cardiac, Tracheo-Esophageal, Renal Limb defects). In particular, the incidence of holo-prosencephaly, a serious and rare malformation occurring naturally in about 1:16 000 births is unclear. Furthermore, these publications do not always include data on other maternal medications, or conditions such as diabetes or hypertension.[30,31]

As the long-term treatment of hyperlipidaemia would not be significantly impaired by discontinuing this medication during pregnancy and lactation, statin use is not routinely recommended during gestation and breastfeeding.

Drugs affecting clotting

Low-dose aspirin

Low-dose aspirin (75–300 mg daily) has been used to prevent thrombosis, mitigate placental damage associated with hypertension in pregnancy, and reduce the risk of miscarriage and other complications in women with anticardiolipin or antiphospholipid antibodies.[67] Aspirin does not increase the incidence of adverse effects in the mother, fetus or neonate when used as thrombosis prophylaxis. Its ability to prevent pre-eclampsia remains controversial.[68]

Warfarin

Between 5 and 10% of fetuses exposed to warfarin or other coumarin derivatives in the first trimester suffer adverse effects. The most common syndrome is chondrodysplasia punctata, in which cartilage and bone formation is abnormal. Increased risk of miscarriage, premature delivery, respiratory distress at birth, and nasal and midface hypoplasia are described.[19,69,70] The fetal effects of warfarin appear to be dose related, as evidenced by a study where fetal effects were not seen in women who required ≤5 mg warfarin daily. In a recent review, the risk of embryopathy was 6.4% (95% confidence interval (CI) 4.6–8.9%) when warfarin was used throughout pregnancy, and this risk was eliminated when oral anticoagulant was replaced by heparin between weeks 6 and 12 of gestation.[71,72]

Exposure to warfarin later in pregnancy may cause repeated small intracerebral haemorrhages. Optic atrophy, microcephaly, mental retardation, agenesis of the corpus callosum and cerebellar atrophy may result. Two fatal cases of fetal intraventricular haemorrhage diagnosed prenatally following maternal warfarin treatment have been reported.[23]

Heparin and related compounds

Heparin does not cross the placenta, due to its high molecular weight and negative charge. The frequency of congenital anomalies, miscarriage, stillbirth and prematurity does not seem to be significantly increased in women treated with standard doses.[19]

Few data are available on the outcome of pregnancies in which low molecular weight heparins (LMWH) have been used. They are less likely to cause maternal complications than unfractionated heparin (UFH). LMWH used for thromboprophylaxis does not seem to cross the placenta and there is no clear evidence of any increased risk of malformation or spontaneous abortion.[73,74]

Overall, heparin is the anticoagulant of choice in pregnancy for most indications where efficacy is established. The combination of low-dose aspirin and LMWH is recommended for the prevention of pregnancy loss in women with antiphospholipid antibodies and previous pregnancy loss. In patients with mechanical prosthetic heart valves, oral anticoagulants throughout pregnancy up to 2 weeks prior to delivery may be considered because of the high risk of thrombotic complications.

Heart valve replacement

Advances in the treatment of congenital heart disease (CHD) have led to an increasing number of females surviving into reproductive age. However, pregnancies in such women may not be risk free, especially if they are complicated by pulmonary hypertension and cyanosis. There is also an increased risk of CHD in their infants, with outflow tract lesions being associated with the highest risk. The optimal type of heart valve replacement and subsequent management of pregnancy remains unresolved.[72] In pregnant women with mechanical prosthetic valves there is a need to maintain a high level of anticoagulation to prevent thromboembolic complications. Currently there is no clear evidence as to which is the most effective anticoagulation regimen that is associated with the lowest maternal and fetal toxicity.

There is evidence that women with mechanical mitral valves have a high rate of pregnancy loss that is associated with warfarin use throughout pregnancy. UFH, although safe from the fetal point of view as it does not cross the placenta, has been associated with valve thrombosis and sometimes death. It is still unclear whether heparin failure is due only to inadequate dosing. Other complications associated with heparin treatment include osteoporosis and heparin-induced thrombocytopenia.[71,72]

LMWH, with longer half-lives and increased bioavailability, have a more predictable anticoagulant effect as well as a better side-effect profile. A pooled analysis of 486 pregnancies in which LMWHs were used (mainly for prophylaxis of venous thrombosis and for treatment of autoantibody-associated pregnancy loss) suggests that they are safe for the fetus,[71] but experience with these agents in women with prosthetic heart valves is limited and the true incidence of valve thrombosis in LMWH-treated pregnant women remains unknown. Over the last 2 years the anticoagulant options for this group of pregnant women have been reviewed in detail.[71,72]

Vitamin K$_1$

Phytomenadione does not seem to cross the placenta and infants are relatively deficient in this vitamin (see Epilepsy section). Vitamin K is used in neonates to prevent haemorrhagic disease of the newborn. Concerns that parenteral vitamin K in neonates may increase the risks of childhood cancers are generally refuted.[19]

Drugs used to treat epilepsy

Adverse effects of untreated epilepsy versus those associated with the most commonly used antiepileptic drugs, as well as folic acid and vitamin K, will be described in this section.

Antiepileptic drugs (AEDs)

Approximately 25% of people with epilepsy will be women of reproductive age, and it is estimated that about 1 in 200 women attending antenatal clinics will be taking AEDs. Where there is concomitant use of oral contraceptives and certain AEDs there is a higher risk of breakthrough bleeding in some women – about 7 per 1000 woman-years – due to accelerated oestrogen metabolism.[75]

Infants of mothers with epilepsy treated with AEDs have an approximately two- to threefold increase in major and minor malformations, resulting in an overall risk of fetal toxicity of about 10%.[76–79] Conversely, there is still at least a 90% chance of having a normal baby, compared with about 98% in the general population. There is no ideal epidemiological technique to separate the effects of the drugs and the disease on the fetus.[77] Multiple AED therapy is associated with a greater risk, but this may be related to the severity of the maternal epilepsy. Although there have been a number of local initiatives to develop guidelines for the treatment of epilepsy in women of childbearing age, national agreement is lacking.[75,80]

In some pregnant women, seizure frequency can increase. Possible causes include hormonal changes, sleep deprivation, and changes in AED clearance and binding. There are equivocal data on whether or not maternal seizures during pregnancy have any impact on the frequency of malformations.[81] Frequent and prolonged uncontrolled maternal fits can cause miscarriage, intracranial haemorrhage, and premature labour. In extreme cases, alterations in placental blood flow and transfer of oxygen and nutrients to the fetus can result in fetal hypoxia with bradycardia and brain damage. Therefore, it is important that AED therapy is continued throughout pregnancy and good seizure control maintained.[75,77,80,82]

Barbiturates, carbamazepine, oxcarbazepine, oxazolidines, phenytoin, primidone, succinimides and valproic acid have all been associated with malformations (see also section on Bipolar Disorder). These include facial dysmorphism – widely spaced eyes, depressed nasal bridge, cleft lip and palate, small jaw, low-set ears and a low hairline; anencephaly and spina bifida; cardiac defects; hypospadias; and limb abnormalities.[75–86] There are growing concerns about the long-term effects on postnatal neurodevelopment.[82,83] Valproic acid seems to be the most potent teratogen, particularly when used in doses exceeding 1 g daily or when plasma concentrations of more than 70 µg/mL are achieved.[79,82]

It is thought that immaturity of the fetal/neonatal epoxide hydrolase (EH) system can affect susceptibility to adverse drug reactions both *in utero* and in the perinatal period.[83–85] Fetal and neonatal EH levels seem to be lower than in adults, and this may be partly responsible for the fetal toxicity seen with carbamazepine and phenytoin, both of which require EH for detoxification. Other mechanisms that have been proposed over the last 15 years for AED teratogenicity are: a) an arene oxide metabolite of phenytoin or other AEDs is the ultimate teratogen; b) a genetic defect in EH which detoxifies arene oxidases increases the risk of fetal toxicity; c) free radicals produced by AED metabolism are cytotoxic; or d) there may be a genetic defect in free-radical scavenging enzyme activity that increases the risk of fetal toxicity.[82,85]

There are insufficient data in human pregnancy on the effects of monotherapy with the newer AEDs such as gabapentin, lamotrigine, levetiracetam, topiramate and vigabatrin to give an adequate estimation of the risk of fetal toxicity.[79]

Folic acid

Folic acid, a B vitamin needed for cell replication and growth, helps form the building blocks of DNA and RNA. The requirement for folic acid increases considerably during pregnancy because rapidly growing tissues such as those of a fetus have a high need for folic acid. Administration of folic acid is not generally associated with side effects (even when taken in overdose).

AEDs can cause folate deficiency, and this has been proposed as a possible cause of teratogenesis. The results of the Medical Research Council trial in 1991 indicated that for women who have already had a child with a neural tube defect, preconception supplementation with folic acid reduced the recurrence risk of neural tube defects such as spina bifida.[86] All pregnant women are now recommended to take folic acid 400 µg (0.4 mg) daily during the first 3 months of pregnancy, when the fetal major organs are forming. Women who have a family history of malformations, especially neural tube defects, or who are in a high-risk category (e.g. suffer from epilepsy) are recommended to take the higher dose of 5 mg daily.[75,77–82,87] There are conflicting views as to whether folic acid should be added to food and whether supplementation before conception is effective in reducing the total incidence of congenital malformations.[77,87,88]

Recently, there have been unsubstantiated claims that taking folate supplements during pregnancy increases the risks of miscarriage,[89] multiple births with more complications and poorer outcomes, and the risks of maternal breast cancer.[87,90,91] There are several methodological flaws in these studies and there seems to be no clear evidence to indicate an increase in any of these endpoints.[87,89,90]

Vitamin K

Vitamin K is needed so that the liver can produce blood clotting factors (e.g. prothrombin) and for the production of some of the proteins needed for bone development (see section on Drugs Affecting Clotting, p. 85). Some AEDs (carbamazepine, phenytoin, phenobarbit, primidone and topiramate) induce liver enzymes and reduce the levels of vitamin-K-dependent clotting factors.[77,82] Infants are relatively deficient in vitamin K, and prenatal exposure to these AEDs has been reported to cause internal bleeding in the neonate, particularly in the cranium, usually within the first 24 hours after delivery. However, accurate prevalence statistics are not available. A prothrombin precursor protein induced by the absence of vitamin K (PIVKA) has been discovered in the serum of mothers taking AEDs. Assays for PIVKA may permit prenatal identification of infants at risk of haemorrhage.

Although there is some placental transfer of vitamin K from the mother to the fetus the mechanism is not well defined and there are conflicting opinions about the benefits of giving maternal supplementation.[82,92] Furthermore, where vitamin K supplementation is recommended, there is often disagreement on the treatment regimen. The commonly used regimens include giving an oral daily dose of either 10 mg or 20 mg to the mother from the 36th week of pregnancy, and usually 1 mg to the newborn at birth, either orally or intramuscularly. The fetal dose is repeated after 12 hours if required. The prothrombin times and levels of vitamin-K-dependent clotting factors should be evaluated, and further vitamin K given as required.[75,77,80,82]

Mental health disorders

Psychiatric disorders are common in women of childbearing age and are associated with higher risks of morbidity and mortality.[93–95] The UK Confidential Enquiry into Maternal Deaths (CEMD) reported that psychiatric disorders contributed to 12% of all maternal deaths. Suicide is the second leading cause of maternal death in the UK after cardiovascular disease.[94]

For every 1000 live births, 100–150 women will suffer a depressive illness and one or two will develop a puerperal psychosis.[96] Failure to treat either disorder may result in prolonged, deleterious effects on the relationship between the mother and baby and on the child's psychological, social and educational development.[97–100] The morbidity of clinical depression or psychosis is often prolonged by a delay in diagnosis or an inadequate course of treatment. Treatment may be withheld or inappropriate doses used because of concerns about the effects of the drug on the developing fetus and in the neonate. Many of the drugs used to treat psychiatric disorders have been associated with congenital malformations and/or neonatal toxicity. Therefore, it is important to balance any risk to the fetus from the drug therapy against the risks to both mother and fetus from failing to treat the maternal illness, particularly if there is a high risk of self-harm.

Adverse effects of drugs use to treat affective disorders and depression will be described below.

Drugs used in the treatment of psychosis

Lithium

Lithium salts are the treatment of choice for bipolar disorders (BDs) in pregnancy. Treatment with AEDs such as sodium valproate or divalproex sodium (semisodium salt of sodium valproate that dissociates to valproic acid in the gastrointestinal tract), carbamazepine and lamotrigine are generally not recommended.[77,78]

Usually, plasma concentrations of lithium in the fetus are similar to or higher than maternal plasma concentrations. The pharmacokinetics of lithium change during pregnancy, resulting in increased clearance. Therefore, prescribing and monitoring need to be adjusted to maintain the concentration within the therapeutic range. Monitoring in the last month of pregnancy is especially important. Dietary factors such as salt intake and other medication taken by the mother should also be reviewed.[94,101,102]

Fetal toxicity can occur at any time during pregnancy and may be related to maternal toxicity. In addition, lithium treatment may increase the risk of cardiovascular defects (CHD) and other abnormalities.[97–100,103–105]

In the 1960s it was alleged that lithium was associated with a significant increase (400-fold) in the incidence of a very rare (1:20 000 live-births) cardiac malformation, Ebstein's anomaly, involving abnormalities of the tricuspid valve. A registry of lithium-exposed pregnancies, established in Denmark in 1968 and later extended internationally, revealed a possible association between lithium exposure and CHD. However, an expert report published in 1995 revealed that the registry data are biased toward the overestimation of adverse outcome.[15] The author concluded that none of the previously published human studies provided sufficient dose–response information for quantitative risk assessment. The results of more recent studies confirm these findings.[97,99,103] It is now estimated that the increased incidence of Ebstein's anomaly is at most 1:1000–1:2000 (0.05–0.1%) of births following first-trimester lithium exposure. Analysis of combined data from several well-designed studies indicates that the overall risk of CHD varies from 0.9 to 12% versus 0.5–1% in the general population.[99] Although the estimated risk of Ebstein's anomaly in lithium-exposed infants is 10–20 times higher than expected, the absolute risk is small (0.05–0.1%).

Rarer adverse effects that have been reported are fetal and neonatal arrhythmias, stillbirth, polyhydramnios after fetal polyuria, neonatal goitre, and neonatal jaundice.[15,97–100,103–105] A 'floppy infant syndrome' of tachypnoea, tachycardia, cyanosis, hypotonia, lethargy and poor sucking response has also been reported. Follow-up data on 95 children with no apparent malformations who were exposed to lithium *in utero* suggest that there are no excessive sequelae up to 5 years of age.[99,103] However, data on longer-term postnatal development are not available.

Overall, in women with severe BD in whom discontinuation of lithium poses a substantial risk of increased morbidity, it may be possible to discontinue therapy temporarily during the first trimester of pregnancy (embryogenesis). Reintroduction of lithium and/or treatment with antipsychotic agents should be considered if clinical deterioration occurs.

However, in women with severe BD in whom discontinuation of lithium poses an unacceptable risk of increased morbidity, it may be necessary to maintain therapy throughout pregnancy. Where lithium exposure has occurred in part of or throughout the first trimester, reproductive genetic risk counselling as early in pregnancy as possible, high-resolution ultrasound examination, and fetal echocardiography at about 20 weeks' gestation to screen for cardiac abnormalities are recommended. Provided that adequate screening tests are done the majority of women who take lithium throughout their pregnancy will deliver a healthy infant. Lithium is arguably the safest currently available mood stabiliser for use in pregnancy.

Antiepileptic drugs

Sodium valproate, carbamazepine or lamotrigine are commonly used in the treatment of bipolar disorders. The recent guidelines from the CSM (Committee on Safety of Medicines), NICE (National Institute for Health and Clinical Excellence) and SIGN (Scottish Intercollegiate Guidelines Network) concerning the teratogenic effects of these drugs have caused considerable concern among clinicians treating affective disorders.[78–80] The choice of drugs to treat pregnant women with BD is very limited, and none is without risk to the mother and fetus. These effects have already been described in the section on treatment of epilepsy.

Antipsychotics (neuroleptics)

The older neuroleptic agents act by blocking cerebral dopamine receptors. This group of drugs includes phenothiazines (low and high potency), thioxanthenes and butyrophenones. Pregnancy outcome is known to be poorer in psychotic women, especially if inadequately treated.[104] There is growing evidence that emotional stress during organogenesis can cause congenital malformations, particularly those of the cranial neural crest cells that are involved in the development of the head, face and heart.[106]

Most data on use during pregnancy are available for phenothiazines and haloperidol. Phenothiazines readily cross the placenta and elimination is much slower by the fetus and the neonate than by adults.

Much less information on use during pregnancy is available for alimemazine, fluphenazine, levomepromazine, pericyazine, perphenazine, prochlorperazine, promazine, thioridazine, trifluoperazine and triflupromazine. The data on pregnancy outcome are conflicting.[107] There have been case reports of malformations such as microcephaly, syndactyly and cardiac defects, but most larger studies have failed to demonstrate a significant risk for congenital malformations.[96,97,99,107] Most information is derived from studies of treatment of hyperemesis gravidarum rather than of psychosis. For this indication smaller doses are used than those needed to treat psychosis, which should be considered when making a risk assessment.

As phenothiazines block the dopamine receptors in the basal ganglia, hypothalamus and limbic system, which may result in extrapyramidal symptoms (EPS), there was concern about their potential effects on the developing fetal CNS. Several case reports have documented transient EPS, including motor restlessness, tremor, hypertonicity, dystonia and parkinsonism in neonates exposed to neuroleptics during pregnancy. These problems have typically been of short duration and have been followed by apparently normal subsequent motor development.[99,107] Risks for potential neurobehavioural or cognitive effects from prenatal exposure to older neuroleptics have also been considered, but the available data remain limited and inconclusive. A longitudinal study in the 1960s that evaluated the general intelligence and behaviour of children exposed to low-potency neuroleptics *in utero* found no evidence of dysfunction or developmental delays up to 5 years.[99] Few or no data are available for the thioxanthenes chlorprothixene, clopenthixol, flupenthixol, perazine, prothipendyl, zotepine and zuclopenthixol.

Among the butyrophenones, most data are available on haloperidol. Much less is available on others in the class, such as benperidol, bromperidol, droperidol, melperone, pipamperone and trifluperidol. Although teratogenic effects were not seen, the data are insufficient to exclude the possibility of an increased risk. Early case reports described limb reduction defects (LRD) following first-trimester exposure to haloperidol, but several other studies have not demonstrated that haloperidol is a major teratogen.[99,107] Withdrawal symptoms have been reported in the neonate after chronic use or use of high doses near delivery (sedation, feeding problems, restlessness).

Although a meta-analysis of studies of low-potency neuroleptic use in pregnancy noted a possible increase in overall risk for congenital malformations following first-trimester exposure, no specific type of malformation was identified. Overall, there is no clear evidence of an increase in absolute teratogenic risk associated with any of the older typical neuroleptics, of either low or high potency.[97,99,107]

In clinical practice, high-potency neuroleptic agents such as fluphenazine, haloperidol, perphenazine and trifluoperazine are recommended because they have lesser autonomic, sedative and cardiovascular side effects than do the low-potency agents. The use of one of the other neuroleptics is not an indication for invasive diagnostic procedures or termination of pregnancy. Fetal ultrasonography may be offered in the 20th week of pregnancy. Neonates should be monitored for EPS and withdrawal symptoms, especially where there has been long-term exposure or when high doses have been used near the time of delivery.

Atypical antipsychotics (ATPs)

The ATPs may be better tolerated and cause fewer EPS than other antipsychotics. They have not been associated with prolactin elevation and are therefore less likely to inhibit ovulation and female fertility (see Chapter 9). However, switching from a prolactin-elevating antipsychotic such as phenothiazine to a newer ATP without such effects can increase the likelihood of becoming pregnant.[108]

Information on the reproductive safety of the newer ATPs such as clozapine, olanzapine, risperidone, quetiapine or ziprasidone remains very sparse. There are no adequate human studies to evaluate the risk for potential teratogenicity.

There have been a number of published case reports between 1993 and 1997 describing 107 children exposed *in utero* to clozapine.[109] A number of diverse pregnancy outcomes were described, including maternal toxicity such as hyperglycaemia and gestational diabetes, as well as fetal and neonatal problems, e.g. 'floppy infant syndrome' and an unexplained seizure. There were five infants with malformations that were not described, but the majority of liveborn infants (79) were healthy. As these pregnancies were not reported in detail, no clear conclusions can be drawn as to whether or not the effects observed were causally related to clozapine.

There are published reports on 18 healthy infants exposed *in utero* to olanzapine. Another 11 retrospective reports describe two infants with

Table 4.6 Summary of main types of fetal and neonatal toxicity associated with drug treatment

Drug group	Clear evidence		
	Congenital malformations	Neonatal withdrawal	Long-term effects
Lithium	Yes	Yes	Yes – limited
Antiepileptics[a] – valproate carbamazepine	Yes	Yes	Limited data
Old antipsychotics – phenothiazines haloperidol	No	Yes	Limited data
ATPs[b] – clozapine, olanzapine, quetiapine	Limited data	Yes – limited	Not known

NB. Exclusion of a drug from this table does not imply safety.

[a] There are insufficient monotherapy data available on lamotrigine and other newer antiepileptic drugs to make an adequate risk assessment.[79]

[b] For most ATPs no data in human pregnancy are available.

congenital malformations (one with a dysplastic kidney and one with trisomy 21), which are unlikely to be causally related, and five with diverse types of neonatal toxicity.[109] The manufacturer has established a registry that includes at least 172 prospective reports of outcomes following prenatal exposure to olanzapine.[110] The majority of infants (120) were healthy and five had congenital malformations, but no pattern of defects was observed. Overall, there is no clear evidence of a causally related increase in fetal toxicity, but experience to date with all these registries for atypical antipsychotic agents remains insufficient to provide for adequate assessment of fetal safety.

Two published reports describe the outcome of 12 pregnancies in which risperidone exposure occurred. There were nine liveborn healthy infants and three therapeutic terminations. No details were available regarding the timing or duration of exposure in these pregnancies.[109] Only one case report was found of a successful pregnancy outcome following treatment with quetiapine throughout pregnancy. The infant was described as doing well at 6 weeks of age.[109]

A summary of the main types of fetal and neonatal toxicity associated with drug treatment of psychosis is given in Table 4.6.

Drugs used in depression

There is sufficient evidence to show that leaving severe depression untreated can have adverse effects on pregnancy outcome, especially if the mother is in danger of self-harm, and can adversely affect the mother–child relationship.[97–100] Treatment with antidepressants may be required throughout pregnancy and the first couple of months or so after the birth. Therefore, it is important to assess the potential adverse effects of medication on the fetus and on the neonate and child, who may continue to be exposed via the breast milk.

Tricyclic antidepressants (TCAs)

There is no epidemiological evidence of an association between therapy with TCAs and an increased incidence of birth defects or other adverse pregnancy outcomes. Occasional suggestions of harm are unsubstantiated.[111–113] Short-term neonatal withdrawal symptoms such as jitteriness, hyperexcitability, myoclonus, convulsions and suckling problems have been reported, especially in premature or small-for-dates infants. Limited data based on 80 preschool children did not indicate any adverse effects on neurodevelopment, such as global IQ, language and behavioural development.[114]

TCA poisoning can cause severe maternal toxicity, including convulsion, coma and cardiac arrhythmia, with consequent fetal harm. Therefore, it is important to treat any maternal toxicity that arises from such exposure as a matter of urgency.

Selective serotonin/noradrenaline reuptake inhibitors (SSRI/SNRI)

Fluoxetine is the only drug in this class that has been extensively studied in pregnancy. The data showed no increase in either the malformation rate or the incidence of spontaneous abortion.[107, 115–120] A report of an association with a higher incidence of three or more minor anomalies lacks clinical data and is difficult to assess.[121] Exposure *in utero* to fluoxetine in 55 preschool children did not affect neurodevelopment.[114] One study of third-trimester fluoxetine exposure on the neonate showed no significant increase in postnatal complications, but chronic use, or the use of SSRIs near term, has been associated with neonatal withdrawal symptoms in some cases. Although fewer data are available on citalopram, fluvoxamine and sertraline, there is no clear evidence of an increased risk of fetal toxicity or other pregnancy complications so far.[118,122,123] Neonatal withdrawal symptoms have been reported with all SSRIs and SNRIs.[121–124] There is increasing concern that the most severe neonatal symptoms are associated with prenatal exposure to paroxetine and venlafaxine.[125]

SSRIs are known to cause bleeding disorders and haematoma in adults (see Chapter 6), and two cases of haemorrhage have been reported in neonates prenatally exposed to fluoxetine and paroxetine, respectively.[117]

Monoamine oxidase inhibitors (MAOIs)

MAOIs have been associated with a high incidence of toxicity in humans. They can exacerbate pregnancy-associated hypertension, which can lead to alterations in placental blood flow, particularly placental hypoperfusion. This may have serious consequences for fetal growth and development. There is a possible interaction with tyramine, which is present in high-protein-content food and drinks, and this may produce an acute hypertensive crisis. There is no clear evidence of fetotoxicity with phenelzine or tranylcypromine.[107,113] A case report discussed the association between cardiac anomalies, hypertelorism and other defects.[126] No data were found on the use of moclobemide in pregnancy. No reports were found describing effects in the neonate specifically related to MAOIs.

Bupropion

Bupropion was initially developed as an antidepressant and has since been marketed as a non-nicotine aid to smoking cessation. It is a weak inhibitor of the neuronal uptake of noradrenaline (norepinephrine), serotonin and dopamine. There are no controlled studies on bupropion exposure during human pregnancy. The manufacturer has set up a Bupropion Registry to monitor outcome of pregnancy data; prospective data suggests that that inadvertent exposure is not associated with an increased risk of fetal toxicity.[127] The data based on 604 pregnancies exposed to bupropion, 481 in the first trimester, indicate no increased risk of either malformations (2.3% vs 2–3% expected) or miscarriages (11.4% vs 10–20% expected). However, among the 12 liveborn infants with congenital malformations, six had cardiac defects (1.7%), which may be cause for concern. At present, caution should be exercised when interpreting these data because cardiac malformations are one of the most common birth defects (0.5–1%) in the general population. Currently, there is no clear evidence to indicate that there is a direct causal relationship between bupropion and an increased risk of malformations in this case series.[127]

In summary, amitriptyline and imipramine remain the drugs of choice for the treatment of depression during pregnancy, based on the length of time that they have been in use and the cumulative data on their lack of fetotoxicity. SSRIs are safer in overdose. Until more data are available, fluoxetine should be reserved for use in pregnant women where amitriptyline or imipramine is ineffective or poorly tolerated, or for women perceived to be at high risk of suicide. The serotonin/noradrenaline reuptake inhibitors and the miscellaneous newer antidepressants should be avoided until more data are available. MAOIs should be avoided if at all possible because of their inherent maternal toxicity and lack of published data on safety in pregnancy. If clinically appropriate, the dose of the antidepressant should be tapered 3–4 weeks before the expected date of delivery to minimise the risk of withdrawal symptoms.

Drugs used in endocrine disorders

Adverse effects of drugs used to treat diabetes and thyroid disorders will be described in this section.

Drugs used in diabetes

Diabetes mellitus

Diabetes mellitus is due to absolute insulin deficiency (type 1, insulin dependent) or partial insulin deficiency (type 2, non-insulin dependent). Both of these conditions will have predated the pregnancy and should be distinguished from gestational diabetes, which only occurs during pregnancy, usually after week 20.[128–130]

Gestational diabetes may be due to changes in insulin metabolism, or to the production of anti-insulin hormones such as human placental lactogen, progesterone, oestrogens and glucocorticoids, which are present in increasing amounts during pregnancy, as the placenta grows. There is some concern that pregnant women who need treatment with atypical antipsychotics (ATPs) may have an increased risk of hyperglycaemia[109] (see section on Mental Health Disorders, p. 90). In most pregnant women the pancreas is able to produce the extra insulin needed to counter insulin resistance, but where the pancreas cannot make enough insulin, gestational diabetes develops. Risk factors include obesity and a family history of diabetes. Some affected women are likely to have had undiagnosed diabetes prior to pregnancy.[128–130]

Women with any type of diabetes and their babies are at an increased risk of a number of pregnancy complications. In contrast to gestational diabetes, prepregnancy type 1 diabetes may be associated with maternal vascular disease, resulting in uteroplacental insufficiency, hypertension and pre-eclampsia (see sections on Statins, p. 84, and Drugs Used to Treat Infections, p. 104). Pregnant women with inadequately controlled diabetes mellitus are at a higher risk (two- to fourfold increase) of miscarriage, intrauterine death or a baby with congenital malformations, e.g. cardiovascular system defects, neural tube defects, bilateral renal agenesis and organomegaly (heart and liver). Increased erythropoiesis, which can lead to fetal hypertension, is also a risk. Significant neonatal morbidity and perinatal mortality (two- to threefold increase) has also been reported.[130–134]

Macrosomia (a large baby) is a common problem where blood glucose control is poor. The fetal pancreas begins to develop during weeks 5–8 post conception. From week 12 of gestation onwards, parenchyma, acini and islets of Langerhans are present and insulin and glucagon are formed.[135] The total pancreatic insulin and glucagon increases with fetal age. Maternal hyperglycaemia can induce hyperglycaemia and pancreatic hyperplasia in the fetus. In response to hyperglycaemia the fetal pancreas produces more insulin, which allows extra glucose to be converted to fat and therefore the fetus is abnormally large. This can make vaginal delivery difficult and necessitate a caesarean section or delivery before full term.

If maternal blood sugar levels are high, especially in the 24 hours before delivery, the neonate may be hypoglycaemic because of residual hyperfunction of neonatal islet cells. The neonate will therefore have high insulin levels but no longer has a glucose supply from its mother, and in some instances may need intravenous administration of glucose. The neonates of women with diabetes often also have hyaline membrane disease or respiratory distress syndrome. Maintaining good normoglycaemic control has been shown to reduce adverse outcomes for both mother and child, and pregnant women are often advised to monitor their blood glucose six to eight times a day.[132–134]

Women with diabetes who are planning a pregnancy should be advised to make sure they achieve tight blood glucose control before conception. Ideally, pregnant women with diabetes should be managed in specialist multidisciplinary antenatal clinics to obtain optimal care. Ultrasound examination to monitor for growth and congenital malformations is recommended.[130–134]

Insulin

Insulin replacement therapy has made it possible for women with diabetes to carry successful pregnancies. Human insulin does not cross the placenta and there is no indication that it is associated with an increased risk of fetal or neonatal toxicity. Where toxicity does occur it is usually associated with suboptimal control of the maternal glucose levels. Therefore, it is important that type 1 diabetes should be optimally controlled with insulin before pregnancy and prenatal counselling given.[128–133] Where gestational diabetes is diagnosed, insulin therapy should be started as early as possible. Human insulin is preferred to that of animal origin because of the possibility of antibody development. In women with diabetes established before pregnancy, insulin needs during pregnancy often increase in the second trimester.[130–133] The overall principles in achieving adequate glucose control are to balance energy supply and consumption and to replace insulin. Some glucocorticoids (e.g. used antenatally to prevent respiratory distress syndrome) and tocolytics (drugs used to suppress uterine contractions and prevent premature labour) decrease maternal carbohydrate metabolism, so if these drugs are used monitoring of metabolic control is advisable.

Oral antidiabetic drugs

Most oral antidiabetic drugs do not cross the placenta. The most commonly used agents, the sulphonylureas (e.g. chlorpropamide, tolbutamide) and the newer second-generation drugs (glibenclamide, gliclazide and glipizide) stimulate the pancreatic beta cells that are still able to function. In contrast, biguanides such as metformin reduce glucose synthesis in the liver. There are few data on the effects in pregnancy of the newer antidiabetic drugs, such as those that stimulate insulin release (e.g. nateglinide and repaglinide) or reduce peripheral insulin resistance (e.g. pioglitazone and rosiglitazone). Therefore a reliable risk assessment of their effects on the fetus cannot be made.

Because oral antidiabetic drugs have not been shown to regulate blood sugar as effectively as insulin, they are generally not considered suitable for treatment of diabetes during pregnancy. Some of these drugs, particularly the sulphonylureas, have been associated with an increased risk of fetal malformations and neonatal hypoglycaemia. However, it is not clear whether this is a direct effect of the drugs or a secondary effect associated with poor glucose control.[128,131,132]

Ideally, pregnant women with type 2 diabetes should be treated with insulin in the same way as those with type 1 diabetes. A fetal ultrasound scan at about 20 weeks is recommended to screen for malformations and assessment of fetal size. The use of insulin or antidiabetic drugs in pregnancy is not an indication for medical termination of pregnancy or the use of invasive diagnostic procedures.

Drugs used to treat thyroid disorders

Maternal thyroid function changes during pregnancy in response to changes in protein binding, hormone production and an increased need for iodine. Both overactivity (hyperthyroidism or thyrotoxicosis) and underactivity (hypothyroidism) of the maternal thyroid gland can have adverse effects on fetal development.[128,136,137]

The thyroid is the first endocrine gland to develop in the fetus, at about week 3–4 post conception, with follicles growing and colloid being produced at 10–12 weeks. The gland begins to function by the end of the third month of pregnancy.[135]

Hyperthyroidism (thyrotoxicosis)

Hyperthyroidism affects up to 0.2% of pregnancies, and if left untreated is associated with increased fetal mortality and morbidity.[137,138] Thus treatment with antithyroid drugs such as propylthiouracil or carbimazole is required. Beta-blockers, such as propranolol, should be reserved for presurgical treatment and immediate control of severe thyrotoxic features[128,136,137,139,140] (see section on Beta-adrenoceptor Antagonists, p. 82).

Propylthiouracil (PTU) is considered to be the drug of choice in pregnancy, especially in the first trimester.[128,136,137] Carbimazole and its active metabolite thiamazole (methimazole) cross the placenta, and can cause hypothyroidism in the fetus or neonate.[128,136,137,141] Close monitoring of thyroid function, approximately once a month, is particularly important because the need for antithyroid therapy often declines through pregnancy, and in the second trimester treatment may occasionally be discontinued.

Both PTU and thiamazole have been implicated in cases of a congenital scalp defect called aplasia cutis, but this has not been confirmed in a review of nearly 50 000 pregnancies.[142,143] In a recent study of 643 neonates born to mothers with Graves' disease there were no cases of aplasia cutis, and congenital malformations were significantly more common in the offspring of women whose thyrotoxicosis was left untreated (3/50 = 6%) compared to those receiving thiamazole (3/593 = 0.5%).[144]

There have been a few case reports of choanal atresia, often with oesophageal atresia, or tracheo-oesophageal fistula; minor facial and skin dysmorphic features; hypoplastic nipples, growth restriction and developmental delay following fetal exposure to thiamazole.[145] This pattern of abnormalities has been called methimazole-induced (MMI) embryopathy and it has been seen after maternal treatment with either carbimazole or thiamazole, but no certain causal relationship has been established.

The use of higher doses of carbimazole in combination with levothyroxine to prevent hypothyroidism (blocking-replacement therapy) should be avoided in pregnancy. There is high placental transfer of carbimazole but not levothyroxine, putting the fetus at risk of intrauterine hypothyroidism, even if the mother's thyroid function has been restored to normal (euthyroid). Also, congenital abnormalities are more common in the babies of women receiving levothyroxine and carbimazole (9.5%) than in those treated with carbimazole alone (4.1%).[136]

Radioiodine

Radioiodine administration also raises a number of concerns.[128,136,137] For hyperthyroidism, the usual dose range of radioiodine is 4–10 millicuries (mCi; unit of radioactivity), depending on the patient's condition. As the fetal thyroid is able to concentrate iodine from about 10–12 weeks' gestation, radioiodine administered later than this may cause ablation of the gland, resulting in fetal and neonatal hypothyroidism with potentially severe and irreversible consequences, including mental retardation.

Parental gonadal exposure may result in genetic effects, and several studies have demonstrated chromosomal damage following radioiodine. However, the increased risk of genetic abnormalities arising from this exposure is low (0.003%) compared to the spontaneous risk of genetic abnormalities in the general population under 35 years of age (0.8%).[136] Studies in Japanese atomic bomb survivors, and in the offspring of those treated with high doses of radioiodine for thyroid cancer, have demonstrated little evidence of genotoxicity and do not suggest that patients who have received radioiodine before conception produce abnormal children. Nevertheless, an interval of at least 4 months is normally advised between maternal radioiodine therapy and conception, and some also apply this interval to a prospective father.[136]

The risk to the fetus of cancer or heritable disease caused by treatment with radioiodine has been estimated at one in 15 000–20 000/mGy (milligray; a measure of the radiation energy absorbed). In early pregnancy, although the risk of cancer induction is not zero it is much lower than at later stages, probably because by then cells have become specialised and damage is more likely to be permanent. Despite the possible risks associated with radiation to the fetus, inadvertent therapy with iodine-131 (^{131}I) does not always adversely affect the fetus if administered before the 10th week of gestation. In patients who received radioiodine in higher doses (e.g. for carcinoma of the thyroid) before conception there was also no increase in fetal malformation, although there was a slightly higher miscarriage rate that may have been due to a change in maternal hormonal status.[136]

The threshold doses for fetal death and fetal malformation are far in excess of those from 'normal' radioiodine therapy for hyperthyroidism. If the irradiation occurs between 8 and 15 weeks there is a chance that mental retardation could result regardless of the dose, but the predicted loss would be 0.03 intelligence quotient points per mGy, which is unlikely to be clinically important with antithyroid drugs.[136]

The effects of maternal ^{131}I radioiodine treatment on the fetal thyroid can be investigated by measuring fetal thyroid-stimulating hormone through umbilical cord sampling, and this may indicate the need for fetal levothyroxine therapy. Unlike therapeutic doses in the millicurie range, diagnostic ^{131}I is used in microcuries (μCi), well below the dose that will impair fetal thyroid function.

Women exposed to antithyroid drugs or radioiodine in early pregnancy need accurate and timely information when deciding whether to proceed with the pregnancy. The best available evidence indicates that the risk to the fetus from exposure to these treatments in early pregnancy is low, lower than is commonly perceived, and less than that of untreated hyperthyroidism.[128,136,137,139,140]

Hypothyroidism

Hypothyroidism affects 9 in 1000 pregnancies and is usually associated with iodine deficiency or autoimmune thyroiditis, but may be due to iatrogenic effects as a result of thyroidectomy or ^{131}I therapy.[138,139] However, clinical diagnosis of hypothyroidism is often difficult. During pregnancy hypothyroidism can impair the mental development of the baby and adversely affect neuropsychological test results. An increase in miscarriages, stillbirths and congenital anomalies has also been reported. Therefore, appropriate treatment is essential for both maternal and fetal wellbeing.

Thyroid hormones such as L-triiodothyronine (T_3) and thyroxine (T_4) that are metabolically active in their free non-protein-bound form are effective treatments. T_3 is the more biologically effective hormone with a short period of activity, whereas T_4 is the less effective prohormone that needs to be deiodinated to T_3 as required. Thyroid hormones are essential for placental development, but placental transfer is limited.

However, where fetal thyroid agenesis occurs there is substantial transfer of maternal T_4 because of the high concentration gradient.

There is no evidence of an increased risk of congenital anomalies following the use of either T_3 or T_4. As for other people with hypothyroidism, when thyroid hormones are required for pregnant women levothyroxine preparations should be used so that the patient retains control over the hormonal activity by controlling the conversion of T_4 to T_3. The dose of levothyroxine is variable, depending on the severity of the underlying disease. Requirements may increase during pregnancy. Therefore, regular monitoring of blood levels during pregnancy to ensure adequate thyroid control is recommended. Iodine should be supplemented as required, but it is important to get the balance right.[128,136–139,146] Low iodine levels are associated with cretinism, but if the mother takes too much iodine, fetal hypothyroidism can be induced.

Drugs used to treat infections

The adverse effects of some of the most commonly used anti-infective drugs, such as the aminoglycosides, tetracyclines, trimethoprim and quinolones, will be described in this section.

Aminoglycosides

Aminoglycosides rapidly cross the placenta and most can damage the fetal auditory nerve and cause congenital hearing loss.[21] It is not possible to predict which fetuses or mothers will be adversely affected. Therefore, aminoglycosides are not recommended for parenteral use in pregnancy unless there is a life-threatening infection. In such cases, maternal serum concentrations should be carefully monitored and the dose adjusted if necessary.

Tetracyclines

Exposure to tetracycline prior to 15 weeks of pregnancy has not been clearly associated with an increased risk of fetal toxicity.[21] Tetracyclines bind strongly to calcium and incorporation into teeth and bones occurs after 15 weeks. Yellow-brown discoloration and banding of the teeth and reversible growth retardation of the long bones can result. In addition, staining of lenses has been reported.[39] Cases of congenital or infantile cataracts have been reported following first-trimester exposure to tetracycline; however, a causal association has not subsequently been confirmed.

Trimethoprim

Trimethoprim is a folate antagonist commonly prescribed for the treatment of urinary tract infections (UTIs). Because of this, many women are inadvertently exposed before their pregnancy is confirmed. Low folate levels have been associated with an increased risk of malformations in some pregnancies and may limit fetal availability of folic acid and impair normal development.[21,147] The sensitive time for neural tube development is within the first 28 days after conception. Trimethoprim should be avoided in women with established folic acid deficiency, low dietary folic acid intake, or who take other folate antagonists, unless a folate supplement is also given. In well-nourished women with normal folate status, therapeutic use of trimethoprim for a short period is unlikely to induce folate deficiency (see section on Folic Acid, p. 89). If there are concerns about folate deficiency in individual patients a folate supplement can be given concomitantly.

Quinolones

The quinolones impair bacterial DNA metabolism by inhibiting DNA gyrase. At normal therapeutic doses they have bactericidal activity, but at higher doses they also have bacteristatic properties by inhibiting bacterial RNA and protein synthesis. Quinolones have a high affinity for cartilage and bone, especially immature cartilage. Most data are available for ciprofloxacin and norfloxacin.

The quinolones cross the placenta and are found in low concentrations in amniotic fluid. Umbilical concentrations of some quinolones, including ciprofloxacin, have been found to be lower than maternal blood concentrations.[21] Use in the first trimester has not been associated with fetal harm.[148,149] They were found not to be teratogenic in preclinical animal studies. However, data from animal studies have shown that quinolones can cause damage to the cartilage of immature animals and the fetus, resulting in joint arthropathies. The sensitivity is highest in the dog. Such effects are dependent on the dose and duration of treatment, and occur only in the sensitive period. Musculoskeletal dysfunction has so far not been found after prenatal exposure in human pregnancies.[21,148]

Because of the possibility of producing these joint arthropathies and the limited safety data available, quinolones are normally contraindicated in human pregnancy. Inadvertent exposure is not a reason for invasive diagnostic techniques or termination of pregnancy. In cases of complicated and resistant infections where other treatments have failed, then treatment with either ciprofloxacin or norfloxacin (most safety data in pregnancy) may be considered. Where exposure to quinolones has occurred, a detailed ultrasound scan at 20+ weeks is recommended.[21,148,149]

Miscellaneous agents

In this section the adverse effects of drugs such as vitamin A derivatives, misoprostol, methotrexate, leflunomide, bisphosphonates and Ecstasy will be described. There are very few data available on the safety of most of these drugs in human pregnancy, making evidence-based risk assessment extremely difficult. This often results in very difficult moral and medico-legal discussions as to whether to terminate much-wanted pregnancies.

Vitamin A derivatives

The overall risks of fetal malformations, craniofacial, thymus and congenital heart defects of liveborn infants exposed to isotretinoin *in utero* following maternal systemic use is estimated to be 20–30%. The incidence of spontaneous abortion is more than 20%. Approximately 30% of infants with no gross malformations have mental retardation, and up to 60% have impaired neuropsychological function.[150] The possible persistence of isotretinoin in maternal fat could increase the risk of embryopathy for days or weeks after treatment.[151] The elimination half-life of isotretinoin's longest-lived metabolite is up to 50 hours, suggesting that most of the drug and its biotransformation products would be gone within 10 days of the last dose. It is currently recommended that a negative pregnancy test is confirmed before treatment starts, and that effective contraception is used. Isotretinoin should be discontinued at least 1 month prior to attempting pregnancy, although the pharmacokinetics suggest little risk after 10 days.[151]

There are few data available to assess the potential fetotoxic effects of topical isotretinoin use, but animal data are reassuring.[152–154] Two well-controlled studies involving a total of 300 women did not indicate an increased incidence of malformations. When used topically the average absorption rate is between 2 and 6% of the usual 0.5% concentration in topical retinoid preparations. Furthermore, a rise in plasma retinoid concentration (2–5 µg/L) does not occur after topical use, which makes teratogenic effects unlikely if the treated area was not large. However, it must be borne in mind that severely inflamed skin or the additional use of antiseptics may increase the absorption rate.

Etretinate is an aromatic derivative of retinoic acid. In the body, etretinate serves as a prodrug for the formation of acitretin. Etretinate is teratogenic in experimental animals at doses similar to or greater than those used in humans. These teratogenic effects are dependent on the dose and time of exposure. Increased frequencies of CNS, craniofacial, skeletal, and other malformations, as well as fetal death, have been reported. Unlike more water-soluble retinoids, such as isotretinoin, etretinate and acitretin/etretinate persist in the human body for an extremely long time after administration. The drug has been detected in the serum or plasma 2 years or more after cessation of therapy. It is not known for how long after discontinuation of etretinate therapy teratogenic effects may occur. In the UK, prior to its being taken off the market, it was recommended that women receiving etretinate did not conceive for 2 years following termination of therapy. The US package labelling recommends that pregnancy should be avoided for 'an indefinite period of time', a recommendation described as too vague to be helpful.

Acitretin was introduced to replace etretinate because, unlike etretinate, acitretin is excreted from the body rapidly (half-life 50–60 hours, compared to 100–120 days for etretinate). However, since the beginning of 1991 it has been known that in some women, especially those who use alcohol, etretinate formation may occur after acitretin administration. Once acitretin therapy is discontinued, contraception for 2 years is commonly recommended, although residual etretinate in body fat has been detected in women as long as 52 months after stopping acitretin. In reality, it is not known for how long after discontinuing etretinate therapy teratogenic effects may occur. It is perhaps most prudent to delay pregnancy until serum etretinate is undetectable. However, such measurements are not readily available. In a series of 36 pregnancies in which the mothers had stopped using acitretin between 6 weeks and 23 months before conception, no defects indicative of retinoid teratogenesis were detected. A more recent report identified 44 infants whose mothers used acitretin between 0 and 2 years before conception. The only birth defect identified in this group of infants was one case of undescended testicle, which is a relatively common anomaly and unlikely to be causally related to acitretin exposure.

Misoprostol

Misoprostol is a synthetic analogue of prostaglandin E_1 which can be given orally for the prophylaxis and treatment of peptic ulcer disease. The drug is also given vaginally or orally to induce cervical ripening and initiate labour near term, or usually in combination with other agents to induce abortion in the first or second trimester of pregnancy. The data on fetotoxicity seem to be associated with failed abortions.

In some countries, such as Brazil, where abortions are illegal, misoprostol, usually obtained on the black market, is widely used as an abortifacient.[155–158] Children of women who attempted unsuccessfully to induce abortion with misoprostol early in pregnancy may have Moebius syndrome (congenital palsies of the sixth and other cranial nerves) and a higher than expected frequency of hydrocephalus, holoprosencephaly, bladder exstrophy, amniotic bands, terminal transverse limb reduction defects and arthrogryposis.[16,159–162] The most common total dose use was 800 µg (range 200–1600 µg) as four tablets for 20 days. It has been suggested that some of these malformations may be the result of vascular disruption.[162] However, other studies have failed to confirm these findings.[163,164] Much of this information has been collected retrospectively in Brazil and may be influenced by maternal and/or physician recall bias. There have been unconfirmed reports from Brazil and South America that in cases where misoprostol-induced abortion failed, herbal and other alternative remedies have also been used, making it difficult to attribute causality to any particular substance taken.

Overall, an increased teratogenic risk after inadvertent therapeutic misoprostol exposure, although probably low, cannot be excluded. Although not approved for any specific indication in pregnancy, it is increasingly used to induce abortion throughout Europe. A pregnancy that continues after a failed abortion attempt with prostaglandins needs detailed risk assessment because teratogenic effects cannot be excluded. High-resolution ultrasonography is recommended at about 20 weeks to assess morphological fetal development. However, cranial nerve palsies may not be detected and may not be apparent until after birth.

Methotrexate

Methotrexate is both a cytotoxic and a disease-modifying antirheumatic drug with folate antagonist effects. The risk of fetal toxicity associated with exposure to methotrexate in pregnancy seems to be dose related.[9,28,165] From the limited data available it has been suggested that maternal doses above 10 mg weekly during the critical period of 6–8 weeks after conception are more likely to be associated with congenital abnormalities. However, the severity of the maternal illness, the duration of exposure and the effects of any concomitant medication also need to be considered. First-trimester exposure is associated with a high rate of miscarriage, and with a very uncommon and characteristic pattern of congenital anomalies, including a large cloverleaf skull with swept-back hair, craniosynostosis, large fontanelles, ocular hypertelorism and skeletal defects. Neural tube defects, hydrocephalus and mental retardation may also occur.[166] Aminopterin, a closely related agent, causes a similar pattern. The effect on the fetus of maternal treatment with methotrexate during the second or third trimester of pregnancy is unknown. No increase in the frequency of congenital anomalies was apparent in over 750 pregnancies in women who had previously been treated with methotrexate for gestational or other neoplasms.[167]

Because of its embryotoxic effects, methotrexate is also used in high doses to terminate ectopic pregnancies.[4] If termination fails, or there is an undetected intrauterine pregnancy as well as an ectopic, then the remaining embryo(s) will be exposed to high concentrations of methotrexate at a very early stage of development. In such situations there is a very high risk of embryo/fetal damage, and a detailed risk assessment is required if the woman wishes to continue with the pregnancy. A scan at about 12 weeks to assess gestational age, viability and detect severe gross abnormalities such as anencephaly is recommended. High-resolution ultrasonography is recommended at about 20 weeks to assess morphological fetal development in more detail. However, some abnormalities and any CNS dysfunction will not be detected and may not be apparent until after birth. Alternative methods of pregnancy termination may need to be considered.

Leflunomide

Leflunomide, an inhibitor of pyrimidine biosynthesis used to treat rheumatoid arthritis, is contraindicated in pregnancy because animal studies show severe embryological damage at low doses.[27] In a small case series of six leflunomide-exposed pregnancies where outcome was known, there were two elective terminations (no fetal data available), one miscarriage (also exposed to methotrexate and etanercept) and three liveborn infants with no malformations.[28] The results of this study have been misquoted in the literature as 'no malformations were observed among the offspring of ten women who were treated with leflunomide during pregnancy in one series'. Although ten women were reported to have been exposed, the report states there were four pregnancies in which the outcome was unknown at the time of publication.

Because of concerns about leflunomide exposure during pregnancy, treatment with colestyramine is recommended for 11 days to enhance drug elimination, and two plasma concentrations 14 days apart should show no detectable drug before a woman attempts to conceive. At present there are insufficient data on which to base a reliable fetal risk assessment. If inadvertent exposure occurs, it is not necessarily an indication for termination of pregnancy or invasive prenatal diagnostic tests. High-resolution ultrasonography at about 20 weeks is recommended.

Bisphosphonates

Animal studies have shown skeletal malformations, the result of the pharmacological effects on bone, following doses far in excess of the human therapeutic doses. Some bisphosphonates have a half-life in bone up to 10 years (manufacturer's data). The fetal skeleton develops throughout gestation, and is therefore at risk. However, the mechanism of action in rats may be different from that in humans. Abnormal outcome in rat pregnancies exposed to bisphosphonates are associated with maternal hypocalcaemia, which does not occur in humans on therapy. There is concern that treatment with bisphosphates in women of reproductive age might result in the release of drug from bone several years after treatment. If the woman became pregnant following treatment this could result in embryo/fetal exposure.

No epidemiological studies of congenital anomalies in infants born to women treated with bisphosphonates during pregnancy have been reported. Two cases have been described in which normal infants were born to women who were treated with alendronate for osteoporosis immediately prior to or throughout pregnancy.[168,169]

Based on the lack of human safety data these drugs cannot be recommended for women of childbearing potential. At present there are insufficient data on which to base a reliable fetal risk assessment. If inadvertent exposure occurs, it is not necessarily an indication for termination of pregnancy or invasive prenatal diagnostic tests. High-resolution ultrasonography at about 20 weeks is recommended.

Ecstasy (methylenedioxymethamfetamine, MDMA)

There are few published data on the teratological effects of Ecstasy in animal or human pregnancy,[11,25,26,170] but structurally related amfetamines increase cardiac malformations in animals.[4]

The National Teratology Information Service (NTIS) has collected prospective follow-up data on 198 pregnancies with 201 outcomes (three sets of twins) referred to us for risk assessment. Ecstasy only was taken by 87 (44%) of the mothers and 111 (56%) took Ecstasy with other drugs, mainly combinations of amfetamine, cannabis, cocaine, ethanol and LSD (lysergide).

There were 123 liveborn babies, nine of whom were premature, 101 (82%) healthy, 16 (13%) with congenital abnormalities, and six (5%) with minor anomalies (normally excluded from general population data). Fetal loss occurred in 78 pregnancies: 18 miscarriages, one intrauterine death and 59 elective terminations (malformations reported in three fetuses, two with multiple defects, one with anencephaly).

Eight infants and one aborted fetus with malformations were exposed to Ecstasy alone; the other eight infants and two aborted fetuses were exposed to multiple drugs. One term neonate exposed *in utero* to heroin and methadone died. The malformations (excluding minor anomalies) in liveborns included CNS (3), septal defects (2), ptosis of the eye (1), talipes equinovarus (4) and other different musculoskeletal defects (6). The miscarriage rate was within the expected range (9% vs 10–20%), but the elective terminations were slightly higher than expected (29% vs 23%).

Overall, the data from this small case series shows that the incidence of congenital malformations, excluding minor anomalies (16/123 livebirths), is four to seven times higher than expected for the general population (13% vs 2–3%). After taking account of the higher prevalence of malformations associated with high-risk pregnancies in the NTIS database (13% vs 6.4%) there is still a twofold increased incidence of malformations associated with exposure to Ecstasy with or without other illicit drugs, which raises concern. However, at present, insufficient data are available to establish whether a single exposure to Ecstasy alone, with no maternal toxicity, increases the risk of malformation. Further research is required.

At present there are insufficient data on which to base a reliable fetal risk assessment. If inadvertent exposure occurs, it is not necessarily grounds for termination of pregnancy or invasive diagnostic techniques. An ultrasound scan at about 20 weeks is recommended.

Summary

The effects of a newly licensed medicine on the developing human fetus are largely unknown, despite the numerous tests demanded by regulators. Drugs can have adverse effects at any stage of pregnancy. Inadvertent exposure still occurs, and many women first realise they are pregnant well after organogenesis has begun. Prescribers should consider whether their prescriptions for women of childbearing age would be safe in the event of pregnancy. Where medication does carry a high risk of fetal toxicity, for example with antiepileptic or retinoid therapy, the risks should be discussed with the patient before they consider becoming pregnant. Healthcare professionals should also be aware of the potential harm to the fetus from substances of abuse.

CASE STUDY 4.1

A GP asks about a patient Mrs A, aged 26, who is delighted that she has just had a positive pregnancy test. Mrs A has suffered from depression for about 10 years and is concerned about whether she can continue her medication. She is being successfully managed on venlafaxine and is feeling well. Several other antidepressants had been prescribed in the past but were ineffective.

The GP asks you:
- Will venlafaxine damage the fetus?
- Which tests should he consider?
- Should he advise her to have a termination?
- If she needs to continue treatment, should he switch to fluoxetine, which he has heard is safe in pregnancy?

Factors to consider:

Other information needed It would be important to estimate the duration of pregnancy, according to date of last menstrual period and to consider the type of fetal toxicity that may have already occurred with the medication involved. Further information about the depressive illness would be helpful (e.g. severity, history of self-harm). Enquire about previous obstetric history – miscarriages, congenital malformations (CM) – any other illness or disability, as these factors may influence the patient's overall risk of an adverse pregnancy outcome. Details of other medicines (including OTC and complementary therapies) should be noted; consider the potential for drug interactions or synergistic effects. Folic acid should be started immediately.

Fetal/neonatal abnormalities associated with venlafaxine? No causal link with structural congenital malformations has been identified to date. There is some evidence that neonatal withdrawal symptoms may occur, and the possibility of CNS dysfunction.

Tests Dating scan at 12 weeks, detailed anomaly scan at 20 weeks. No prenatal diagnostic tests for CNS dysfunction.

Elective termination of pregnancy There are no medical grounds on the basis of the drug exposure.

Should venlafaxine be stopped? The patient has a long history of depression that has not responded to other therapies. Changes in treatment and drug

→

CASE STUDY 4.1 (continued)

concentrations during the changeover period could exacerbate her depression. There may be more risk associated with withholding therapy or switching to another drug. As the patient's depression is now well managed it may be appropriate to continue venlafaxine, although data on pregnancy outcome are extremely limited. Fluoxetine may be an appropriate alternative (data on 1500+ pregnancies with no evidence of increased risk of congenital malformations). As with all antidepressants there is the possibility of neonatal withdrawal symptoms. The potential risks should be discussed with the patient to allow her to make an informed choice.

CASE STUDY 4.2

Mrs B is a 40-year-old nulliparous woman with a poor obstetric history involving periods of infertility and several miscarriages. She has insulin-dependent diabetes mellitus (IDDM) complicated with hypertension and hyperlipidaemia. Her current, effective treatment regimen includes insulin, captopril and atorvastatin. During a routine check at the diabetic clinic it was discovered that she was about 12 weeks pregnant.

- Should Mrs B be advised to stop taking her medication, apart from insulin?
- Will captopril and atorvostatin have damaged the fetus?
- Alpha-fetoprotein testing (AFP) and a dating scan have been booked; what other specific diagnostic tests should be considered? Should elective termination be considered?
- How should the patient's drug therapy now be managed?

Factors to consider:

Other information needed   Is this an unplanned pregnancy? Determine the stage of pregnancy and assess the type of fetal toxicity that may have already occurred. At about 12 weeks embryogenesis is almost complete. Has any other medication been taken? Consider drug interactions or synergistic effects. A full medical and obstetric history should be taken – miscarriages, congenital malformation. Should folate be started? (in this case too late for prevention of neural tube defects). It may be beneficial if other folate antagonist drugs are taken (e.g. trimethoprim for UTI).

→

CASE STUDY 4.2 (continued)

The background risk of congenital malformations at 40 years should be considered.

Fetal/neonatal abnormalities associated with captopril Although the major adverse effects associated with ACE inhibitors have been reported after second- and third-trimester exposure, evidence is accumulating to indicate that these effects are initiated in the first trimester.

Fetal/neonatal abnormalities associated with atorvastatin There are equivocal data as to whether there is a causal relationship between statin exposure and congenital malformations.

Should medication be stopped/changed? Consider the potential adverse effects of uncontrolled diabetes, hypertension and hyperlipidaemia on the mother and fetus. It may be possible to stop atorvastatin without compromising maternal or fetal health. Hypertensive treatment should be reviewed and, if clinically possible, change ACE inhibitor to either methyldopa or long-acting nifedipine; consider a diuretic. It is important to keep blood pressure well controlled.

Tests Tight maternal glucose and blood pressure monitoring. A fetal nuchal scan at about 16 weeks and a detailed anomaly scan at 20 weeks to monitor fetal development, especially if treatment with an ACE inhibitor and a statin continues. Depending on the results of these scans chorionic villus sampling could be considered, but this invasive procedure does carry a small risk of miscarriage. There are no prenatal diagnostic tests for CNS dysfunction. Elective termination of pregnancy is not indicated on the grounds of drug exposure alone. However, if prenatal diagnostic tests indicate abnormalities, termination may need to be considered.

References

1. Peters P, Schaefer CH. General commentary to drug therapy and drug risks in pregnancy. In: Schaefer Ch, ed. *Drugs During Pregnancy and Lactation.* Amsterdam: Elsevier, 2001: 1–13.
2. Wilson JG. Current status of teratology. In: Wilson JG, Clarke FC, eds. *Handbook of Teratology*, Vol. 1. New York: Plenum Press, 1977: 47–74.
3. McElhatton PR. The principles of teratogenicity. *Curr Obstet Gynaecol* 1999; 9: 163–169.
4. Schardein JL. *Chemically Induced Birth Defects*, 3rd edn. New York: Marcel Dekker, 2000.
5. Loebstein R, Lalkin A, Koren G. Pharmacokinetic changes during pregnancy and their clinical relevance. *Clin Pharmacokinet* 1997; 33: 328–343.
6. McElhatton PR. Drug use in Pregnancy Part 1. *Pharm J* 2003; 270: 270–272.

7. Sullivan FM. Mechanisms of teratogenesis. In: Richards DJ, Rondel RK, eds. *Adverse Drug Reactions. Their Prediction, Detection and Assessment*. London: Churchill Livingstone, 1972: 19–25.

8. Buttar H. An overview of the influence of ACE inhibitors on fetal–placental circulation and perinatal development. *Mol Cell Biochem* 1997; 176: 61–71.

9. Lloyd ME, Carr M, McElhatton P, Hall GM, Hughes RA. The effects of methotrexate in pregnancy, fertility and lactation. *Q J Med* 1999; 92: 551–563.

10. Borgatta L, Burnhill MS, Tyson J, *et al.* Early medical abortion with methotrexate and misoprostol. *Obstet Gynecol* 2001; 97: 11–16.

11. McElhatton PR. Fetal effects of substance abuse. *J Toxicol Clin Toxicol* 2000; 38: 194–195.

12. Royal College of Physicians Tobacco Advisory Group. *Nicotine Addiction in Britain*. London: Royal College of Physicians, 2000.

13. Thomas SHL, McElhatton PR. Fetal effects of maternal alcohol exposure. *J Toxicol Clin Toxicol* 2000; 38: 192–193.

14. Astley SJ, Clarren SK. Diagnosing the full spectrum of fetal alcohol-exposed individuals: Introducing the 4-digit diagnostic code. *Alcohol Alcoholism* 2000; 35: 400–410.

15. Moore JA. An assessment of lithium using the IEHR evaluative process for assessing human developmental and reproductive toxicity of agents. *Reprod Toxicol* 1995; 9: 175–210.

16. Orioli IM, Castilla EE. Epidemiological assessment of misoprostol teratogenicity. *Br J Obstet Gynaecol* 2000; 107: 519–523.

17. Schardein JL. Miscellaneous drugs. In: Schardein JL, ed. *Chemically Induced Birth Defects*, 3rd edn. New York: Marcel Dekker, 2000: 763–795.

18. Deka P, McElhatton PR, Thomas SHL. Outcome of pregnancy following maternal treatment with retinoids. *J Toxicol Clin Toxicol* 2005; in press.

19. Reuvers M. Anticoagulant and fibrinolytic drugs. In: Schaefer Ch, ed. *Drugs During Pregnancy and Lactation*. Amsterdam: Elsevier, 2001: 85–92.

20. Saji H, Yamanaka M, Hagieara A, Ijiri R. Losartan and fetal toxic effects. *Lancet* 2001; 357: 363.

21. Garbis H, Reuvers M, Rost van Tonningen M. Anti-infective agents. In: Schaefer Ch, ed. *Drugs During Pregnancy and Lactation*. Amsterdam: Elsevier, 2001: 58–84.

22. McElhatton P. Heart and circulatory system drugs. In: Schaefer Ch, ed. *Drugs During Pregnancy and Lactation*. Amsterdam: Elsevier, 2001: 116–131.

23. Ville Y, Jenkins E, Shearer MJ, *et al.* Fetal intraventricular haemorrhage and maternal warfarin. *Lancet* 1993; 341: 1211.

24. Ornoy A, Patlas N, Pinto T, Golomb G. The transplacental effects of alendronate on the fetal skeleton in rats. *Teratology* 1998; 57: 242.

25. McElhatton PR, Bateman DN, Evans C, Pughe KR, Thomas SHL. Congenital anomalies after pre-natal Ecstasy exposure. *Lancet* 1999; 354: 1441–1442.

26. McElhatton P, Hedgley C, Thomas S. Congenital anomalies after prenatal Ecstasy exposure. BPS meeting Newcastle University, 20–22 December 2004. *Br J Clin Pharmacol* 2005 (in press); http://www.pA2online.org/Vol2Issue4 abst183P.html

27. Brent RL. Teratogen update: reproductive risks of leflunomide (Arava); a pyrimidine synthesis inhibitor: counselling women taking leflunomide before

or during pregnancy and men taking leflunomide who are contemplating fathering a child. *Teratology* 2001; 63: 106–112.

28. Chakravarty EF, Sanchez-Yamamoto D, Bush TM. The use of disease modifying antirheumatic drugs in women with rheumatoid arthritis of childbearing age: a survey of practice patterns and pregnancy outcomes. *J Rheumatol* 2003; 30: 241–246.

29. Mondello C, Giorgi R, Nuzzo F. Chromosomal effects of methotrexate on cultured human lymphocytes. *Mutat Res* 1984; 139: 67–70.

30. Manson JM, Freyssinges C, Ducrocq MB, Stephenson WP. Postmarketing surveillance of lovastatin and simvastatin exposure during pregnancy. *Reprod Toxicol* 1996; 10: 439–466.

31. Edison RJ, Muenke M. Central nervous system and limb anomalies in case reports of first-trimester statin exposure. *N Engl J Med* 2004; 350: 1579–1582.

32. Marín R, Gorostidi M, Portal CG, *et al.* Long-term prognosis of hypertension in pregnancy. *Hypertens Pregnancy* 2000; 19: 199–209.

33. Abalos E, Duley L, Steyn DW, Henderson-Smart DJ. Antihypertensive drug therapy for mild to moderate hypertension during pregnancy. Cochrane Database of Systematic Reviews 2001; Issue 1.

34. Allen VM, Joseph KS, Murphy KE, Magee LA, Ohlsson A. The effect of hypertensive disorders in pregnancy on small for gestational age and stillbirth: a population based study. *BMC Pregnancy and Childbirth* 2004; 4–17.

35. Hayman R. Hypertension in pregnancy. *Curr Obstet Gynaecol* 2004; 14: 1–10.

36. Steer PJ, Little MP, Kold-Jensen T, Chapple J, Elliott P. Maternal blood pressure in pregnancy, birth, weight, and perinatal mortality in first births. *Br Med J* 2004; 329: 1312–1314.

37. Vreeburg SA, Jacobs DJ, Dekker GA, *et al.* Hypertension during pregnancy in South Australia, Part 2: risk factors for adverse maternal and/or perinatal outcome – results of multivariable analysis. *Aust NZ J Obstet Gynaecol* 2004; 44: 410–418.

38. Schaefer Ch, Peters P. Diuretics. In: Schaefer Ch, ed. *Drugs During Pregnancy and Lactation.* Amsterdam: Elsevier, 2001: 113–115.

39. Briggs GG , Freeman RK, Yaffe SJ. *Drugs in Pregnancy and Lactation*, 6th edn. Baltimore: Lippincott Williams and Wilkins, 2002: 242–245.

40. Moar CA, Jeffries MA. Neonatal head circumference and the treatment of maternal hypertension. *Br J Obstet Gynaecol* 1978; 85: 933–937.

41. Pearson G, Bradley S. Pharmacologic management of hypertension in pregnancy. *On Continuing Practice* 1993; 20: 38–44.

42. Smith GN, Piercy WN. Methyldopa hepatotoxicity in pregnancy: a case report. *Am J Obstet Gynecol* 1995; 172: 222–224.

43. Kean L. Managing hypertension in pregnancy. *Curr Obstet Gynaecol* 2002; 12: 104–110.

44. Magee LA, Elran E, Bull SB, Logan A, Koren G. Risks and benefits of beta-receptor blockers for pregnancy hypertension: overview of the randomized trials. *Eur J Obstet Gynecol Reprod Biol* 2000; 88:15–26.

45. Magee LA, Duley L. Oral beta-blockers for mild to moderate hypertension during pregnancy. Cochrane Database of Systematic Reviews 2003, Issue 3.

46. World Health Organization. *Review: Labetalol for the Treatment of Hypertension in Pregnancy.* 15 December 2004. Geneva: WHO.

47. Lip GY, Beevers M, Churchill D, Shaffer LM, Beevers DG. Effect of atenolol on birth weight. *Am J Cardiol* 1997; 79: 1436–1438.
48. Lydakis C, Lip GY, Beevers M, Beevers DG. Atenolol and fetal growth in pregnancies complicated by hypertension. *Am J Hypertens* 1999; 12: 541–547.
49. von Dadelszen P, Ornstein MP, Bull SB, *et al*. Fall in mean arterial pressure and fetal growth restriction in pregnancy hypertension: a meta-analysis. *Lancet* 2000; 355: 87–92.
50. Bayliss H, Churchill D, Beevers M, Beevers DG. Anti-hypertensive drugs in pregnancy and fetal growth: evidence for 'pharmacological programming' in the first trimester. *Hypertens Pregnancy* 2002; 21: 161–174.
51. Wagenvoort AM, Van Vugt JMG, Sobotka M, Van Geijn HP. Topical timolol therapy in pregnancy: is it safe for the fetus? *Teratology* 1998; 58: 258–262.
52. Magee LA, Schick B, Sage SR, *et al*. The safety of calcium channel blockers in human pregnancy: a prospective, multicenter cohort study. *Am J Obstet Gynecol* 1996; 174: 823–828.
53. Casele HL, Windley KC, Prieto JA, Gratton R, Laifer SA. Felodipine use in pregnancy. Report of three cases. *J Reprod Med* 1997; 42: 378–381.
54. Papatsonis DNM, Van Geijn HP, Ader HJ, *et al*. Nifedipine and ritodrine in the management of preterm labor: a randomized multicenter trial. *Obstet Gynecol* 1997; 90: 230–234.
55. Blomström-Lundqvist C, Scheinman MM, Aliot EM, *et al*. ACC/AHA.ESC Guidelines for the management of patients with supraventricular arrhythmias–executive summary. A report of the American College of Cardiology/American Heart Association Task Force on practice guidelines and the European Society of Cardiology Committee for practice guidelines. ACC/AHA/ESC Practice Guidelines 2003.
56. Lambot MA, Vermeylen D, Noël JC. Angiotensin II-receptor inhibitors in pregnancy. *Lancet* 2001; 357: 1619–1620.
57. Hinsberger A, Wingen A-M, Hoyer PF. Angiotensin II-receptor inhibitors in pregnancy. *Lancet* 2001; 357: 1620.
58. Chung NA, Lip GYH, Beevers M, Beevers DG. Angiotensin II-receptor inhibitors in pregnancy. *Lancet* 2001; 357: 1620–1621.
59. Martinovic J, Benachi A, Laurent N, Daïkha-Dahmane F, Gubler MC. Fetal toxic effects and angiotensin-II-receptor antagonists. *Lancet* 2001; 358: (correspondence 21 July).
60. Salameh WA, Mastrogiannis DS. Maternal hyperlipidaemia in pregnancy. *Clin Obstet Gynecol* 1994; 37: 66–77.
61. Jay RH, Sturley RH, Stirling C, *et al*. Effects of pravastatin and cholestyramine on gonadal and adrenal steroid production in familial hypercholesterolaemia. *Br J Clin Pharmacol* 1991; 32: 417–422.
62. Travia D, Tosi F, Negri C, *et al*. Sustained therapy with 3-hydroxy-3-methylglutaryl-coenzyme-A reductase inhibitors does not impair steroidogenesis by adrenals and gonads. *J Clin Endocrinol Metab* 1995; 80: 836–840.
63. Edison RJ, Muenke M. Evidence for human teratogenicity of statins. *Birth Defects Res (Part A)* 2003; 67: 318.
64. Ghidini A, Sicherer S, Willner J. Congenital abnormalities (VATER) in baby born to mother using lovastatin. *Lancet* 1992; 339: 1416.
65. Rosa F. Anti-cholesterol agent pregnancy exposure outcomes. *Reprod Toxicol* 1994; 8: 445–446.

66. Hayes A, Gilbert A, Lopez G, Miller WA. MEVACORr – a new teratogen? *Am J Hum Genet* 1995; 57(Suppl 4): A92.
67. CLASP Collaborative Group. CLASP: a randomized trial of low-dose aspirin for the prevention and treatment of preeclampsia among 9634 pregnant women. *Lancet* 1994; 343: 619–629.
68. Heyborne KD. Preeclampsia prevention, lessons from the low-dose aspirin therapy trials. *Am J Obstet Gynecol* 2000; 183: 523–528.
69. Hall JG, Pauli RM, Wilson KM. Maternal and fetal sequelae of anticoagulation during pregnancy. *Am J Med* 1980; 68: 122–140.
70. Bates SM, Ginsberg JS. Anticoagulants in pregnancy: fetal effects. *Baillieres Clin Obstet Gynaecol* 1997; 11: 479–488.
71. Ginsberg JS, Chan WS, Bates SM, Katz S. Anticoagulation of pregnant women with mechanical heart valves. *Arch Intern Med* 2003; 163: 694–698.
72. Yu-Ling Tan J. Cardiovascular disease in pregnancy. *Curr Obstet Gynaecol* 2004; 14: 155–165.
73. Sanson B-J, Lensing AWA, Prins MH, *et al.* Safety of low-molecular-weight heparin in pregnancy: A systematic review. *Thromb Haemost* 1999; 81: 668–672.
74. Bar J, Cohen-Schaler B, Hod M, *et al.* Low molecular-weight heparin for thrombophilia in pregnant women. *Int J Gynecol Obstet* 2000; 69: 209–213.
75. Duncan S, Fairey A, Gomersall S, *et al.* Primary care guidelines for the management of females with epilepsy. London: Royal Society of Medicine Press, 2004.
76. Canger R, Battino D, Canevini MP, *et al.* Malformations in offspring of women with epilepsy: a prospective study. *Epilepsia* 1999; 40: 1231–1236.
77. Robert E, Reuvers M, Schaefer C. Antiepileptics. In: Schaefer Ch, ed. *Drugs During Pregnancy and Lactation*. Amsterdam: Elsevier, 2001: 46–57.
78. Anticonvulsants – Committee on Safety of Medicines and Medicines and Healthcare products Regulatory Agency. Current Problems in Pharmacovigilance. Volume 29, September 2003.
79. National Institute for Clinical Excellence. *Newer Drugs for Epilepsy in Adults.* Technology Appraisal 76 March 2004.
80. Scottish Intercollegiate Guidelines Network. *Diagnosis and Management of Epilepsy in Adults. A National Clinical Guideline.* October 2004.
81. Kaneko S, Battino D, Andermann E, *et al.* Congenital malformations due to antiepileptic drugs. *Epilepsy Res* 1999; 33: 145–148.
82. Yerby MS, Kaplan P, Tran T. Risks and management of pregnancy in women with epilepsy. *Cleveland Clin J Med* 2004; 71(Suppl 2): S25–S37.
83. Meador KJ, Zupanc ML. Neurodevelopmental outcomes of children born to mothers with epilepsy. *Cleveland Clin J Med* 2004; 71(Suppl 2): S38–S41.
84. Ornoy A, Cohen E. Outcome of children born to epileptic mothers treated with carbamazepine during pregnancy. *Obstet Gynecol Surv* 1997; 52: 472–474.
85. Ginsberg G, Hattis D, Miller R, Sonawane B. Pediatric pharmacokinetic data: implications for environmental risk assessment for children. *Pediatrics* 2004; 113: 973–983.
86. Medical Research Council Vitamin Research Group. Prevention of neural tube defects: results of the Medical Research Council vitamin study. *Lancet* 1991; 338: 131–137.
87. Oakley GP, Mandel JS. Folic acid fortification remains an urgent health priority. *Br Med J* 2004; 329: 1376.

88. Kalter H. Folic acid and human malformations: a summary and evaluation *Reprod Toxicol* 2000; 14: 463–476.
89. Gindler J, Li Z, Zheng J, *et al.* Folic acid supplements during pregnancy and risk of miscarriage. *Lancet* 2001; 358: 796–800.
90. Li Z, Gindler J, Wang H, *et al.* Folic acid supplements during early pregnancy and likelihood of multiple births: a population-based cohort study. *Lancet* 2003; 361: 380–384.
91. Charles D, Ness AR, Campbell D, Davey Smith G, Hall MH. Taking folate in pregnancy and risk of breast cancer. *Br Med J* 2004; 329: 1375–1376.
92. Kaaja E, Kaaja R, Matila R, Hiilesmaa V. Enzyme-inducing antiepileptic drugs in pregnancy and the risk of bleeding in the neonate. *Neurology* 2002; 58: 549–553.
93. Murray CJ, Lopez AD. Evidence-based health policy-lessons from the Global Burden of Disease Study. *Science* 1996; 274: 740–743.
94. Royal College of Obstetricians and Gynaecologists. *Why Mothers Die 1997–1999: the Fifth Report of the Confidential Enquiries into Maternal Deaths in the United Kingdom.* London: RCOG; 2001.
95. Mortality Statistics. Cause. Review of the Registrar General on deaths by cause, sex and age, in England and Wales, 2003. London: Office for National Statistics. Series DH2 no.30.
96. American Academy of Pediatrics. Committee on Drugs. Use of psychoactive medication during pregnancy and possible effects on the fetus and newborn. *Pediatrics* 2000; 105: 880–887.
97. Ward RK, Zamorski MA. Benefits and risks of psychiatric medications during pregnancy. *Am Fam Phys* 2002; 66: 629–636.
98. Postnatal Depression and Puerperal Psychosis. Section 4: prescribing issues in pregnancy and lactation. Scottish Intercollegiate Guidelines Network Publication No. 60. June 2002.
99. Viguera AC, Cohen LS, Baldessarini RJ, Nonacs R. Managing bipolar disorder during pregnancy: weighing the risks and benefits. *Can J Psychiatry* 2002; 47: 426–436.
100. Cantwell R, Cox JL. Psychiatric disorders in pregnancy and the puerperium. *Curr Obstet Gynaecol* 2003; 13: 7–13.
101. Williams K, Oke S. Lithium and pregnancy. *Psychiatr Bull* 2000; 24: 229–231.
102. REPROTEXT database, MICROMEDEX 2005.
103. Jacobson SJ, Jones K, Johnson K, *et al.* Prospective multicentre study of pregnancy outcome after lithium exposure during first trimester. *Lancet* 1992; 339: 530–534.
104. Jablensky AV, Morgan V, Zubrick SR, Bower C, Yellachich L. Pregnancy, delivery, and neonatal complications in a population of women with schizophrenia and major affective disorders. *Am J Psychiatry* 2005; 162: 79–91.
105. Bipolar Affective Disorder. Scottish Intercollegiate Guidelines Network, September 2004.
106. Hansen D, Lud HC, Olsen J. Serious life events and congenital malformations: a national study with complete follow up. *Lancet* 2000; 356: 875–880.
107. Garbis H, McElhatton PR. Psychotropic, sedative–hypnotic and Parkinson drugs. In: Schaefer Ch, ed. *Drugs During Pregnancy and Lactation.* Amsterdam: Elsevier, 2001: 182–191.
108. Gregoire A, Pearson S. Risk of pregnancy when changing to atypical antipsychotics. *Br J Psychiatry* 2002; 180: 83–84.

109. The National Teratology Information Service (NTIS) *Minipreg Summaries on Clozapine, Olanzapine, Quetiapine and Risperidone.* 2002.

110. Eli-Lilly and Company Ltd. Olanzapine Worldwide Pharmacovigilance Database 30.9.2001.

111. McElhatton PR, Garbis HM, Elefant E, *et al.* The outcome of pregnancy in 689 women exposed to therapeutic doses of antidepressants. A collaborative study of the European Network of Teratology Information Services (ENTIS). *Reprod Toxicol* 1996; 10: 285–294.

112. Ericson A, Kallen B, Wiholm BE. Delivery outcome after the use of antidepressants in early pregnancy. *Eur J Clin Pharmacol* 1999; 55: 503–508.

113. McElhatton P. Use of antidepressants in pregnancy and lactation. *Prescriber* 1999; 10: 101–111.

114. Nulman I, Rovet J, Stewart DE, *et al.* Neurodevelopment of children exposed in utero to antidepressant drugs. *N Engl J Med* 1997; 336: 258–262.

115. Chambers CD, Johnson KA, Dick LM, Felix RJ, Lyons Jones K. Birth outcomes in pregnant women taking fluoxetine. *N Engl J Med* 1996; 335: 1010–1015.

116. Goldstein DJ, Marvel DE. Psychotropic medications during pregnancy. Risk to the fetus. *JAMA* 1993; 270: 2177.

117. Mhanna MJ, Bennet JB II, Izatt SD. Potential fluoxetine chloride (Prozac) toxicity in a newborn. *Pediatrics* 1997; 100: 158–159.

118. Addis A, Koren G. Safety of fluoxetine during the first trimester of pregnancy: A meta-analytical review of epidemiological studies. *Psychol Med* 2000; 30: 89–94.

119. Zeskind PS, Stephens LE. Maternal selective serotonin reuptake inhibitor use during pregnancy and newborn behaviour. *Pediatrics* 2004; 113: 368–375.

120. Yaris F, Kadioglu M, Kesim M, *et al.* Newer antidepressants in pregnancy: prospective outcome of a case series. *Reprod Toxicol* 2004; 19: 235–238.

121. Goldstein DJ. Effects of third trimester fluoxetine exposure on the newborn. *J Clin Psychopharmacol* 1995; 15: 417–420.

122. Mattson SN, Eastvold AD, Jones KL, *et al.* Neurobehavioral follow-up of children prenatally exposed to fluoxetine. *Teratology* 1999; 59: 376.

123. Heikkinen T, Ekbald U, Kero P, Ekbald S, Laine K. Citalopram in pregnancy and lactation. *Clin Pharmacol Ther* 2002; 72: 184–191.

124. Sanz E, De-las-Cuevas C, Kiuru A, Bate A, Edwards R. Selective serotonin reuptake inhibitors in pregnant women and neonatal withdrawal syndrome: a database analysis. *Lancet* 2005; 365: 482–487.

125. National Institute for Clinical Excellence. *Depression: Management of Depression in Primary and Secondary Care.* NICE Clinical Guideline 23, December 2004.

126. Kennedy DS, Evans N, Wang I, Webster WS. Fetal abnormalities associated with high dose tranylcypromine in two consecutive pregnancies. *Teratology* 2000; 61: 441.

127. The Bupropion Pregnancy Registry. Interim report 1 September 1997–31 August 2004. Issued December 2004.

128. Scialli A, Rost van Tonningen M. Hormones. In: Schaefer Ch, ed. *Drugs During Pregnancy and Lactation.* Amsterdam: Elsevier, 2001: 132–148.

129. De Swiet M, ed. *Medical Disorders in Obstetric Practice*, 4th edn. Oxford: Blackwell Science, 2002.

130. Temple R, Aldridge V, Greenwood R, *et al*. Association between outcome of pregnancy and glycaemic control in early pregnancy in type 1 diabetes: population based study. *Br Med J* 2002; 325: 1275–1276.
131. Walkinshaw SA. Type 1 and type 2 diabetes and pregnancy. *Curr Obstet Gynaecol* 2004; 14: 375–386.
132. Tuffnell DJ, West J, Walkinshaw SA. Treatment for gestational diabetes in impaired glucose tolerance in pregnancy (Review). Cochrane Collaboration 2005. Chichester: John Wiley and Sons Ltd, 2005.
133. Turok D, Ratcliffe S, Baxley E. Management of gestational diabetes mellitus. *Am Fam Phys* 2003; 68: 1767–1772; 1775–1776.
134. Moses RG, Webb AJ, Lucas EM, Davis WS. Twin pregnancy outcomes for women with gestational diabetes mellitus compared with glucose tolerant women. *Aust NZ J Obstet Gynecol* 2003; 43: 38–40.
135. Moore KL, Persaud PVN. *The Developing Human: Clinically Orientated Embryology*. London: WB Saunders, 2003.
136. O'Doherty MJ, McElhatton PR, Thomas SHL. Treating thyrotoxicosis in pregnant and potentially pregnant women. *Br Med J* 1999; 318: 5–6.
137. Girling JC. Thyroid disorders in pregnancy. *Curr Obstet Gynaecol* 2003; 13: 45–51.
138. Shillingford AJ, Weiner S. Maternal issues affecting the fetus. *Clin Perinatol* 2001; 28: 31–70.
139. McElhatton PR. Drug use in pregnancy. Part 2. *Pharm J* 2003; 270: 305–307.
140. Dale J, Frankly J. The drug treatment of thyroid disorders. *Prescriber* 2002; 13: 50–68.
141. Wing DA, Millar LK, Koonings PP, Montoro MN, Mestman JH. A comparison of propylthiouracil versus methimazole in the treatment of hyperthyroidism in pregnancy. *Am J Obstet Gynecol* 1994; 170: 90–95.
142. Van Dijke CP, Heydendael RJ, de Kleine MJ. Methimazole, carbimazole and congenital skin defects. *Ann Intern Med* 1987; 106: 60–61.
143. Vogt T, Stolz W, Landthaler M. Aplasia cutis congenita after exposure to methimazole: a causal relationship? *Br J Dermatol* 1995; 1333: 994–996.
144. Momotani N, Ito K, Hamada N, *et al*. Maternal hyperthyroidism and congenital malformation in the offspring. *Clin Endocrinol* 1984; 20: 695–700.
145. Clementi M, di Gianantonio E, Pelo E, *et al*. Methimazole embryopathy: delineation of the phenotype. *Am J Med Genet* 1999; 83: 43–46.
146. Diav-Citrin O, Ornoy O. Teratogen update: antithyroid drugs – methimazole, carbimazole, and propylthiouracil. *Teratology* 2002; 65: 38–44.
147. Hernández-Díaz S, Werler MM, Walker AM, Mitchell AA. Folic acid antagonists during pregnancy and the risk of birth defects. *N Engl J Med* 2000; 343: 1608–1614.
148. Schaefer C, Amoura-Elefant E, Vial T, *et al*. Pregnancy outcome after prenatal quinolone exposure. Evaluation of a case registry of the European Network of Teratology Information Services (ENTIS). *Eur J Obstet Gynecol Reprod Biol* 1996; 69: 83–89.
149. Loebstein R, Addis A, Ho E, *et al*. Pregnancy outcome following gestational exposure to fluoroquinolones: A multicenter prospective controlled study. *Antimicrob Agents Chemother* 1998; 42: 1336–1339.
150. Adams J, Lammer EJ. Neurobehavioral teratology of isotretinoin. *Reprod Toxicol* 1993; 7: 175–177.

151. Teratology Society. Recommendations for isotretinoin use in women of child-bearing potential. *Teratology* 1991; 44: 1–6.

152. Jensen BK, McGann LA, Kachevsky V, Franz TJ. The negligible availability of retinoids with multiple and excessive topical application of isotretinoin 0.05% gel (Isotrex) in patients with acne vulgaris. *J Am Acad Dermatol* 1991; 24: 425–428.

153. Chen C, Jensen BK, Mistry G, *et al.* Negligible systemic absorption of topical isotretinoin cream: implications for teratogenicity. *J Clin Pharmacol* 1997; 37: 279–284.

154. Van Hoogdalem EJ. Transdermal absorption of topical anti-acne agents in man; a review of clinical pharmacokinetic data. *J Eur Acad Dermatol Venereol* 1998; 11: S13–S19; S28–S29.

155. Christin-Maitre S, Bouchard P, Spitz IM. Medical termination of pregnancy. *N Engl J Med* 2000; 342: 946–956.

156. Kahn JG, Becker BJ, Maclsaa L, *et al.* The efficacy of medical abortion: A meta-analysis. *Contraception* 2000; 61: 29–40.

157. Newhall EP, Winikoff B. Abortion with mifepristone and misoprostol: Regimens, efficacy, acceptability and future directions. *Am J Obstet Gynecol* 2000; 183: S44–S53.

158. Song J. Use of misoprostol in obstetrics and gynecology. *Obstet Gynecol Surv* 2000; 55: 503–510.

159. Sitruk-Ware R, Davey A, Sakiz E. Fetal malformation and failed medical termination of pregnancy. *Lancet* 1998; 352: 323.

160. Pastuszak AL, Schuler L, Speck-Martins CE, *et al.* Use of misoprostol during pregnancy and Mobius' syndrome in infants. *N Engl J Med* 1998; 338: 1881–1885.

161. Coelho K-EFA, Sarmento MvF, Veiga CM, *et al.* Misoprostol embryotoxicity: Clinical evaluation of fifteen patients with arthrogryposis. *Am J Med Genet* 2000; 95: 297–301.

162. Vargus FR, Schuler-Faccini L, Brunoni D, *et al.* Prenatal exposure to misoprostol and vascular disruption defects: A case–control study. *Am J Med Genet* 2000; 95: 302–306.

163. Castilla EE, Orioli IM. Teratogenicity of misoprostol: Data from the Latin-American Collaborative Study of Congenital Malformations (ECLAMC). *Am J Med Genet* 1994; 51: 161–162.

164. Schuler L, Pastuszak A, Sanseverino MTV, *et al.* Pregnancy outcome after exposure to misoprostol in Brazil: A prospective, controlled study. *Reprod Toxicol* 1999; 13: 147–151.

165. Lewden B, Vial T, Elefant E, *et al.* Low dose methotrexate in the first trimester of pregnancy: results of a French collaborative study. *J Rheumatol* 2004; 31: 2360–2365.

166. Donnenfeld AE, Pastuszak A, Noah JS, *et al.* Methotrexate exposure prior to and during pregnancy. *Teratology* 1994; 49: 79–81.

167. Woolas RP, Bower M, Newlands ES, *et al.* Influence of chemotherapy for gestational trophoblastic disease on subsequent pregnancy outcome. *Br J Obstet Gynaecol* 1998; 105: 1032–1035.

168. Harsch IA, Hubner RH, Hahn EG, Hensen J. Osteoporosis and multiple pregnancy – a case report with positive outcome. *Med Klin (Munich)* 2001; 96: 402–407.

169. Rutgers-Verhage AR, deVries TW, Torringa MJ. No effects of bisphosphonates on the human fetus. *Birth Defects Res A Clin Mol Teratol* 2003; 67: 203–204.
170. van Tonningen-van Driel MM, Garbis Berkvens JM, Reuvers Lodewijks WB. Zwangerschapsuitkomst na ecstacygebruik; 43 gevallen gevolgd door de Teratologie Informatie Service van het RIVM. *Ned Tijdschr Geneeskd* 1999; 143: 27–31.

Further reading

De Swiet M ed., *Medical Disorders in Obstetric Practice*, 4th edn. Oxford: Blackwell Science, 2002.
Lee A, Inch S, Finnegan D eds. *Therapeutics in Pregnancy and Lactation*. Oxford: Radcliffe Medical Press, 2000.
McElhatton P. The effects of drug misuse in pregnancy. In: Philips R, ed. *Children Exposed to Substance Misuse – Implications for Family Placement*. London: BAAF, 2004: 43–72.
Schaefer C ed., *Drugs During Pregnancy and Lactation*. Amsterdam: Elsevier, 2001.

Glossary

Agenesis Defective development or absence of part(s) of the body.

Arthrogryposis The state of a persistent flexure or contracture of a joint. In arthrogryposis multiplex congenita there is a congenital generalised fibrous ankylosis of the joints of the upper and lower extremities.

Atresia Imperforation; absence or closure of a normal opening.

Holoprosencephaly Impaired midline cleavage of the embryonic forebrain, the most extreme form being cyclopia.

Hydrocephaly A condition characterised by abnormal increase in the amount of cerebral fluid accompanied by dilation of the cerebral ventricles.

Hypertelorism Abnormal distance between two organs or parts; commonly used to describe increased interpupillary distance.

Hypocalvaria/acalvaria Hypoplasia of the membrane bones of the skull. The brain is usually relatively normal, the standard being that the bones are absolutely small for age. It is usually defined as the absence of calvarial bones, dura mater and associated muscles in the presence of a normal skull base and facial bones. Hypocalvaria/acalvaria probably results from a postneurulation event.

Hypospadias The congenital opening of the urethra on the undersurface of the penis; may also refer to the opening of the urethra into the vagina.

Microencephaly Abnormal smallness of the head.

NTD Neural tube defect.

Philtrum The vertical groove in the medial portion of the upper lip, extending from beneath the nose to the outer surface of the upper lip.

Phocomelia In its extreme form, direct attachment of the hands or feet to the trunk. The term may also be applied to cases of partial absence of any proximal region of the limbs.

Polydactyly A developmental anomaly characterised by the presence of super-numerary digits on the hands or feet.

Syndactyly A condition in which two or more fingers or toes are partially or completely adherent owing to fusion of the skin or fusion of skin and bone. Cutaneous syndactyly of the second and third toes is a very common genetic finding in the general population, and is also noted in various syndromes.

Talipes equinovarus A deformity of the foot in which the heel is turned inward from the midline of the leg and the foot is plantarflexed. This is associated with the raising of the inner border of the foot and displacement of the anterior part of the foot so that it lies medially to the vertical axis of the leg. With this type of foot the arch is higher and the foot is in equinus. This is a typical form of clubfoot.

Tetralogy of Fallot The most common form of cyanotic congenital heart disease, consisting of pulmonic stenosis, ventricular septal defect, dextroposition of the aorta, and right ventricular hypertrophy.

5

Drug-induced skin reactions

Anne Lee and John Thomson

Introduction

Cutaneous drug eruptions are one of the most common types of adverse reaction to drug therapy, with an overall incidence rate of 2–3% in hospitalised patients.[1-3] Almost any medicine can induce skin reactions, and certain drug classes, such as non-steroidal anti-inflammatory drugs (NSAIDs), antibiotics and antiepileptics, have drug eruption rates approaching 1–5%.[4] Although most drug-related skin eruptions are not serious, some are severe and potentially life-threatening. Serious reactions include angio-oedema, erythroderma, Stevens–Johnson syndrome and toxic epidermal necrolysis. Drug eruptions can also occur as part of a spectrum of multiorgan involvement, for example in drug-induced systemic lupus erythematosus (see Chapter 11). As with other types of drug reaction, the pathogenesis of these eruptions may be either immunological or non-immunological. Healthcare professionals should carefully evaluate all drug-associated rashes. It is important that skin reactions are identified and documented in the patient record so that their recurrence can be avoided. This chapter describes common, serious and distinctive cutaneous reactions (excluding contact dermatitis, which may be due to any external irritant, including drugs and excipients), with guidance on diagnosis and management.

A cutaneous drug reaction should be suspected in any patient who develops a rash during a course of drug therapy. The reaction may be due to any medicine the patient is currently taking or has recently been exposed to, including prescribed and over-the-counter medicines, herbal or homoeopathic preparations, vaccines or contrast media. Remember that the non-drug components of a medicine, i.e. the pharmaceutical excipients, may cause hypersensitivity reactions in some patients.

Classification and mechanism

Cutaneous drug reactions may be caused by several different mechanisms, but in many cases the precise mechanism is unknown. Many drug eruptions are the result of a hypersensitivity reaction with an underlying immune mechanism. Skin reactions as a result of non-immunological causes are more common and include cumulative toxicity, overdose, photosensitivity, drug interactions, and metabolic alterations.[5]

The term hypersensitivity is applied when the immune response to an agent (immunogen) results in an increased or exaggerated response. Drugs, or their metabolites, act as haptens by covalently binding to peptides and modifying them to become immunogenic, inducing a specific cell-mediated or humoral immune response. All of the four Coombs' and Gell immune mechanisms may be involved (Table 5.1). Recent immunological research suggests that combined involvement of different immune mechanisms may feature in some reactions, and that T cells are involved in all four types of reaction.[6] It has also been postulated that some drugs have structural

Table 5.1 Immunological (hypersensitivity) reactions

Type I reactions are caused by the formation of drug/antigen-specific IgE that cross-links with receptors on mast cells and basophils. This leads to immediate release of chemical mediators, including histamine and leukotrienes. Clinical features include pruritus, urticaria, angio-oedema and, less commonly, bronchoconstriction and anaphylaxis. The drugs most commonly responsible for type I hypersensitivity are aspirin, opioids, penicillins and some vaccines.

Type II or cytotoxic reactions are based on IgG or IgM-mediated mechanisms. These involve binding of antibody to cells with subsequent binding of complement and cell rupture. This mechanism accounts for blood cell dyscrasias such as haemolytic anaemia and thrombocytopenia.

Type III reactions are mediated by intravascular immune complexes. These arise when drug antigen and antibodies, usually of IgG or IgM class, are both present in the circulation, with the antigen present in excess. Slow removal of immune complexes by phagocytes leads to their deposition in the skin and the microcirculation of the kidneys, joints and gastrointestinal system. Serum sickness and vasculitis are examples of type III reactions.

Type IV reactions are mediated by T cells causing 'delayed' hypersensitivity reactions. Typical examples include contact dermatitis or delayed skin tests to tuberculin. Drug-related delayed-type hypersensitivity reactions include Stevens–Johnson syndrome and toxic epidermal necrolysis (TEN). Recent work has proposed that type IV reactions be divided into four subtypes based on the T-lymphocyte subset and cytokine expression profile involved.[5]

Ig, immunoglobulin.

features allowing direct interaction with T cells, a concept termed pharmacologic interaction with immune receptors (p-I concept).[5] The clinical manifestations of drug hypersensitivity depend on various factors, including the chemical or structural features of a drug, the genetic background of the affected individual, and the specificity and function of the drug-induced immune response.

Different types of immune effector mechanism can produce diverse clinical patterns of hypersensitivity reaction,[4] for example, penicillins, as the classic drugs acting as haptens, are reported to cause type 1 IgE-mediated (immediate-type) hypersensitivity reactions as well as non-IgE mediated reactions, including morbilliform eruptions, erythema multiforme and Stevens–Johnson syndrome.[7,8]

It is especially important that allergic skin reactions are correctly identified, as subsequent exposure to the drug may cause a more severe reaction. Patients with a reliable history of drug allergy should always be carefully monitored when any new medicine is started, as 10% of patients with drug hypersensitivity reactions react to more than one structurally distinct compound.[5] The route of administration is a factor in drug allergy; in general, topical application has the greatest propensity to induce allergy, followed by parenteral then oral administration.[9]

Certain patient groups appear to be predisposed to cutaneous adverse drug reactions (ADRs).[10] There is a high incidence of hypersensitivity reactions in patients with altered immune status, for example due to viral infections (Epstein–Barr virus or HIV). A well-documented example is the increased risk of co-trimoxazole hypersensitivity in HIV patients. As with ADRs in general, altered drug handling due to organ impairment or genetic factors may play a part; for example, slow-acetylator status may predispose to sulfonamide reactions. The role of atopy in predisposing to drug reactions is controversial.[11] It may be important in reactions to iodinated contrast material, but not in those to penicillins or during anaesthesia.[12] The term multiple drug allergy syndrome has been used to describe patients who have a propensity to react against different, chemically unrelated drugs.[13]

Diagnosis

It can be difficult to diagnose a drug eruption with confidence. Most drugs are associated with a spectrum of skin reactions, although some agents seldom cause skin reactions (Table 5.2).[6,14] Some types of skin rash are very rarely drug induced, for example eczema. Many drug reactions cannot be distinguished from naturally occurring eruptions, and so misdiagnosis is

Table 5.2 Drugs rarely causing cutaneous eruptions (rates estimated to be 3 cases per 1000)

Antacids	Muscle relaxants
Antihistamines (oral)	Nitrates
Atropine	Nystatin
Benzodiazepines	Oral contraceptives
Corticosteroids	Propranolol
Digoxin	Spironolactone
Ferrous sulphate	Theophylline
Insulin	Thyroid hormones
Laxatives	Vitamins
Local anaesthetics (other than topical)	

common. For example, there may be uncertainty about whether a morbilliform rash is due to a viral infection or an antibiotic, and this may unnecessarily limit the future use of a particular medication. Furthermore, patients may be taking several medicines, making it difficult to establish the one responsible. Some drugs are more likely to be the cause of a particular type of eruption than others. For example, if a patient taking both demeclocycline and chlorpromazine develops a photosensitivity reaction the chances are that demeclocycline is the cause, although both drugs are capable of producing the reaction. However, if the patient develops skin hyperpigmentation then chlorpromazine is more likely to be implicated.

The timing of skin reactions is often a useful diagnostic tool. In general, the onset occurs within a few weeks of the introduction of the causative drug. If a medicine has been taken for many years without a problem then it is less likely to be responsible. When examining a list of medicines taken by a patient with a rash, new drugs taken within the previous month are the most likely cause. There are some notable exceptions to this rule. Hypersensitivity reactions to penicillins can occur several weeks after the drug has been discontinued, and the typical psoriasiform skin eruption seen with the beta-blocker practolol (withdrawn in the 1970s) generally occurred after many months of treatment. Gold can also cause very late reactions.

Drugs suspected of causing skin reactions should usually be withdrawn and not used again in that patient, although the risk–benefit potential needs to be considered before discontinuing any necessary medicines. Symptomatic treatment may be needed. Calamine lotion or systemic antihistamines may relieve pruritus and topical corticosteroids may help inflammation and itch. For more serious reactions, systemic corticosteroids may be indicated. The main clinical features that are suggestive of a severe reaction include mucous membrane involvement, blisters or skin detachment, high fever, angio-oedema or tongue swelling, facial oedema, skin necrosis, lymphadenopathy or dyspnoea. In most cases drug eruptions are reversible, resolving gradually after the causative drug is withdrawn. Knowledge of the half-lives of the implicated medicines can be important; for medications with long half-lives, the time to resolution may be several weeks or more.

Although skin-prick or blood tests may be used in the diagnosis of some reactions (e.g. those dependent on IgE, such as immediate-type reactions to penicillin), they are not usually helpful in skin manifestations of an allergy.[7,15] Skin-prick tests are not risk free and should only be carried out close to intensive care facilities. Rechallenge is not normally advised in the diagnosis of skin reactions because of the inherent risks to the patient.

Management points

When a patient may have experienced a drug eruption:

*   Take an accurate medication history. Note details of all current and recent medication, including over-the-counter medicines, herbal (e.g. St John's Wort, echinacea) and homoeopathic preparations, and injections, including vaccines or contrast media.
*   Note the times when each medicine was first taken relative to the onset of the reaction, and check whether the patient has taken these medicines previously.
*   Some skin reactions, particularly urticaria, may be due to sensitivity to pharmaceutical excipients. If this type of reaction is present, it is worth noting the proprietary (brand) names of medicines taken as well as the generic name.
*   Ask the patient if they have a previous history of drug sensitivity, contact dermatitis, connective tissue disease or atopic disease with asthma or eczema.
*   Examine the rash to determine what type it is and whether it appears to be a drug eruption.
*   Record clearly in the patient's notes any known or suspected ADR, with details of the presumed cause. Tell the patient or relatives, and preferably give a written note so that future exposure can be avoided.
*   Take great care in prescribing for the patient subsequently. Check prescribing information (e.g. the *British National Formulary*) for

potential cross-reactions if you are not sure. Clarify that compound preparations do not contain potentially harmful constituents.

- Notify suspected ADRs to the relevant regulatory authority. This information is essential for identifying new drug safety hazards and enables the study of factors associated with ADRs.

Exanthematous (erythematous) reactions

Exanthema is an umbrella term for skin reactions that literally burst forth on the skin. Enanthematous reactions similarly occur on the mucous membranes. Typical characteristics of skin exanthemas include erythema (redness), or morbilliform (resembling measles) or maculo-papular lesions. Macules are small, distinct, flat areas and papules are small, raised lesions. This is the most common type of drug-induced cutaneous reaction. The eruption often starts on the trunk; the extremities and intertriginous areas are often involved, but the face may be spared. The rash is usually bright red in colour and the skin may feel hot, burning or itchy.

These reactions can occur with almost any medicine at any time, usually up to a month after treatment is started, but they are most common in the first 10 days. If the causative drug is continued, exfoliative dermatitis may develop. These eruptions usually resolve rapidly when the causative drug is stopped, and occasionally while it is still being taken. Penicillins and sulfonamides frequently cause these rashes. With all the penicillins almost every type of exanthematous eruption may occur; a generalised morbilliform eruption is common with ampicillin and amoxicillin. Viral infections may increase the incidence of morbilliform drug reactions. Ampicillin almost always causes a severe morbilliform eruption when given to a patient with infectious mononucleosis. The exact mechanism involved is unknown. Ampicillin and its derivatives should be avoided in these patients.

Drugs that commonly cause exanthematous reactions are shown in Table 5.3.

Erythroderma and exfoliative dermatitis

A widespread confluent erythematous rash (erythroderma), often associated with desquamation (exfoliative dermatitis), is one of the most severe patterns of cutaneous drug reaction. There may be systemic symptoms, such as fever, lymphadenopathy and anorexia. Possible complications

Table 5.3 Some drugs that commonly cause exanthematous reactions

Allopurinol
Antimicrobials: cephalosporins, penicillins, chloramphenicol, erythromycin,
    gentamicin, amphotericin, antituberculous drugs, nalidixic acid, nitrofurantoin,
    sulfonamides
Barbiturates
Captopril
Carbamazepine
Furosemide
Gold salts
Lithium
Phenothiazines
Phenylbutazone
Phenytoin
Thiazides

include hypothermia, fluid and electrolyte loss, and infection. The main drugs implicated are sulfonamides, chloroquine, penicillin, phenytoin and isoniazid.

Fixed drug eruption

A fixed drug eruption is due to exogenous drugs or chemicals are the sole cause. It consists of erythematous round or oval lesions of a reddish, dusky purple or brown colour, sometimes featuring blisters, either bullae or vesicles. Initially, one lesion appears, although others may follow. The patient may complain of itching or burning in the affected area, but systemic involvement is usually absent. The eruption can appear within a day to a few weeks of ingesting the causative drug and can occur on any part of the skin or mucous membranes. The hands, feet, tongue, penis or perianal areas are most frequently affected. The site of the eruption is fixed, i.e. whenever the individual takes the causative drug the eruption occurs within hours at exactly the same site. Healing occurs over 7–10 days after the causative drug is stopped, although residual hyperpigmentation may be slow to resolve.[2,16,17] The pathogenesis of fixed drug eruption is not well understood. Familial cases have been reported and genetic susceptibility may have a role. There are many known causes, including food additives and pharmaceutical excipients. Sulfonamides, tetracyclines and NSAIDs are frequently implicated. Because phenolphthalein has been removed from most laxatives, it is much less often

Table 5.4 Some common causes of fixed drug eruption

ACE inhibitors
Allopurinol
Antimicrobials: co-trimoxazole, sulfonamides, tetracyclines, cephalosporins,
    penicillin, clindamycin, trimethoprim, metronidazole
Barbiturates
Benzodiazepines
Calcium channel blockers: amlodipine, diltiazem
Carbamazepine
Dextromethorphan
Diltiazem
Fluconazole
Lamotrigine
NSAIDs, including aspirin
Paclitaxel
Paracetamol
Phenolphthalein
Proton pump inhibitors: omeprazole, lansoprazole
Quinine
Salicylates
Terbinafine

ACE, angiotensin-converting enzyme.

the culprit than in past years. Where a fixed drug eruption is suspected, oral challenge to confirm the diagnosis is accepted and safe practice. Topical corticosteroids may help reduce the intensity of the reaction. Table 5.4 lists the most common drug causes.

Urticaria and angio-oedema

Drug-induced urticaria is the second most common form of cutaneous drug reaction after exanthematous reactions. Urticaria is seen in association with anaphylaxis, angio-oedema or serum sickness. The clinical appearance of drug-induced urticaria is indistinguishable from that from other causes, but is often more severe and may be accompanied by hypotension, breathing difficulties, shock, and even death. Urticaria lesions, sometimes known as nettle rash or hives, present as raised, itchy, red blotches or weals that are pale in the centre and red around the outside. Drug-induced urticaria may occur after the first exposure to a drug or after many previously well-tolerated exposures. The onset is more rapid than with other drug eruptions; lesions usually develop within 36 hours of initial drug exposure. Individual lesions rarely persist for more than 24 hours. On rechallenge, lesions may develop within minutes. Urticaria is characterised as acute when it lasts 6 weeks or less and chronic when it persists beyond this. Drugs are the cause of a minority of cases of chronic urticaria, and in this situation it may be difficult to establish the cause.[18] Acute anaphylaxis and anaphylactoid reactions typically present with angio-oedema, urticaria, dyspnoea and hypotension.

Serum sickness begins 6–14 days after the initial exposure to foreign protein and has distinctive skin findings. Erythema first occurs on the sides of the fingers, toes and hands, before a more widespread morbilliform eruption occurs in about two-thirds of patients. About half the cases of serum sickness have systemic symptoms such as fever, arthralgia and arthritis.

Angio-oedema is a vascular reaction resulting in increased permeability and fluid leakage, leading to oedema of the deep dermis, subcutaneous tissue or submucosal areas. It is rarer than urticaria. The tongue, lips, eyelids or genitalia are generally affected, and the oedema may be either unilateral or symmetrical. Angio-oedema of the upper respiratory tract can result in serious acute respiratory distress, airway obstruction and death.

The mechanisms involved in this spectrum of urticarial reactions are believed to be immunological, mediated by IgE; mediated by circulating immune complexes (serum sickness); and non-immunological. The latter group may involve complement activation, release of cutaneous mast cell mediators, or altered chemical pathways such as arachidonic acid metabolism.[2,18,19] Table 5.5 shows some drugs that may cause urticarial reactions, with their associated mechanisms.

It is essential to take a detailed medication history when a patient presents with urticaria, remembering that pharmaceutical excipients may be a trigger. It can be especially difficult to identify the causative drug in patients taking several medicines, all started at about the same time. The problem for which the patient is being treated, such as infection, may be the cause or may exacerbate a pre-existing urticaria. Specialist skin testing (e.g. radioallergenosorbent test (RAST), skin testing, leukocyte histamine release, tryptase measurement) may help identify the cause. Positive rechallenge is required to confirm that urticaria is caused by a particular drug, but most physicians remain wary of the potential risks and is rarely justified.

Management of urticarial reactions involves stopping the causative agent and treatment with an oral antihistamine. Where there is a systemic

Table 5.5 Some drugs that may cause urticaria/angioedema

Mechanisms of drug-induced urticaria

Mechanism	*Example drugs*
Drugs acting through IgE receptors to the drug on mast cells triggering degranulation	Antibiotics (penicillins, cephalosporins, sulfonamides, tetracyclines), antiepileptics
Drugs that cause mast cell degranulation	Codeine, opioids, tubocurarine, atropine, hydralazine, pentamidine, quinine, radiocontrast media, vancomycin, dextran
Drugs that pharmacologically promote or exacerbate urticaria	Aspirin, NSAIDs, ACE inhibitors, monoclonal antibodies
Immune complex formation precipitation and activation of complement	Penicillin, sulfonamides, thiouracils, cholecystographic dyes, aminosalicylic acid
Excipients in the medication that provoke allergic or pseudoallergic reactions	Benzoic acid, butylated hydroxytoluene, sulfites, aspartame, colourings, tartrazine, preservatives

Ig, immunoglobulin.
Adapted from ref. 18.

involvement, hypotension, respiratory problems, or serum sickness, a short course of oral corticosteroids may be necessary.[2,18] Where urticaria or angio-oedema are a component of anaphylaxis or an anaphylactoid reaction, resuscitation guidelines should be followed.[20] When these reactions occur they should always be reported to the appropriate regulatory authority.

Angiotensin-converting enzyme (ACE) inhibitors are one of the most common causes of angio-oedema. The estimated incidence is 0.1–1% in Caucasians, but may be higher in people of African-American origin.[21,22] In most cases the reaction occurs in the first week of treatment, often within hours of the initial dose. However, in some cases it has developed after prolonged therapy of up to several years, and it may recur intermittently while the drug is continued.[22–24] It has been shown that continuing use of ACE inhibitors after the first episode of angio-oedema results in a markedly increased rate of recurrence, with serious morbidity. ACE inhibitors should therefore be withdrawn immediately in any patient who presents with angio-oedema, and they are contraindicated in patients with a history of idiopathic angio-oedema.

The mechanism of ACE-inhibitor-induced angio-oedema is thought to involve increased levels of bradykinin. For this reason it has been presumed that the use of angiotensin-II receptor antagonists, which theoretically do not affect bradykinin, should not present a risk for patients who had this complication while taking ACE inhibitors. However, angiotensin-II receptor antagonists have recently been implicated as a cause of angio-oedema,[25-27] and their safety for use in this situation is now debated. Cicardi *et al.* carried out a retrospective analysis of 64 patients who had experienced angio-oedema while taking an ACE inhibitor.[22] An angiotensin-II receptor antagonist seemed to sustain angio-oedema in only two of 26 patients subsequently switched to this drug class. An angiotensin-II antagonist may be tolerated in patients with ACE-inhibitor-induced angio-oedema, but caution is needed as angio-oedema can have serious consequences.

Aspirin and other NSAIDs are another common cause of urticarial reactions, with an estimated prevalence of 0.1–0.3%.[28] Facial angio-oedema is the most frequent adverse skin reaction associated with NSAIDs. These reactions seem to be more common in children and young adults, and patients with a history of chronic urticaria. Some, but not all, patients show a mixed clinical pattern of cutaneous and respiratory symptoms (e.g. rhinitis, breathlessness). Some patients react to NSAIDs belonging to different chemical classes ('cross-reactors'), whereas others experience problems with agents in only one particular NSAID chemical group ('single reactors'), suggesting that the underlying mechanisms may be respectively pseudoallergy and IgE.

Acne

Some drugs can cause or exacerbate acne. The term acneiform is applied to drug eruptions that resemble acne vulgaris. The lesions are papulopustular but comedones are usually absent.[29] Corticotropin (ACTH), corticosteroids, androgens (in females), oral contraceptives, haloperidol, isoniazid, phenytoin and lithium are among the most frequently implicated drugs.

Psoriasis and psoriasiform eruptions

Psoriasiform eruptions are similar to idiopathic psoriasis and typically consist of erythematous plaques surmounted by large dry silvery scales. A number of drugs can induce psoriasis in patients with no previous history, and some can worsen pre-existing psoriasis, although many reports are anecdotal and causality is unknown. One definite trigger is lithium, which can unveil psoriasis in susceptible patients or aggravate existing psoriasis.[30] The time course between initiation of the causative agent and exacerbation or formation of the eruption varies between drugs, from less than 1 month to more than 3 months.[2]

Several investigators have confirmed that interferon alfa may either induce or worsen psoriasis.[31,32] The lesions were shown to improve on drug withdrawal and to recur on rechallenge. In patients with pre-existing psoriasis symptoms usually developed within the first month of interferon treatment, but in those with no previous history they developed after at least 2 months' treatment. Other interferons have also been implicated.[33,34] Terbinafine can also cause or exacerbate psoriasis.[35–37] The eruption tended to develop within 2 months after starting treatment and generally resolved on discontinuation of the drug.

The effect of chloroquine and hydroxychloroquine on psoriasis is variable: in some studies most patients treated noted no change in their condition,[38] whereas in others symptoms worsened in a large proportion of patients.[39] It is clear that psoriasis may worsen in some patients, and this may make choice of therapy difficult in some situations, such as malaria prophylaxis in a patient with psoriasis. Care should be taken with the use of hydroxychloroquine in patients with psoriatic arthropathy.

Over the past 20 years, skin eruptions have been described with numerous beta-blockers. Practolol was withdrawn worldwide following a serious syndrome termed the oculomucocutaneous syndrome, featuring a psoriasiform rash, xerophthalmia due to lachrymal gland fibrosis, otitis media, sclerosing peritonitis and a lupus-like syndrome.[40] The pathogenesis of this problem remains unknown, but it appears to have been unique to practolol. Psoriasiform eruptions have since been reported with several beta-blockers,[30] including ophthalmic preparations (e.g. timolol).[41] Cross-reactivity within the class has also been noted.

Beta-blockers may also transform psoriasis into pustular or erythrodermatous psoriasis. The time to onset of the reaction can vary from days to up to a year after initiation of therapy. The underlying mechanism is unknown, but it is notable that beta$_2$ receptors are present in the epidermis.

Drug-associated or -exacerbated psoriasis is typically resistant to treatment indicated for idiopathic psoriasis. The causative agent should ideally be stopped or the dose reduced. Most cases begin to improve within days without the need for specific treatment, and lesions have usually cleared within weeks. Topical treatments such as corticosteroids or calcipotriol may accelerate resolution.

Table 5.6 Drugs that may cause psoriasiform eruptions or exacerbate psoriasis

ACE inhibitors	Interferons
Beta-blockers	Lithium
Chloroquine and hydroxychloroquine	NSAIDs
Digoxin	Penicillamine
Gold	Terbinafine
Granulocyte colony-stimulating factor (G-CSF)	Tetracyclines
	TNF-alpha antagonists

TNF, tumour necrosis factor.

Purpura

Purpura describes small cutaneous extravasations of blood. It is an occasional feature of drug-induced skin eruptions, and in some cases it is the main characteristic. The main causes are thrombocytopenia or platelet dysfunction (drug-induced thrombocytopenia and platelet dysfunction are discussed in Chapter 12). However, a similar picture can be caused by damage to small blood vessels, either by immunological mechanisms or by changes in vascular permeability. Tests of haemostasis, including platelet function, are usually within normal limits. Drugs associated with non-thrombocytopenic purpura include aspirin, quinine, sulfonamides, atropine and penicillin.

Vasculitis

The term vasculitis refers to inflammation of the blood vessels. The vasculitides comprise a diverse group of conditions that may be manifest mainly as a systemic or cutaneous disorder; both types may be due to drug therapy.[42] Several drugs can induce both systemic vasculitis with cutaneous manifestations and cutaneous vasculitis without other organ involvement. About 10% of cases of acute cutaneous vasculitis are believed to be drug induced. The precise mechanism is unknown; however, it appears to be a type III hypersensitivity reaction with immune complex deposition in postcapillary blood vessels. Cutaneous vasculitis commonly presents with raised purpuric (purple) lesions on the legs, ranging in size from a pinpoint to several centimetres. Characteristically the margins are irregular or stellate. Other lesions include erythematous macules, haemorrhagic blisters and ulceration. Occasionally the buttocks, upper extremities, or even the trunk may be involved. Systemic symptoms, such as malaise, arthralgia and fever, are less common.

The most common type of cutaneous vasculitis is leukocytoclastic. Skin biopsy may be required for accurate diagnosis. The histopathological picture is characterised by necrosis of cutaneous blood vessel walls, neutrophil infiltration and haemorrhage.[2] Henoch–Schönlein purpura is a type of vasculitis which frequently involves the skin, joints, gastrointestinal system, kidneys, heart and central nervous system (CNS). It may be associated with aspirin, gold, penicillins or quinidine. Other types of vasculitis that may be drug induced include polyarteritis nodosa-like vasculitis, pustular hypersensitivity vasculitis and pigmented purpuric dermatoses.

Vasculitic lesions typically develop within several weeks of the initiation of the causative drug. The skin lesions may persist for up to 4 weeks or longer, and in some cases become yellow-brown upon healing. It is often difficult to identify the cause of cutaneous vasculitis; infection, malignancy and connective tissue disease need to be excluded. Drug therapy should be stopped at the first suspicion and the condition usually subsides thereafter.[43] Systemic corticosteroids and immunosuppressants may be of some benefit in severe cases.

Propylthiouracil is associated with a hypersensitivity syndrome that typically manifests as a vasculitis involving one or more organ systems.[44] In some cases the clinical features may be limited almost entirely to the skin, although joint involvement has frequently been noted. The time to onset of the reaction varies between 1 week and several years. Most affected patients recover quickly when the drug is withdrawn, but some require prolonged treatment with high-dose corticosteroids and immunosuppressants. Some drugs frequently implicated in cutaneous vasculitis are shown in Table 5.7.

Table 5.7 Some drugs that may cause cutaneous vasculitic reactions

Allopurinol	Hydralazine
Aspirin	Interferons
Beta-lactam antibiotics	Methotrexate
Carbamazepine	Minocycline
Carbimazole	NSAIDs
Co-trimoxazole	Penicillamine
Diltiazem	Propylthiouracil
Erythromycin	Retinoids
Furosemide	Sulfasalazine
Gold	Sulfonamides
Haemopoietic growth factors	Thiazides
(G-CSF and GM-CSF)	Thrombolytic agents

GM, granulocyte-macrophage.

Erythema multiforme, Stevens–Johnson syndrome and toxic epidermal necrolysis

Erythema multiforme (EM), Stevens–Johnson syndrome (SJS) and toxic epidermal necrolysis (TEN) are considered by many to represent variants within a continuous spectrum of disease.

EM can result from several underlying causes. Most cases are due to herpes virus infection, but up to 20% are drug-induced. As the name implies, it can present in a variety of patterns. Patients typically present with fever and a flu-like syndrome before developing the skin eruption. The classic pattern affects the hands, feet and limbs more than the trunk. There may be blisters, papular lesions or erythematous areas. A characteristic lesion is one of concentric rings, variously described as target, iris or bull's-eye shaped. Involvement of the mucosa is common, so the mouth, eyes and genitalia may be affected, when the condition is usually called SJS.

Infections are a more common cause of EM than drugs, and many cases have been wrongly blamed on drugs. EM may be due to vaccination, a variety of topical medications, and some environmental substances (e.g. nickel).[1,45] When the condition is suspected all medicines, especially those introduced within the past month, should be discontinued as there is a risk of progression to SJS or TEN. Table 5.8 lists some drugs that are commonly implicated in EM and SJS.

SJS comprises fever, malaise, myalgia, arthralgia, and extensive erythema multiforme of the trunk and face. It is frequently drug induced. There may be skin blistering and mucosal erosion covering up to 10% of the body surface area. This syndrome is distinct from TEN, but there is a degree of overlap as severe forms of SJS can evolve into TEN and several drugs can produce both entities.[46–48] The estimated

Table 5.8 Some drugs that may cause erythema multiforme or Stevens–Johnson syndrome

Barbiturates	Macrolides
Beta-lactam antibiotics	Mefloquine
Carbamazepine	NSAIDs
Chlorpropamide	Phenothiazines
Co-trimoxazole	Phenytoin
Gold	Rifampicin
Histamine H_2-antagonists	Sulfonamides
Lamotrigine	Tetracyclines
Leflunomide	Thiazides

incidence of SJS ranges between 1.2 and 6 per million population per year. In about 50% of cases the cause is not known. The fatality rate is believed to be about 5%.

A large number of drugs have been implicated as a cause of SJS. Penicillins, tetracyclines, sulfonamides and NSAIDs are among the most common. Patients with HIV infection seem to be at increased risk of developing SJS with co-trimoxazole.[49] Drugs that may be responsible for the reaction should be stopped immediately. Bachot and Roujeau[48] examined the impact of the date of drug withdrawal in a large series of patients with SJS or TEN, and noted that the mortality rate was lower in patients whose drug therapy was stopped early than in those who continued to use suspect drugs after the onset of blisters. Management involves systemic corticosteroids, fluid replacement and antibiotics, if required. Drug rechallenge is never justified.

Toxic epidermal necrolysis

Toxic epidermal necrolysis (TEN), or Lyell's syndrome, is a medical emergency. The disorder is characterised by widespread full-thickness epidermal necrosis with involvement of more than 30% of the body surface area. Commonly, there is severe involvement of the mucous membranes (oropharynx, eyes and genitalia). The estimated incidence ranges from 0.4 to 1.2 per million population per year.[46] It has a high associated mortality approaching 40%. The main cause in adults is drugs (Table 5.9). Patients with HIV infection, systemic lupus erythematosus and bone marrow transplant recipients seem to be predisposed to this disorder.[48,49] Elderly patients and those with extensive TEN have a worse prognosis. Drug-induced TEN is rare in children, in whom the diagnosis must be distinguished from staphylococcal 'scalded skin syndrome'.[46,50]

TEN presents with a prodromal period of nausea, vomiting, conjunctivitis, pharyngitis, sore throat, chest pain, myalgia and arthralgia.

Table 5.9 Some drugs that may cause toxic epidermal necrolysis

Allopurinol	Nitrofurantoin
Antituberculous drugs	NSAIDs (especially
Barbiturates	oxicam derivatives)
Carbamazepine	Penicillins
Gold	Phenytoin
Griseofulvin	Salicylates
Lamotrigine	Sulfonamides
Leflunomide	Tetracyclines

These symptoms may last up to 14 days. The acute phase consists of persistent fever and a burning or painful skin rash. The rash generally begins on the face or upper trunk and is characterised by poorly defined erythematous or dark-coloured macules, irregular target-like bullae, or diffuse ill-defined erythema. The affected skin may develop flaccid bullae or may detach irregularly, sometimes in large sheets. The lesions generally progress and extend in waves over a 3–4-day period, but can progress rapidly in a few hours. The conjunctivae are commonly affected 1–3 days before the appearance of skin lesions. Buccal, nasopharyngeal and pulmonary tract desquamation and erosion may be present. The oesophageal and perianal mucosae are affected less often. The consequences of such a massive loss of epidermis include dehydration, increased energy expenditure, and local or systemic infection such as septicaemia. In severe cases, other organ systems can be involved: hepatocellular damage, pneumonia, nephritis and myocardial damage may occur.

The mechanisms responsible for TEN are unknown, although a hypersensitivity–immunological basis is suspected.[6,48] Identification of the causative drug is often difficult. In general, most drugs causing TEN have been given in the previous 1–3 weeks. Drugs started less than 7 days or more than 2 months before the onset of the reaction are unlikely to be responsible. Phenytoin-induced TEN can occur at any time between 2 and 8 weeks after initiation of therapy, and may progress despite discontinuation of the drug.

There has been debate about where this serious condition should be managed. Most experts now agree that management in a specialist burns unit is preferred. Treatment involves the careful protection of exposed dermis and eroded mucosal surfaces, managing fluid and electrolyte balance, nutritional support, and close monitoring for evidence of infection. Fluid rehydration is essential because epidermal loss results in massive fluid shifts and dehydration. Antibiotic therapy should be given at the first sign of sepsis, rather than prophylactically. The place of systemic corticosteroids in the management of TEN is controversial. The best available data suggest that corticosteroids should be avoided in the most severe cases.[48] The benefits of short-term high doses of steroids prior to skin blistering have not been determined in prospective trials.[51] High doses of intravenous immunoglobulins have been used in small numbers of TEN patients, with apparent success,[48,52] but the potential benefits of this treatment require further evaluation. Immunosuppressive agents such as cyclophosphamide have also been given to some patients, with claimed benefits.

The antiepileptic lamotrigine causes serious skin reactions.[53] About 1:1000 adults treated develop these reactions, including SJS and TEN.

Children are at increased risk; the frequency of these problems may be as high as 1:300–1:100. Factors increasing the risk include the use of higher than recommended doses, rapid dose escalation, and concomitant use of valproate. Most of these problems have developed within 8 weeks of starting lamotrigine and resolved upon withdrawal, but deaths have occurred.[54,55]

Blistering drug eruptions

Idiopathic pemphigus and bullous pemphigoid are autoimmune disorders. Idiopathic pemphigus typically features superficial flaccid blisters, although sometimes erythema, crusting and scaling are the major clinical signs. Idiopathic bullous pemphigoid is characterised by large tense blisters developing on an erythematous base. The fluid within is often haemorrhagic. A number of drugs, most of which contain a thiol (or sulphydryl) group in their molecular structure, such as penicillamine or captopril, have been implicated in causing a disorder closely resembling these idiopathic conditions (Table 5.10).[56] Cicatricial pemphigoid is a rare variant in which mouth ulcers, eye problems and other complications may develop, with subsequent scarring. Linear IgA disease results from a deposition of IgA along the basement membrane zone. There are two somewhat different conditions, one affecting childhood and one adults. In the adult form the trunk is almost always affected but lesions can occur elsewhere.

Blistering drug eruptions consist of drug-induced pemphigus and pemphigoid, linear IgA bullous dermatosis and pseudoporphyria cutanea tarda.[2,6] The clinical presentation may comprise widely scattered large, firm bullae, classical but with fewer lesions, scarring plaques, an erythema multiforme-like picture or a pemphigus-like picture. About half of all cases

Table 5.10 Some causes of blistering drug eruptions

Type of eruption	Causative drugs
Pemphigus	Captopril, cephalosporins, penicillin, penicillamine, piroxicam, gold/sodium aurothiomalate
Bullous pemphigoid	Furosemide, ACE inhibitors (captopril, enalapril), penicillin, penicillamine, chloroquine, sulfasalazine
IgA bullous dermatosis	Captopril, ceftriaxone, co-trimoxazole, furosemide, G-CSF, interleukin-2, lithium, NSAIDs, penicillin, rifampicin, vancomycin
Pseudoporphyria cutanea tarda	NSAIDs, tetracycline, thiazides, furosemide

have oral involvement. In general, affected patients are younger than those with idiopathic disease. The mechanism is unknown; the presence of autoantibodies similar to those occurring in idiopathic pemphigus has been demonstrated.

The entire clinical spectrum of pemphigus has been reported in association with penicillamine. As many as 7% of patients taking it for more than 6 months develop a blistering eruption. This is thought to be a cutaneous manifestation of the autoimmunogenic properties of the drug. The condition usually improves when penicillamine is stopped, but may persist for many years.

Treatment for all forms of drug-induced blistering eruptions starts with discontinuation of the causative agent. This leads to resolution or improvement in most cases. Many patients benefit from oral corticosteroids until signs of active disease remit, often many weeks later. Immuno-suppressants are required rarely. In a minority of patients the lesions persist, or new lesions develop after stopping the causative drug. These patients should be given conventional treatment for idiopathic pemphigus.

Photosensitivity

Photosensitivity denotes a reaction occurring when a photosensitising agent in or on the skin reacts to normally harmless doses of ultraviolet or visible light. It may be due to topical or systemic drugs (Table 5.11). Up to 8% of cutaneous drug reactions are photosensitivity eruptions.

Table 5.11 Some drugs associated with photosensitivity reactions

Frequent	Less frequent
Amiodarone	Antidepressants (tricylic, MAOIs)
NSAIDs	Antifungals
Phenothiazines (particularly chlorpromazine)	Antimalarials
Retinoids	Benzodiazepines
Sulfonamides	Beta-blockers
Tetracyclines (particularly demeclocycline)	Carbamazepine
Thiazides	Griseofulvin
	Oral contraceptives
	Quinine
	Quinolones
	Retinoids
	St John's Wort
	Sulphonylureas

MAOI's, monoamine oxidase inhibitors.

Drug-induced photosensitivity is classified as either phototoxic or photoallergic.[57] Some drugs may induce photosensitivity by precipitating porphyria (e.g. hepatic damage from oral contraceptives) or lupus erythematosus (e.g. hydralazine). Patients who report photosensitivity should be questioned about the medications they are taking and the products they are applying to the skin. Sunscreens, fragrances, and occasionally soaps may cause photoallergic reactions. Phototoxic and photoallergic reactions occur in sun-exposed areas of skin, including the face, neck, hands and forearms. A widespread eruption suggests exposure to a systemic photosensitising agent, whereas a localised eruption indicates a reaction to a locally applied topical photosensitiser.

Phototoxic reactions are common and can be produced in most individuals given a high-enough dose of drug and sufficient light exposure. The eruption is usually evident within 5–20 hours of exposure, and resembles exaggerated sunburn with erythema, oedema, blistering, weeping and desquamation. The rash is confined to areas exposed to light. Hyperpigmentation may remain after other features have subsided. Patients taking potent photosensitising agents on a long-term basis should be warned of the problem and counselled on the need to avoid direct sunlight, to wear protective clothing and to use sunblocks.[57,58] In most cases of phototoxic drug eruption it is not necessary to stop the medication provided protection from the sun is possible. Several antibiotic classes are associated with photosensitive reactions, including the sulfonamides, tetracyclines and quinolones.[59]

Amiodarone is associated with a 30–50% incidence of photosensitivity. Symptoms develop within 2 hours of sun exposure, as a burning sensation followed by erythema. A small number of affected patients develop slate-grey pigmentation on light-exposed areas. Light sensitivity may persist for up to 4 months after the drug is stopped. Cutaneous pigmentation slowly fades after amiodarone is stopped, but may persist for months to years. The problem is related to both the dosage and the duration of drug therapy. Skin cells and cells of other organs in affected patients have been found to contain myelin-like lysosomal structures and membrane-bound granules. This generalised derangement of lysosomal storage may be the basis for other adverse effects of amiodarone, such as interstitial alveolitis, acute hepatitis and disturbed thyroid function.[60,61]

Chlorpromazine may cause a phototoxic response when given in high doses. The reaction is characterised by a burning, painful erythema within minutes of exposure to sunlight, either directly or through windowpanes. Erythema may persist for more than 24 hours. Occasionally, a golden-brown or slate-grey pigmentation, predominantly of exposed sites, may be seen. Photoallergy is less common than phototoxicity and may occur after exposure to chlorpromazine powder.[57]

Photoallergic drug reactions occur when ultraviolet energy causes the drug to bind as a hapten to protein on epidermal cells, creating an antigen that sensitises nearby lymphocytes.[6] It occurs in predisposed individuals who have been previously sensitised. After cessation of the drug, the reaction develops after re-exposure. These are delayed-type hypersensitivity reactions and their onset is often delayed by as long as 24–72 hours after exposure to the drug and light. Unlike phototoxic reactions, the reaction may spread beyond irradiated areas. The reaction usually manifests as a pruritic eczematous eruption. Erythema and vesiculation are present in the acute phase. The incidence of photoallergic reactions is less than that of phototoxic reactions. Most systemic drugs causing photoallergy also cause phototoxicity. These reactions may occur as a result of local photocontact dermatitis to a topical photoallergen, or of systemic drug therapy. Medications suspected of causing photoallergic drug reactions should be discontinued, as even minimal amounts of further sun exposure can lead to reactions of increasing severity.

Lichenoid drug eruptions

Lichenoid drug eruptions (LDE) are so called because of their resemblance to idiopathic lichen planus. The first drugs reported to cause lichenoid skin reactions were arsenicals used in the treatment of syphilis. Several causative drugs are now known (Table 5.12), although LDE are quite rare in comparison with other drug-induced skin reactions. The lesions can be described as small, shiny, purplish polygonal papules, sometimes with a network of white lines known as Wickham's striae. They are usually itchy, but can be asymptomatic. The surrounding skin

Table 5.12 Some drugs that may cause lichenoid eruptions

ACE inhibitors	Interferon alfa
Antihistamines	Lithium
Antimalarials	Methyldopa
Beta-blockers	NSAIDs
Captopril	Penicillamine
Carbamazepine	Phenothiazines
Furosemide	Phenytoin
Gold	Proton pump inhibitors
Hydroxycarbamide	Sulphonylureas

is completely normal. LDE can rarely affect the buccal mucosa; a characteristic white lace pattern may be present.[62] Idiopathic lichen planus has a predilection for the flexor aspects of the forearms and legs, whereas a lichenoid drug eruption typically has a more symmetric involvement of the trunk and extremities.[2,6]

LDE tend to be extensive and may be linked with, or develop into, an exfoliative dermatitis. LDE can also result from contact dermatitis in photographic workers who handle certain p-phenylenediamines.[63] The clinical course of LDE has been investigated in many studies. The mechanism is thought to have an immunological basis. The time to onset of the reaction ranges from weeks to months after initiation of therapy. In most patients the symptoms cleared spontaneously within weeks to months of drug withdrawal. Postinflammatory hyperpigmentation can be significant and prolonged. In prolonged or severe cases, topical or systemic corticosteroids may be used.[63]

Pigmentary disorders

Many skin diseases are followed by changes in skin colour. In particular, after lichenoid eruptions and fixed drug eruptions there may be residual pigmentation. Drug-induced alteration in skin colour may result from increased (or more rarely decreased) melanin synthesis, increased lipofuscin synthesis, or cutaneous deposition of drug-related material (Table 5.13). Sometimes the exact nature of the pigment is unknown. The pigmentation may be widespread or localized, and pigment deposits occasionally occur in internal organs.

A brown patchy pigmentation on light-exposed areas may be a result of prolonged administration of phenytoin. It occurs in about 10% of patients, and women are more likely to be affected. The pigmentation is similar to chloasma, affecting mainly the face, neck and arms.

Pigmentary changes develop in about 25% of patients receiving antimalarials for more than 3 or 4 months. The shins and pretibial area are

Table 5.13 Some drugs that may cause pigmentation

Amiodarone (slate grey)	Imatinib
Chloroquine (blue-grey or brown)	Mepacrine (yellow)
Chlorpromazine (blue-grey)	Minocycline
Cytotoxic agents	Oral contraceptives (brown)
Gold (blue-grey)	Phenytoin (brown)
Hydroxychloroquine	

most commonly affected. Irregular patches from grey to blue-black in colour are seen. Patients who develop this pigmentation should undergo an eye examination, as corneal depositions and retinal damage frequently coexist. Antimalarials should preferably be discontinued in affected patients, as the retinal damage is irreversible.

Hyperpigmentation has been described after long-term use of minocycline and imipramine,[64] and more recently with the use of imatinib.[65-67]

Alopecia

Many drugs have been reported to cause hair loss (Table 5.14). The human scalp has about 100 000 hairs, 100 of which are shed daily. Human hair follicles undergo three cyclical stages: the actively growing phase of anagen, which lasts about 3 years and features 80–90% of the scalp's follicles; the brief involutionary phase of catagen; and the resting phase of telogen, which lasts about 3 months. The telogen phase culminates in the shedding of the hair shaft and at the same time new growth in the hair follicle begins.[68-70] Hair follicles produce two types of hair according to the area of the body. Vellus hair is soft and colourless, covering the body surface apart from palms and soles. Terminal hair is the large, coarse, pigmented hair that occurs on the scalp, eyebrows, axillae etc.

Drugs that induce hair loss may be classified according to the phase of the hair follicle cycle that is affected. In anagen effluvium, drugs induce an abrupt cessation of active anagen growth and the hairs are shed within days or weeks, with tapered and broken roots. Anagen hair loss is an expected pharmacological effect of cytotoxic chemotherapy and is often dose related. The hair loss is almost always reversible, but a delay of several weeks is common before regrowth begins. Alopecia is associated with alkylating agents such as cyclophosphamide, cytotoxic antibiotics such as

Table 5.14 Some drugs that may cause alopecia

Amfetamines	Interferons
Anticoagulants (warfarin, heparin, heparinoids)	Leflunomide
Antidepressants	Lithium
Antithyroid drugs	Oral contraceptives
Beta-blockers	Phenytoin
Carbamazepine	Retinoids
Cimetidine	Tamoxifen
Cytotoxic agents	Valproate
Hypolipidaemics	

bleomycin, vinca alkaloids, and platinum compounds. Scalp hypothermia may be useful to partially prevent hair loss in patients undergoing chemotherapy.

Telogen hair loss may be a consequence of drug therapy or events such as severe illness, and it can be difficult to establish the cause. It features a conversion in the hair root from the anagen phase to the telogen phase. Drug-induced telogen effluvium usually becomes evident 2–4 months after the treatment is started. Alopecia may or may not be noticeable, depending on the proportion of follicles involved. Hair loss is usually confined to the scalp, although the eyebrows, axillary and pubic regions may be affected. Spontaneous regrowth of hair at the follicle usually occurs within 2–5 months after the causative drug is discontinued. It can be very difficult to establish whether or not a particular drug is the cause of the hair loss. Alopecia is a well recognised sign of hypothyroidism and can occur when the disorder is drug induced (see Chapter 9).

Idiopathic androgenic alopecia (male pattern baldness) presents in several ways but often as a bitemporal recession of the hairline. In women, a diffuse thinning over the top of the scalp with preservation of the anterior hairline occurs. Drugs with androgenic activity may cause this problem, such as danazol, metyrapone and anabolic steroids. It can also occur with the oestrogen receptor antagonist tamoxifen.

Hair gain

There are two patterns of unwanted increase in hair growth, both of which may be associated with drug administration. Hirsutism is an excessive growth of coarse hair with masculine characteristics in a female. This is a consequence of androgenic stimulation of hormone-sensitive hair follicles. Drugs commonly responsible include testosterone, danazol, corticotropin, anabolic steroids and glucocorticoids. Patients with drug-induced hirsutism may also present with other dermatological signs of virilisation, such as acne.

Hypertrichosis is the growth of terminal and/or vellus hair on areas of the body where the hair is usually short, such as the forehead and cheeks. Table 5.15 shows some drugs that have been associated with the development of hypertrichosis. The problem is usually dose related and is reversible after drug withdrawal. Ciclosporin may produce hypertrichosis in 50% of transplant recipients, with the excess growth being most marked on the face and upper back. The problem is less frequent in conditions where lower doses of ciclosporin are used. Minoxidil causes

Table 5.15 Some drugs that may cause hypertrichosis

Androgens	Nifedipine
Ciclosporin	Penicillamine
Diazoxide	Phenytoin
Methoxsalen	Verapamil
Minoxidil	

Table 5.16 Some drugs that may cause nail disorders

Captopril	Lithium
Chloramphenicol	Methoxsalen
Chlorpromazine	Penicillamine
Cytotoxic agents	Phenytoin
Fluoroquinolones	Retinoids
Gold	Tetracyclines
	Thiazides

some degree of hypertrichosis in nearly all patients; this effect has led to its therapeutic use as a topical treatment for male pattern baldness.

Nail disorders

A large number of drugs of different classes can be responsible for the development of nail changes.[71,72] Such changes usually involve several or all of the nails, and appear within a few weeks of drug administration. Nail problems can be asymptomatic or associated with pain and impaired digital function. They are usually reversible on drug discontinuation. Nail abnormalities include Beau's lines (horizontal notches in the nail plate), brittle nails, onycholysis (separation of the nail plate from the nail bed), onychomadesis (separation of the nail plate from the matrix area, with progression to shedding) and paronychia (erythematous and tender nail folds). The nail can be considered to be homologous to hair and the same drugs frequently affect both tissues.[68] The pathogenesis of drug-induced nail abnormalities is not well understood, but most cases are thought to involve a toxic effect of the drug on the nail epithelia. Other potential factors may be drug deposition in the nail plate, leading to nail discoloration and impaired digital perfusion, causing necrosis of the nail apparatus or damage to the nailbed blood vessels. Some drugs that may cause nail disorders are shown in Table 5.16.

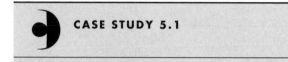

A 62-year-old man presented at the Accident and Emergency department with unilateral swelling of the face, lips, jaw line and cheek. About 24 hours ago he had noticed some swelling of his cheek, and since then it had gradually progressed and there was now massive swelling of his lips and face. He described having experienced several previous episodes of localised swelling of the face over the last 6–12 months. Medical history included hypertension and depression.

Current drug therapy:

- Enalapril   10 mg daily
- Bendroflumethiazide   2.5 mg daily
- Citalopram   20 mg daily

He had been taking all of these medicines for at least 5 years and had not taken any others recently.

What condition do the symptoms suggest?

The symptoms suggest angio-oedema, which is characterised by well demarcated non-pitting oedema commonly involving the face, lips, tongue, pharynx and neck. Occasionally the hands, feet, genitalia and mucous membranes of the gastrointestinal tract may be involved. In some instances it may cause respiratory distress due to laryngeal obstruction.

Which of the patient's medicines is most likely to be responsible?

Angio-oedema is a known adverse effect of ACE inhibitors, with an overall incidence of 0.1–0.5%.[23–25] Most patients develop the problem within the first week of treatment, but recent case reports indicate that delayed-onset angio-oedema, occurring after many years of treatment, is more common than was previously thought.[22] It has been suggested that the incidence may be as high as 1% for patients taking ACE inhibitors for more than 10 years. The precise mechanism for the reaction is unclear; increased bradykinin availability has been postulated, but other factors may be involved.[74] Predisposing factors for the development of angio-oedema include being of African origin, having a previous history of angio-oedema or complement C1 esterase inhibitor deficiency, and possibly poor compliance.

How should the problem be managed?

The management of acute angio-oedema depends on its severity at presentation. Any drug therapy suspected to be the cause should be discontinued immediately. Patients should be carefully examined for any evidence of respiratory compromise, such as stridor, dyspnoea, tongue swelling or

→

CASE STUDY 5.1 (continued)

dysphagia. Patients with respiratory symptoms should receive subcutaneous or intramuscular adrenaline (epinephrine) and the airway must be maintained. Antihistamines and corticosteroids should be given until upper airway swelling has resolved. The patient's blood pressure should be monitored, and once the acute problem has settled a drug from another class of antihypertensive should be prescribed. Angiotensin-II receptor antagonists appear to be much less likely to cause angio-oedema, although the problem has been reported and a minority of patients may develop the problem with drugs from either class.[22] All serious suspected reactions should be reported to the Committee for Safety of Medicines (CSM) on a yellow card, even if well recognised.

CASE STUDY 5.2

Ms B, a 34-year-old woman, presented to her GP with a painful pruritic rash on her arms, legs and neck. The rash had begun within a day or so of sun exposure and was not completely confined to sun-exposed areas. The affected skin was erythematous, with some blistering vesicles. Ms B had no recent use of any new skincare products or cosmetics. There was no significant medical history. Her only prescribed medication was the combined oral contraceptive pill, which she had been taking for the past 10 years. Ms B also reported taking ibuprofen when required for painful periods; she had been taking it over the last 48 hours.

What type of drug eruption do the symptoms suggest?

The symptoms suggest drug-induced photosensitivity. With phototoxic reactions the eruption is usually evident within 5–20 hours of exposure. It resembles exaggerated sunburn with erythema, oedema, blistering, weeping and desquamation. The rash is confined to areas exposed to light. Photoallergic reactions occur in individuals who have been previously sensitised. The reaction develops after re-exposure to the causative drug. The onset is often delayed by as long as 24–72 hours after exposure to the drug and light. There is a latent period during which sensitisation occurs, and the reaction generally develops within 24 hours of re-exposure. The skin beyond irradiated areas may be

→

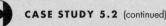

involved. This reaction usually manifests as a pruritic eczematous eruption, with erythema and vesiculation in the acute phase. Photoallergic reactions are less common than phototoxic reactions (see Table 5.11 for a list of drugs causing these reactions).

How should the patient be managed?

The features suggest a photoallergic reaction, so the suspect drug should be discontinued as even minimal amounts of further sun exposure can lead to reactions of increasing severity. In phototoxic drug eruptions it is not always necessary to stop the medication, provided protection from the sun is possible.

NSAIDs are a known cause of photosensitivity reactions. Oral contraceptives have also rarely been linked with photosensitivity,[73] but in this case ibuprofen seems a more likely cause. Photosensitive eruptions vary in severity. Mild cases may be managed with antihistamines and topical steroids. In severe cases hospital admission may be required. The GP advised Ms B to use paracetamol instead of ibuprofen as an analgesic in the meantime, and to continue her oral contraceptive. She prescribed a short course of cetirizine and hydrocortisone 1% cream. The patient was advised to use high-factor sunscreens regularly when outdoors.

One month later Ms B was referred to the dermatology clinic in the local hospital. She described a continued worsening skin rash despite somewhat irregular sunscreen use. She underwent patch and phototesting and completed a detailed questionnaire on photosensitisers. The questionnaire revealed that Ms B had been taking St John's Wort intermittently over the last 6 months for premenstrual mood swings.

Could St John's Wort be implicated as a cause of photosensitivity?

Photosensitivity has been associated with herbal medicines rarely; St John's Wort is the most commonly implicated herb.[75-77] Ms B had not mentioned its use to the GP, as she believed 'natural' products to be completely safe. Phototesting indicated that Ms B was markedly photosensitive in the UVA and UVB range. She was advised to stop taking St John's Wort. At follow-up 4 months later she reported no symptom recurrence. This case illustrates the importance of a complete medication history for the prompt identification and management of ADRs. The patient was unaware that complementary therapies could have significant side effects. Diagnosis was further complicated by concurrent use of two other medicines that can cause this type of skin eruption.

References

1. Breathnach SM, Hintner H. *Adverse Drug Reactions and the Skin.* Oxford: Blackwell Scientific, 1992.
2. Crowson AN, Brown TJ, Magro CM. Progress in the understanding of the pathology and pathogenesis of cutaneous drug eruptions. *Am J Clin Dermatol* 2003; 4: 407–428.
3. Wolkenstein P, Revuz J. Drug-induced severe skin reactions. *Drug Safety* 1995; 13: 56–68.
4. Bigby M. Rates of cutaneous reactions to drugs. *Arch Dermatol* 2001; 137: 765–770.
5. McKenna JK, Leiferman KM. Dermatologic drug reactions. *Immunol Allergy Clin North Am* 2004; 24: 399–423.
6. Pichler WJ. Immune mechanism of drug hypersensitivity. *Immunol Allergy Clin North Am* 2004; 24: 373–397.
7. Friedmann PS, Lee MS, Friedmann AC, *et al.* Mechanisms in cutaneous drug hypersensitivity reactions. *Clin Exp Allergy* 2003; 33: 861–872.
8. Park MA, Li JTC. Diagnosis and management of penicillin allergy. *Mayo Clin Proc* 2005; 80: 405–410.
9. Elias SS, Patel NM, Cheigh NH. Drug-induced skin reactions. In: DiPiro JT, Talbert RL, Yee GC, *et al.*, eds. *Pharmacotherapy: A Pathophysiologic Approach*, 5th edn. New York: McGraw-Hill, 2002: 1705–1716.
10. Nigen S, Knowles SR, Shear NH. Drug eruptions: approaching the diagnosis of drug-induced skin diseases. *J Drugs Dermatol* 2003; 3: 278–299.
11. Revuz J. New advances in severe adverse drug reactions. *Dermatol Clin* 2001; 19: 697–709.
12. Vervloet D, Durham S. ABC of allergies. Adverse reactions to drugs. *Br Med J* 1998; 316: 1511–1513.
13. Khoury L, Warrington R. The multiple drug allergy syndrome: a matched-control retrospective study in patients allergic to penicillin. *J Allergy Clin Immunol* 1996; 98: 462–464.
14. Jick H, Derby LE. Is co-trimoxazole safe? *Lancet* 1995; 345: 1118–1119.
15. DeLeo VA. Skin testing in systemic cutaneous drug reactions. *Lancet* 1998; 352: 1488–1490.
16. Mahboob A, Haroon TS. Drugs causing fixed eruptions: a study of 450 cases. *Int J Dermatol* 1998; 37: 833–888.
17. Savin JA. Current causes of fixed drug eruption in the UK. *Br J Dermatol* 2001; 145: 667–668.
18. Shipley D, Ormerod AD. Drug-induced urticaria. *Am J Clin Dermatol* 2001; 2: 151–158.
19. Grattan C, Powell S, Humphreys F. Management and diagnostic guidelines for urticaria and angioedema. *Br J Dermatol* 2001; 144: 708–714.
20. Resuscitation Council Project Team. *The Emergency Medical Treatment of Anaphylactic Reactions for First Medical Responders and for Community Nurses.* Resuscitation Council (UK) Revised January 2002 (originally published July 1999). http://www.resus.org.uk/pages/AtoZindx. Accessed 1/5/05
21. Howes L, Tran D. Can angiotensin receptor antagonists be used safely in patients with previous ACE inhibitor-induced angioedema? *Drug Safety* 2002; 25: 73–76.

22. Cicardi M, Zingale LC, Bergamischini L, *et al.* Angio-oedema associated with angiotensin-converting enzyme inhibitor use. *Arch Intern Med* 2004; 164: 910–913.
23. Vleeming W, van Amsterdam JGC, Stricker BHC, *et al.* ACE inhibitor-induced angioedema. *Drug Safety* 1998; 18: 171–188.
24. Sabroe RA, Black AK. Angiotensin-converting enzyme (ACE) inhibitors and angioedema. *Br J Dermatol* 1997; 136: 153–158.
25. Pylypchuk GB. ACE inhibitor- versus angiotensin II blocker-induced cough and angioedema. *Ann Pharmacother* 1998; 32: 1060–1066.
26. Rivera JO. Losartan-induced angioedema. *Ann Pharmacother* 1999; 33: 933–935.
27. Cha YJ, Pearson VE. Angio-oedema due to losartan. *Ann Pharmacother* 1999; 33: 936–938.
28. Sanchez-Borges M, Capriles-Hulett A, Caballero-Fonseca F. NSAID-induced urticaria and angioedema. A reappraisal of its clinical management. *Am J Clin Dermatol* 2002; 3: 599–607.
29. Chu TC. Acne and other facial eruptions. *Medicine* 1997; 25: 30–33.
30. Tsankov N, Kazandjieva J, Drenovska K. Drugs in exacerbation and provocation of psoriasis. *Clin Dermatol* 1998; 16: 333–351.
31. Wolfe JT, Singh A, Lessin SR, Jaworsky C, Rook AH. De novo development of psoriatic plaques in patients receiving interferon alfa for treatment of erythrodermic cutaneous T-cell lymphoma. *J Am Acad Dermatol* 1995; 32: 887–893.
32. Vial T, Descotes J. Drugs acting on the immune system. In: Dukes MNG, ed. *Meylers Side Effects of Drugs*, 13th edn. Amsterdam; Elsevier Science, 1996: Chapter 37.
33. Kowalzick L. Psoriasis flare caused by recombinant interferon beta injections. *J Am Acad Dermatol* 1997; 36: 501.
34. Webster G. Psoriasis flare caused by recombinant interferon beta injections. *J Am Acad Dermatol* 1997; 36: 501.
35. Gupta AK, Lynde CW, Lauzon GJ, *et al.* Cutaneous adverse effects associated with terbinafine therapy: 10 case reports and a review of the literature. *Br J Dermatol* 1998; 138: 529–532.
36. Wilson NJ, Evans S. Severe pustular psoriasis provoked by oral terbinafine. *Br J Dermatol* 1998; 139: 168.
37. Pauluzzi P, Boccucci N. Inverse psoriasis induced by terbinafine. *Acta Dermato-Venereol* 1999; 79: 389.
38. Katugampola G, Katugampola S. Chloroquine and psoriasis. *Int J Dermatol* 1990; 29: 153–154.
39. Kuflik EG. Effects of antimalarial drugs on psoriasis. *Cutis* 1980; 26: 153–158.
40. Wright P. Untoward effects associated with practolol administration: oculo-mucocutaneous syndrome. *Br Med J* 1975; 1: 595–598.
41. Puig L, Goni FJ, Roque AM, *et al.* Psoriasis induced by ophthalmic timolol preparations. *Am J Ophthalmol* 1989; 108: 455–456.
42. Jain KK. Drug-induced cutaneous vasculitis. *Adverse Drug React* 1993; 12: 263–276.
43. Mackel SE. Treatment of vasculitis. *Med Clin North Am* 1982; 66: 941–954.
44. Chastain MA, Russo GG, Boh EE, *et al.* Propylthiouracil hypersensitivity: Report of two patients with vasculitis and review of the literature. *J Am Acad Dermatol* 1999; 41: 757–764.

45. Smith AG. Important cutaneous adverse drug reactions. *Adv Drug React Bull* 1994; 167: 631–634.
46. Wolkenstein PE, Roujeau JC, Revuz J. Drug-induced toxic epidermal necrolysis. *Clin Dermatol* 1998; 16: 399–408.
47. Roujeau JC, Stern RS. Severe adverse cutaneous reactions to drugs. *N Engl J Med* 1994; 331: 1272–1285.
48. Bachot N, Roujeau JC. Physiopathology and treatment of severe drug eruptions. *Curr Opin Allergy Immunol* 2001; 1: 293–298.
49. Rotunda A, Hirsch R, Scheinfeld N, *et al*. Severe cutaneous reactions associated with the use of human immunodeficiency virus medications. *Acta Dermatol Venereol* 2003; 83: 1–9.
50. Becker DS. Toxic epidermal necrolysis. *Lancet* 1998; 351: 1417–1420.
51. Smoot EC. Treatment issues in the care of patients with toxic epidermal necrolysis. *Burns* 1999; 25: 439–442.
52. Roujeau JC. Treatment of severe drug eruptions. *J Dermatol* 1999; 26: 718–722.
53. Committee on Safety of Medicines. Lamotrigine (Lamictal). Increased risk of serious skin reactions in children. *Curr Probl Pharmacovigilance* 1997; 23: 8.
54. Messenheimer J, Mullens EL, Giorgi L, *et al*. Safety review of adult clinical trial experience with lamotrigine. *Drug Safety* 1998; 18: 281–296.
55. Schlienger RG, Shapiro LE, Shear NH. Lamotrigine-induced severe cutaneous adverse reactions. *Epilepsia* 1998; 39(Suppl 7): S22–S26.
56. Vassileva S. Drug-induced pemphigoid: bullous and cicatricial. *Clin Dermatol* 1998; 16: 379–387.
57. Ferguson J, Katsambas A. Photosensitivity disorders. *Medicine* 1997; 25: 34–36.
58. Allen JE. Drug-induced photosensitivity. *Clin Pharm* 1993; 12: 580–587.
59. Vassileva SG, Mateev G, Parish LC. Antimicrobial photosensitive reactions. *Arch Intern Med* 1998; 158: 1993–2000.
60. Chalmers RJ, Muston HL, Srinivas V, *et al*. High incidence of amiodarone-induced photosensitivity in North-West England. *Br Med J* 1982; 285: 341.
61. Zachary CB, Slater DN, Holt DW, *et al*. The pathogenesis of amiodarone-induced pigmentation and photosensitivity. *Br J Dermatol* 1984; 110: 451–456.
62. Highet AS. Lichen planus and lichenoid eruptions. *Medicine* 1997; 25: 75.
63. Ellgehausen P, Elsner P, Burg G. Drug-induced lichen planus. *Clin Dermatol* 1998; 16: 325–332.
64. Ming ME, Bhawan J, Stefanato CM, *et al*. Imipramine-induced hyperpigmentation: Four cases and a review of the literature. *J Am Acad Dermatol* 1999; 40: 159–166.
65. Tsao AS, Kantarjian H, Cortes J, *et al*. Imatinib causes hypopigmentation in the skin. *Cancer* 2003; 98: 2483–2487.
66. Tanvetyanon T, Nand S. Overcoming recurrent cutaneous reactions from imatinib using once-weekly dosing. *Ann Pharmacother* 2003; 37: 1818–1820.
67. Arora A, Kumar L, Sharma A, *et al*. Pigmentary changes in chronic myeloid leukaemia patients treated with imatinib mesylate. *Ann Oncol* 2004; 15: 358–359.
68. Smith AG. Drug-induced disorders of hair and nails. *Adv Drug React Bull* 1995; 173: 655–658.
69. Tosti A, Misciali C, Piraccini BM, *et al*. Drug-induced hair loss and hair growth. Incidence, management and avoidance. *Drug Safety* 1994; 10: 310–317.

70. Gautam M. Alopecia due to psychotropic medications. *Ann Pharmacother* 1999; 33: 631–637.
71. Piraccini BM, Tosti A. Drug-induced nail disorders. *Drug Safety* 1999; 21: 187–201.
72. Piraccini BM, Iorizzo M, Tosti A. Drug-induced nail abnormalities. *Am J Clin Dermatol* 2003; 4: 31–37.
73. Cooper SM, George S. Photosensitivity reaction associated with use of the combined oral contraceptive. *Br J Dermatol* 2001; 144: 641–642.
74. Dykewicz MS. Cough and angio-oedema from angiotensin-converting enzyme inhibitors: new insights into mechanisms and management. *Curr Opin Allergy Clin Immunol* 2004; 4: 267–270.
75. Schulz V. Incidence and clinical relevance of the interactions and side effects of hypericum preparations. *Phytomedicine* 2001; 8: 152–160.
76. Ernst E, Rand JI, Barnes J, *et al.* Adverse effects profile of the herbal antidepressant St Johns Wort. *Eur J Clin Pharmacol* 1998; 54: 589–594.
77. Lane-Brown MM. Photosensitivity associated with herbal preparations of St John's Wort (*Hypericum perforatum*). *Med J Aust* 2000; 172: 302.

Further reading

Becker DS. Toxic epidermal necrolysis. *Lancet* 1998; 351: 1417–1420.
Breathnach SM, Hintner H. *Adverse Drug Reactions and the Skin*. Oxford: Blackwell Scientific, 1992.
Crowson AN, Brown TJ, Magro CM. Progress in the understanding of the pathology and pathogenesis of cutaneous drug eruptions. *Am J Clin Dermatol* 2003; 4: 407–428.
Elias SS, Patel NM, Cheigh NH. Drug-induced skin reactions. In: DiPiro JT, Talbert RL, Yee GC, *et al.*, eds. *Pharmacotherapy: A Pathophysiologic Approach*, 5th edn. New York: McGraw-Hill, 2002: 1705–1716.
Ernst E. Adverse effects of herbal drugs in dermatology. *Br J Dermatol* 2000; 143: 923–929.
McKenna JK, Leiferman KM. Dermatologic drug reactions. *Immunol Allergy Clin North Am* 2004; 24: 399–423.
Smith AG. Important cutaneous adverse drug reactions. *Adv Drug React Bull* 1994; 167: 631–634.

6

Gastrointestinal disorders

Nicholas Bateman and Sheena Kerr

Introduction

Gastrointestinal (GI) disorders account for about 20% of documented adverse drug reactions (ADRs).[1,2] A study of hospital admissions related to ADRs indicated that death from GI bleeding was the commonest ADR-related fatality, accounting for 15 of 28 deaths recorded.[3] In this study GI bleeding was the most common single adverse event: for example, 157 (72%) of all adverse reactions associated with aspirin were of this type. The high frequency of reporting of suspected GI ADRs partly reflects the widespread use of aspirin and non-steroidal anti-inflammatory drugs (NSAIDs), whose gastrotoxic properties are renowned. These drugs can cause lesions anywhere in the GI tract, from oesophagus to colon. Most drugs can affect the gut in some patients, and the potential effects vary in severity from dyspepsia to life-threatening GI haemorrhage.

Many patients will experience GI complaints related to prescribed or over-the-counter (OTC) medicines; NSAIDs, in particular, are increasingly bought OTC. GI symptoms are an important cause of non-compliance. Healthcare professionals should be familiar with the medicines that frequently cause troublesome GI symptoms, especially where they may be a precursor of more serious toxicity.

The mouth

Taste disorders

Chemosensory nerves mediate the senses of taste and smell, and any changes to these senses are often interrelated.[4] Taste may be distorted (dysgeusia; e.g. sweet things taste sour), blunted (hypogeusia), lost completely (ageusia), or perverted (parageusia) e.g. a sense of foul or spoiled food instead of a normal sense of taste.[5] Taste disturbance may be a feature of acute or chronic disease, but many drugs can alter taste by mechanisms that are unclear. This can lead to non-compliance with medicines and occasionally weight loss through poor appetite.[6] Drug-induced taste disturbance usually occurs after taking the medicine concerned for prolonged periods, and often the patient is taking more than one medicine suspected of causing taste disturbances.

Patients with dysgeusia sense an excessively sweet, bitter, salty or metallic taste while eating. This may be as a result of infection, underlying disease or occupational toxic exposure, but is also the most common drug-induced taste disorder. Increased zinc loss has been accepted as a mechanism for causing dysgeusia. Drugs that contain a sulphydryl group, such as captopril and penicillamine, increase the chelation and elimination of zinc and copper, respectively. Both are associated with bitter or metallic dysgeusia. Captopril is considered to be the medicine most commonly associated with dysgeusia; about 2–4% of patients treated with captopril are affected.[7] Although this is believed to be due to the presence of the sulphydryl group, the problem has been reported with angiotensin-converting enzyme (ACE) inhibitors without a sulphydryl group, although the incidence is much less. Penicillamine is also reported to cause transient taste loss and dysgeusia, often in the first 6 weeks of treatment. Patients receiving treatment for rheumatoid disease are more likely to be affected than those with Wilson's disease.[8] Metallic taste has also been reported with gold compounds, metronidazole, metformin and zopiclone.[9] Patients taking acetazolamide have described it as making carbonated drinks taste bitter.[10]

Hypogeusia is a markedly increased threshold for a taste and is common in acutely ill patients as well as those recovering from prolonged illness. This problem has also been reported after general anaesthesia (as has ageusia). A blunting of the taste of sweet substances may be the result of drug-induced zinc deficiency, either through increased clearance of zinc or decreased systemic absorption. Treatment of a taste disturbance with zinc is ineffective unless a true zinc deficiency exists. Complete loss of taste (ageusia) from any cause is very rare. It has been reported with losartan, bleomycin, etidronate and clopidogrel.[11,12] Partial loss of taste may be the result of orofacial surgery or dental procedures.

Medicines commonly reported to cause taste disturbances are listed in Table 6.1. Taste disturbances may be managed by reducing the dose of the causative drug, switching to another medicine, or treating with a zinc supplement (if there is zinc deficiency).[4]

Gingival overgrowth

Gingival enlargement is characterised by an inflammatory overgrowth (hypertrophy) of the soft tissue between the teeth. The enlarged gingival

Table 6.1 Some drugs that can cause taste disturbance

Taste disturbance	Metallic taste
ACE inhibitors	Allopurinol
Acetazolamide	Amiodarone
Calcium channel blockers	Betalactam antibiotics
Clopidogrel	Gold compounds
Etidronate	Lithium
Griseofluvin	Metformin
Isotretinoin	Metronidazole
Levodopa	Penicillamine
Omeprazole	Tetracycline
Penicillamine	Zopiclone
Propylthiouracil	
Terbinafine	

Table 6.2 Some drugs that can cause gingival overgrowth

Barbiturates
Calcium channel blockers (e.g. nifedipine, amlodipine)
Carbamazepine
Ciclosporin
Phenytoin
Valproic acid

tissue develops a characteristic thickened and lobulated appearance. Associated symptoms include pain, tenderness or bleeding of the gums. Drug-induced gingival enlargement usually develops in susceptible individuals within 1–3 months of starting the causative medication. The problem tends to be more severe in areas where plaque accumulates. In some affected patients the gingival changes can be extensive, causing interference with speech, eating and tooth eruption. The underlying mechanism differs depending on the drug implicated.[13,14]

The medicines most commonly implicated are phenytoin, ciclosporin and dihydropyridine calcium channel blockers (Table 6.2). Phenytoin was the first medicine recognised to cause gingival overgrowth; the problem may occur to some degree in up to 50% of patients treated. Ciclosporin has been reported to cause the effect in between 13 and 85% of patients treated. With calcium channel blockers the reported incidence varies, from 3% with amlodipine to 38% with nifedipine.[15]

Table 6.3 Some drugs that can cause pigmentation in the mouth

Chloroquine	Minocycline
Chlorpromazine	Oral contraceptives
Hydroxychloroquine	Zidovudine

Drug-induced gingival overgrowth is difficult to manage. Mild cases may be improved by better oral hygiene together with professional cleaning of the teeth. Gingival enlargement that is a cosmetic or functional problem may require changes to the medication regimen, periodontal surgery to remove excess tissue, or a combination of the two. Patients on chronic therapy with phenytoin, ciclosporin or dihydropyridine calcium channel blockers should be counselled about the importance of good oral hygiene. A dentist's opinion may be helpful in patients with suspected drug-induced gingival changes.

Pigmentation

Abnormal pigmentation in the mouth has been associated with several medicines, including minocycline and some antimalarial agents (Table 6.3).[16,17] The mechanism for pigmentation changes may involve the accumulation of melatonin, iron or drug metabolite in the mucosa to discoloration of the bone.[11,17] The problem may be managed by stopping the causative drug or reducing the dose.

Dry mouth (xerostomia)

Xerostomia is a sensation of oral dryness. The secretion of saliva is regulated by the autonomic nervous system, with the parasympathetic system regulating the volume of secretion and the sympathomimetic system regulating salivary composition.[18] A loss or reduction in saliva secretion can interfere with speech, eating and swallowing food, can increase the risk of mucosal infections, may alter taste sensation, and can result in caries and periodontal disease.[19] Anticholinergic medicines with activity against M3 muscarinic receptors are a common cause of xerostomia. Other drugs implicated in this adverse effect are listed in Table 6.4.[20]

It is important to warn patients starting treatment with anticholinergic agents, tricyclic antidepressants and phenothiazines that they may

Table 6.4 Some drugs that may cause xerostomia

Bupropion	Anticholinergic drugs, including:
Didanosine	Tricyclic antidepressants
H$_2$ antagonists	Antihistamines
Lithium	Oxybutynin
Omeprazole	Tamsulosin
Opioids	Sympathomimetic drugs, including:
Phenothiazines	SSRIs
Protease inhibitors	Antihypertensives
	Tiotropium

SSRIs, selective serotonin reuptake inhibitors.

experience a dry mouth. Affected patients may obtain some relief by chewing sugar-free gum, using a sialogogue such as pilocarpine, or using mouthwashes to alleviate the oral discomfort. Artificial saliva products are available but most are only effective for short periods.[19]

Ptyalism

Excessive flow of saliva (ptyalism or sialorrhoea) may be caused by parasympathomimetic agents such as pilocarpine.[18] Other medicines that have been reported to cause sialorrhoea include clozapine and risperidone. Nocturnal sialorrhoea can be a particular problem, as in patients with impaired swallowing it may cause choking.

Stomatitis and mouth ulcers

Inflammation of the oral mucosa (stomatitis) and/or tongue (glossitis) is often painful and may lead to difficulty speaking, eating and swallowing, with negative effects on a patient's quality of life. Patients typically complain of tingling, burning or severe pain in the mouth. Contact stomatitis can occur when irritant or allergenic substances come into contact with the oral mucosa. It occurs within minutes to hours, and no previous exposure to the causative agent is required. Medicines causing irritant stomatitis include aspirin and vitamin C (Table 6.5).[21] Allergic contact stomatitis requires previous exposure to an allergen. On subsequent exposure to the allergen there is typically a delay of at least 48 hours before the onset of symptoms. Commonly used preservatives such as parabens and propylene glycol can cause allergic contact stomatitis.

Table 6.5 Some drugs that may cause irritant stomatitis

ACE inhibitors
Ascorbic acid
Aspirin
Pancreatic enzyme preparations
Potassium chloride

Table 6.6 Some drugs that may cause ulceration/stomatitis

Antimicrobials	Isoniazid
Aspirin	Leflunomide
Auranofin	Linezolid
Azathioprine	Losartan
Barbiturates	Methotrexate
Beta-blockers	Metronidazole
Carbimazole	Nicorandil
Ciclosporin	Nicotine lozenge and gum
Clarithromycin	NSAIDs
Didanosine	Olanzapine
Fluoxetine	Penicillamine
Foscarnet	Quinidine
Griseofluvin	Ritonavir
Indinavir	Sertraline
Interferons	Sulfonamides

Mouth ulcers (or aphthous ulcers) are most commonly caused by local trauma or stress. A wide range of medicines has been implicated in causing oral ulceration, but the underlying mechanism is often unclear. Cytotoxic chemotherapy is commonly associated with mouth ulcers, most likely as a result of accelerated detachment of oral epithelial cells. Many medicines alter the normal flora of the oral cavity or depress the patient's immune system, increasing susceptibility to oral infections. These infections usually present as painful erosions or ulcerations involving any part of the oral cavity.[22] Fixed drug eruption can manifest as mouth ulceration, particularly on repeated exposure to the causative agent. Drugs implicated include barbiturates, sulfonamides and tetracyclines (Table 6.6).[23]

Lichen planus is a papulosquamous disorder involving the skin and mucous membranes which can develop into erosions and ulcerations of the mouth. A number of drugs have been implicated in lichen planus-like eruptions, including NSAIDs and ACE inhibitors.[22]

The mucous membranes of the mouth are commonly involved in erythema multiforme, and in the severe form, Stevens–Johnson syndrome, massive mucous membrane ulceration can occur throughout the gut (see Chapter 5).

The oesophagus

Drug-induced oesophageal injury is a common cause of oesophageal complaints, including oesophageal ulceration, perforation, stricture and oesophagitis. Up to 20% of benign oesophageal strictures can be attributed to medication consumption. Oesophageal injury may present as mid-chest pain, heartburn, odynophagia (pain on swallowing), dysphagia (difficulty in swallowing), or a perception that food or a tablet is stuck in the throat.[24] Patients may report a sudden onset of burning and retrosternal chest pain aggravated by swallowing, which may lead to a total cessation of swallowing.[25] Occasionally the pain is severe enough to be misdiagnosed as angina or myocardial infarction. The diagnosis is confirmed by radiography or endoscopy.[26,27] Other conditions associated with the development of ulcers in the upper or mid oesophagus include reflux oesophagitis, Crohn's disease and herpes oesophagitis. Where there is a diagnosis of oesophageal ulceration it is important to consider drug therapy as the possible cause.

Patients with drug-induced oesophageal injury typically have a history of taking their medication with little or no water just before or while lying down. Most affected patients have no predisposing factors, but potential contributing factors include (1) the presence of gastro-oesophageal reflux disease and hiatus hernia, which tend to increase oesophageal transit time and decrease lower oesophageal sphincter pressure; (2) pre-existing oesophageal stricture or an enlarged left atrium, which increase the risk by impeding the passage of a bolus; and (3) alcohol, which may impair oesophageal function. Pharmaceutical risk factors include acidic formulations and agents with fast dissolution times that can result in high concentrations of the medication in the oesophagus. Gelatin capsules, which are 'stickier' than tablets, and sustained-release preparations, which tend to be relatively large, are more likely to become lodged in the oesophagus.

Tetracyclines are one of the drug classes most commonly reported to cause oesophageal ulceration, particularly doxycycline capsules. This may be due to either the capsule sticking to the oesophageal wall or to the fast dissolution of the capsule in the oesophagus, leading to a highly concentrated solution of the drug in a small limited area. Bisphosphonates, particularly alendronate, have been reported to cause oesophagitis and ulceration. Oesophageal ulceration due to alendronate has tended to be more severe than that caused by other medicines. Possible mechanisms for the mucosal damage include prolonged contact with oesophageal tissue, or alendronate that has reached the stomach refluxing back into the oesophagus. Alendronate should be used with caution in patients with upper GI problems, and in those taking NSAIDs or aspirin. There are occasional reports of potassium chloride, quinidine and NSAIDs causing oesophageal stricture, and potassium chloride and quinidine have rarely caused deep oesophageal ulceration complicated by haemorrhage, perforation or death. Table 6.7 shows some drugs that may cause oesophageal injury.

Patients taking medicines known to cause oesophageal injury should be counselled to take them while sitting or standing, with sufficient fluid (at least 100 mL) and not to lie down for at least 10–15 minutes afterwards. In the case of alendronate this should be increased to 30 minutes. Where drug-induced oesophageal injury has occurred, the offending medicine should be stopped and the damage will generally resolve within 3–4 days.[25] Analgesia may be required for the acute erosive stages of damage, and sucralfate may also help.

Dysphagia may be a feature of drug-induced parkinsonism or tardive dyskinesia. Antipsychotics, including both medium- to high-potency neuroleptics and atypical agents, can induce symptoms that mimic Parkinson's disease, including dysphagia. Long-term therapy with typical antipsychotics has been reported to cause tardive dyskinesia (see Chapter 15), which may consist of involuntary tongue, lip and jaw movements that can result in dysphagia.

Nausea and vomiting

Nausea is the unpleasant, painless subjective feeling that vomiting is imminent. Vomiting describes the preprogrammed series of motor and

Table 6.7 Some drugs that may cause oesophageal injury[28]

Alendronate	Penicillin
Ascorbic acid	Potassium chloride
Aspirin	Quinidine
Ciprofloxacin	Tetracyclines
Clindamycin	Theophylline
Ferrous sulphate	Zidovudine
NSAIDs	

autonomic responses that result in the forceful expulsion of gastric contents through the mouth. The causes of nausea and vomiting are numerous, including GI disorders such as gastroparesis or pancreatitis, central nervous system disorders such as migraine, endocrine or metabolic disorders such as uraemia, and other causes, such as myocardial infarction.[29] Although nausea and vomiting commonly co-present, they may occur independently.

Almost all medicines can induce nausea or vomiting; over half of the Summaries of Product Characteristics accessible on the electronic Medicines Compendium list nausea as an undesirable effect, and over a third list nausea and vomiting. The pathophysiology of nausea and vomiting is poorly understood, but most drugs are thought to cause the problem through effects on the chemoreceptor trigger zone (CTZ) or the vomiting centre. In practice, it is important to know which drugs frequently cause these symptoms (e.g. most cytotoxics, levodopa, opioids). With drugs that act on the CTZ, these symptoms will often resolve with continued use, although concurrent antiemetics may be required. If nausea and vomiting is severe, the causative drug may need to be stopped. In patients undergoing cancer chemotherapy severe nausea may result in the phenomenon of 'anticipatory vomiting' before subsequent treatment is administered. It is important to avoid this problem by giving appropriate antiemetic pretreatment with highly emetic regimens. For some drugs with a narrow therapeutic range (e.g. digoxin, theophylline), nausea and vomiting may be an indicator of toxicity in clinical use.

The incidence and severity of this problem can sometimes be minimised by delaying the rate of absorption, by advising that the medicine is taken with or after food, or by giving it together with an agent that delays gastric emptying. Some medicines cause nausea by direct gastric irritation (e.g. iron salts, potassium chloride). The mechanism by which antibiotics cause nausea is unclear, although macrolides (e.g. erythromycin) alter GI motility. Drugs that are a common cause of nausea and vomiting are shown in Table 6.8.

Table 6.8 Some drugs that commonly cause nausea and/or vomiting

Bromocriptine	Levodopa
Cytotoxics	Oestrogens (high-dose)
Digoxin	Opioids
Ergot alkaloids	Selective serotonin reuptake inhibitors
Erythromycin	Theophylline
Iron salts	

Stomach and duodenum

The stomach plays an important physiological role in controlling the rate at which food enters the small intestine. Drugs that alter gastric motility may cause a variety of symptoms, and be responsible for adverse drug reactions. Gastric emptying is delayed by opioids and anticholinergics, and increased by promotility agents such as metoclopramide. Drugs that delay gastric emptying may cause symptoms such as bloating, whereas an increased rate of gastric absorption may lead to acute adverse effects that are directly related to the plasma concentration, such as drowsiness with central nervous system (CNS) depressants. The most important upper GI adverse effect is peptic ulceration, most frequently due to NSAIDs.

NSAID gastrotoxicity

Non-steroidal anti-inflammatory drugs, including aspirin, are one of the most widely used classes of medicine in the world. In the UK, prescribers write millions of prescriptions for them each year, and they are widely available OTC. Their potential to damage the GI tract is their biggest disadvantage, and such damage is the most prevalent category of ADR. Aspirin-induced gastric bleeding was confirmed by gastroscopy in 1938, and cases of melaena and GI haemorrhage were first described in the 1950s.[30] NSAID-related GI side effects range in severity from asymptomatic mucosal damage revealed on endoscopy, symptoms such as abdominal pain, heartburn and dyspepsia, to serious GI complications such as bleeding or perforating ulcers requiring hospitalisation. All these adverse effects involve various degrees of damage to the gastric mucosa resulting from inhibition of prostaglandins, the primary site of action of NSAIDs. All NSAIDs inhibit the enzyme cyclooxygenase (COX) and so reduce the synthesis of prostaglandins.[31] Prostaglandins have a physiological role in protecting the gastric mucosa. Inhibition of prostaglandin synthesis and, to a lesser extent, topical irritant effects on the gastric epithelium are responsible for the gastrotoxicity of NSAIDs.[32] Attempts to improve the safety profile of NSAIDs have led to the introduction of a class of drugs that selectively target the COX-2 isoform, COX-2 inhibitors (see section on Pathophysiology, p. 168). All NSAIDs have been found to cause gastric toxicity. That this is due to a systemic rather than a local effect is borne out by the fact that severe GI toxicity occurs after parenteral or rectal as well as oral administration.[33] Selective COX-2 inhibitors are also associated with gastrotoxicity, although the risk is less than with conventional NSAIDs. Although NSAID use is primarily associated with upper

GI problems, such as bleeding, gastric ulcers and perforations, lower GI problems such as inflammation, haemorrhage, perforation and stricture formation have been reported and are discussed below.

Epidemiology

Estimates of the prevalence of NSAID-induced GI complications vary widely. In general, at least 10–20% of patients have dyspepsia while taking an NSAID, although the reported prevalence ranges from 5 to 50%. The overall prevalence of endoscopically confirmed gastric lesions arising during treatment is about 15–30%.[34] Within a 6-month treatment period 5–15% of patients with rheumatoid arthritis (RA) can be expected to discontinue NSAID therapy because of dyspepsia.[35]

In the USA, the Food and Drug Administration estimates that symptomatic GI ulcers, bleeding and perforation occur in about 2–5% of patients using NSAIDs for 1 year.

In the UK it is estimated that in excess of 40% of the more than 8500 episodes of ulcer bleeds in those over 60 years of age, and 40% of the 981 associated deaths, are causally related to NSAID use.[36] Studies have used odds ratios, relative risks and risk ratios to express the risk of NSAID-related events relative to that in a control population.[37–41] An odds ratio of 4.5 for peptic ulceration and bleeding due to NSAIDs and a risk ratio of 3.9 for hospitalisation have been reported.[40,41] In a meta-analysis of 40 studies published between 1975 and 1990, the overall odds ratio for serious NSAID-induced GI complications was 2.74 and the odds ratio for GI surgery was 7.75.[42]

Prospective data from the US Arthritis, Rheumatism and Aging Medical Information System (ARAMIS) indicate that 15 of every 1000 RA patients who take NSAIDs for 1 year have a serious GI complication. This equates to a relative risk of 5.49 compared to that in patients not taking NSAIDs. The corresponding figure for serious complications in osteoarthritis patients is 7.3 per 1000 patients per year (relative risk versus patients not taking NSAIDs = 2.51).[35]

The rate of serious GI complications requiring hospitalisation appears to be declining, presumably owing to increased awareness as a result of efforts to educate prescribers about the magnitude of the problem. The mortality rate among patients hospitalised for NSAID-induced upper GI bleeding in the 1980s was about 5–10%.[43] In a 2004 UK study of 18 820 hospital admissions, 15 of 28 deaths were attributed to serious GI toxicity due to aspirin or NSAIDs.[3] ARAMIS data suggest that the relative risk of death due to GI toxicity in RA patients taking NSAIDs is

4.21 times that in patients not using NSAIDs. Although the annual mortality rate (0.22%) in these patients may not seem high, the lifetime risk for patients with chronic arthritis is substantial. There are difficulties in estimating prevalence from morbidity data in specific patient groups because of the effects of co-prescribed gastroprotective agents.[44,45]

US data suggest that there are at least 107 000 hospital admissions each year due to serious GI complications of NSAIDs, with associated costs in excess of $1 billion.[35] The total number of deaths is believed to be similar to the number of deaths from HIV complications. Furthermore, these data do not take into account usage of OTC NSAIDs. The UK data indicate a similar health burden.[3]

Another cause for concern is the evidence that many regular NSAID users are unaware of or unconcerned about possible GI complications. In a survey of 4799 Americans, 807 had taken NSAIDs (prescribed or OTC) at least once in the past year for five or more consecutive days. About 45% of NSAID users reporting taking them for five or more consecutive days at least once a month, and 40% took both OTC and prescribed NSAIDs. Nearly 75% of regular users were either unaware of or unconcerned about possible GI complications. A large proportion of users indicated that they would expect warning signs before the development of a serious GI problem. This contrasts with the available evidence showing that only a minority of patients who develop such problems (<20%) report any antecedent dyspepsia.[46]

Pathophysiology

Gastroduodenal mucosal injury develops when the normal defensive properties of the mucosa are overwhelmed by the damaging effect of gastric acid. Inhibition of prostaglandin (PG) synthesis by NSAIDs leads to a decrease in epithelial mucus, bicarbonate secretion, mucosal blood flow, epithelial perforation and mucosal resistance to injury. The consequent impairment in mucosal resistance permits injury by a range of endogenous toxins, including acid, pepsin and bile salts, as well as exogenous factors such as NSAIDs. Topical injury caused by NSAIDs may contribute to the development of gastroduodenal mucosal injury, but systemic effects appear to have the predominant role. Thus the use of enteric-coated aspirin preparations, and parenteral or rectal administration of NSAIDs in order to prevent topical damage, has failed to prevent the development of ulcers.

The metabolism of arachidonic acid to prostaglandins is catalysed by the cyclooxygenase pathway. Two related but unique isoforms of

cyclooxygenase, designated cyclooxygenase 1 (COX-1) and cyclooxygenase 2 (COX-2) have been demonstrated.[47,48] The expression of COX-2
can be induced by inflammatory stimuli in many tissues, and the anti-
inflammatory properties of NSAIDs appear to be mediated through
COX-2 inhibition. COX-1 functions as a 'housekeeping' enzyme in most
tissues, including the gastric mucosa, the kidneys and the platelets. Adverse
effects such as gastrotoxicity and platelet dysfunction with conventional
NSAIDs occur via effects on COX-1. COX-2-selective NSAIDs were
developed in an attempt to obtain the beneficial anti-inflammatory effects
without GI toxicity.[48] Producing minimal inhibition of COX-1 function
at therapeutic doses, these agents were designed to exert anti-inflammatory
and analgesic effects without the gastrotoxicity or platelet dysfunction that
are characteristic of conventional NSAIDs. In a study comparing one
selective COX-2 inhibitor, lumiracoxib (400 mg daily), with naproxen
(50 mg twice daily) and high doses of ibuprofen (800 mg three times daily)
in patients with osteoarthritis not taking aspirin, the differential effects on
gastrotoxicity were to a large extent lost with low-dose aspirin coprescrip-
tion. These data suggest that the theoretical benefit of selective COX-2
inhibition is real in humans, but that aspirin in low dose can offset any
benefit.[49]

NSAID-induced GI damage can be categorised into three groups:

- Superficial damage, such as mucosal haemorrhages and erosions,
  which may cause symptoms but not ulcer formation;
- Endoscopically diagnosed non-symptomatic ('silent') ulcers;
- Symptomatic ulcers, including complications such as GI
  haemorrhage.

There are currently no definitive data that precisely correlate endoscopic
findings, often in clinical trials of NSAID safety, with resultant GI haemorrhage, perforation or obstruction. However, it appears likely that all
agents that increase the frequency of endoscopically defined ulcers will
impose an increased risk of GI haemorrhage. Available data suggest that
selective COX-2 inhibitors seem to be associated with reduced GI toxicity in patients not taking concomitant aspirin, but the risk–benefit
profile of these drugs requires further study.[50,51]

In the majority of patients, NSAID-induced gastroduodenal mucosal
injury is superficial and self-limiting. However, peptic ulceration does
develop in some patients and may lead to gastroduodenal haemorrhage,
perforation and death. The spectrum of NSAID-related gastroduodenal
injury includes subepithelial haemorrhage, erosion and ulceration that
are often referred to as NSAID gastropathy. No area of the stomach is

resistant to mucosal injury: the most frequent and severely affected site is the gastric antrum. Duodenal mucosal injury is less common than gastric damage, but the incidence of bleeding and perforation from the two sites is similar.[39]

Risk factors

Because serious GI events occur frequently in patients taking NSAIDs who have not experienced any warning symptoms, it is important to identify factors that increase the risk of serious GI complications and to consider how the risk can be reduced. Advanced age has been consistently found to be a primary risk factor; the risk increases linearly with age.[46,52] It was previously thought that the risk of problems was greatest early in the course of treatment, but a recent study suggests that the risk of GI haemorrhage remains constant over an extended period of observation.[53] *Helicobacter pylori* infection is an independent risk factor for peptic ulcer formation. This is confirmed by a meta-analysis showing an increased risk of bleeding with *H. pylori* infection of 1.79, but of 4.85 with NSAID use. When combined, the risk rose to 6.13. The authors therefore suggest synergy between these two factors, and suggest that ulcer disease is rare in *H. pylori*-negative non-NSAID users.[54]

In contrast, some drugs may protect from bleeding risk, and one study has suggested a decreased risk of bleeding (odds ratio 0.6) with both antisecretory therapy and *nitroso* vasodilators.[55] Recognised risk factors for NSAID-induced gastrotoxicity are shown in Table 6.9.

Relative safety

All conventional NSAIDs have been shown to cause the full spectrum of GI side effects, but there are differences between them with respect to the frequency of side effects, mucosal damage and serious GI complications. The rate of reporting of serious upper GI effects to the Committee on

Table 6.9 Risk factors for NSAID-induced ulcer

Age over 60 years	Hepatorenal dysfunction
Alcohol consumption (possible)	High NSAID dosage
Cigarette consumption (possible)	Previous history of GI problems
Concomitant corticosteroids	(e.g. peptic ulcer, GI bleeding)
Concomitant warfarin	Serious systemic disorder

Safety of Medicines (CSM) (corrected for annual reporting trends) was used in 1994 to group the implicated drugs in order of increasing frequency of their GI side effects.[56] Ibuprofen was associated with the lowest risk. Diclofenac, naproxen and indometacin all had a similar GI risk, greater than that of ibuprofen. Ketoprofen and piroxicam were associated with a greater risk. The rate was highest for azapropazone. This ranking is consistent with the findings of two large case–control studies and several epidemiological studies.[40,41] The Medicines and Healthcare products Regulatory Agency (MHRA) has subsequently re-evaluated its position and continues to believe this categorisation is correct.[57] It also stressed that COX-2 inhibitors should be contraindicated in patients with active peptic ulcer disease.

Aspirin causes significant GI toxicity even at the low doses used for cardiovascular prophylaxis.[3, 34] Patients should be prescribed the lowest effective dose (usually 75 mg daily) in order to reduce the incidence of GI complications.[58] There is no evidence that at these doses the risk of clinically significant GI bleeding is reduced by using enteric-coated or modified-release formulations.[59] The combination of a COX-2-selective NSAID with low-dose aspirin increases ulcer risk.

Treatment of NSAID-related dyspepsia

Symptoms associated with NSAIDs, such as dyspepsia or heartburn, are common and can generally be treated empirically with a histamine H_2-receptor antagonist (H2A) or a proton pump inhibitor. However, the risk of serious GI complications was found to be higher in RA patients with no GI symptoms who were taking antacids or H2As than in those taking no prophylaxis.[53] The reason for this finding is unknown, but it may be explained by the masking of dyspeptic symptoms associated with mucosal injury.

In general, if a gastroduodenal ulcer develops in a patient taking an NSAID the safest approach is to discontinue the NSAID and switch to a simple analgesic such as paracetamol. If treatment with the NSAID must be continued, a proton pump inhibitor should be prescribed concurrently, as these drugs have been shown to heal ulcers at the same rate, whether or not NSAID therapy is continued.

Prevention of GI complications

Because of the prevalence and severity of GI complications, recent efforts have been directed at the prevention of gastrotoxicity. A useful approach before prescribing an NSAID is to ascribe risk categories, as follows:[60]

- Low risk: no risk factors
- Moderate risk: one or two risk factors
- High risk: multiple risk factors or concomitant low-dose aspirin, steroids or anticoagulant
- Very high risk: history of complications.

An endoscopic study compared omeprazole and ranitidine in the prevention of recurrent gastroduodenal ulcers in a large number of patients with arthritis in whom NSAID therapy could not be discontinued.[61] After 6 months 16.3% of patients treated with ranitidine had gastric ulcers and 4.2% had duodenal ulcers. In the omeprazole group 5.2% of patients had gastric ulcers and 0.5% had duodenal ulcers. H2As are only effective in the prevention of NSAID-induced duodenal ulcers and are less effective than proton pump inhibitors, so their use cannot be recommended.

Misoprostol can be used for the prevention of NSAID-induced ulcers (gastric and duodenal) and has been shown to protect against clinically important complications.[62,63] It must be taken at least three times a day to provide adequate prophylaxis. In the MUCOSA study (Misoprostol Ulcer Complications Outcomes Safety Assessment) concomitant treatment with misoprostol achieved a 40% reduction in the overall rate of NSAID-induced complications compared with placebo. Patients at particular risk of complications who require continued NSAID administration may benefit from prophylaxis with misoprostol or a proton pump inhibitor. Misoprostol is teratogenic, and may cause diarrhoea.

NSAID-induced GI complications account for a considerable number of hospital admissions and deaths, and GI bleeding is the commonest adverse drug reaction associated with hospital admission in the UK. A significant number of these complications could be prevented if simple guidelines on NSAID use were followed, and millions of pounds saved.[3] Healthcare professionals have an important role in minimising the occurrence of these problems (Table 6.10).

Other drugs

Weil and colleagues[34] studied the risk of GI bleeding in a large cohort and found that concomitant anticoagulation, treatment of heart failure, oral corticosteroid use, and treatment for diabetes mellitus were all associated with increased risk, which was in turn further increased by

Table 6.10 Minimising the risk of non-steroidal anti-inflammatory drug (NSAID)-induced gastrotoxicity

- No more than one NSAID should be taken at any one time
- If an NSAID is indicated, one of the less toxic agents should be first choice
- The lowest effective dose should be used
- The maximum recommended dose should not be exceeded
- Patients at particular risk of GI complications (including those over 65 years old) should receive prophylaxis with misoprostol or a proton pump inhibitor
- Patients on long-term repeat prescription should be reviewed regularly to avoid unnecessary prolonged treatment, especially the elderly
- Patients should receive appropriate counselling. They should be advised not to take more than the recommended dose, and to consult their doctor immediately if they have any bloodstained vomit, black tarry stools or other signs of internal bleeding.

NSAID use. Taken together with smoking and a history of previous peptic ulcer disease, it was estimated that NSAID use accounted for 80% of all predisposing risk factors. In this analysis calcium channel antagonists were not associated with an increased risk of bleeding. Other studies also indicate calcium channel blockers are not generally associated with gastrotoxicity.[34,64–67]

Corticosteroids

There has been much debate about whether oral corticosteroids cause peptic ulcers. Several studies have suggested such a link, but most have weaknesses in their methodology. A large case–control study confirmed that patients taking steroids had twice the risk of developing a peptic ulcer, but this increased risk was confined to patients on concurrent NSAIDs.[68] It seems likely that corticosteroids do not increase the risk of haemorrhage *per se*, rather that they delay rates of healing of established ulcers.

Selective serotonin reuptake inhibitors

Published case reports and case–control studies have suggested an association between selective serotonin reuptake inhibitors (SSRIs) and bleeding disorders, ranging from ecchymoses, purpura, epistaxis and prolonged bleeding time to more serious conditions such as GI, genitourinary tract and intracranial bleeding. Release of serotonin by platelets plays an important role in haemostasis. Because platelets are not capable of synthesising serotonin, depletion of serotonin stores could induce haemorrhagic complications. A recently published cohort study examined the risk of upper GI bleeding with antidepressant medication.[69] The results suggested that SSRIs increase the risk of upper GI bleeding, and this effect is potentiated by concurrent use of NSAIDs or low-dose aspirin. An increased risk of upper GI bleeding could not be attributed to other types of antidepressant. Further study is needed, but in the meantime caution is essential in patients taking SSRIs together with other drugs known to affect platelet function, and in those with a history of bleeding disorders.

Clopidogrel

Clopidogrel is an antiplatelet drug that irreversibly inhibits adenosine diphosphate (ADP) receptor function. For the secondary prevention of thrombotic vascular events, in comparative studies with low-dose aspirin clopidogrel was marginally more effective and resulted in a moderately lower rate of GI bleeding. A recent study compared clopidogrel with aspirin plus proton pump inhibitor in 320 patients who had previously experienced aspirin-induced ulcer bleeding.[70] Over a 1-year follow-up period, the patients in the clopidogrel group had an increased rate of recurrent upper GI ulcer bleeding (8.6% vs 0.7%, $P = 0.001$). The findings indicate that the use of clopidogrel in patients with major GI intolerance of aspirin may be harmful, and that it should not be regarded as a safe alternative to aspirin.

Small intestine

Ulceration and perforation

The healthy small intestine, from the duodenum to the caecum, facilitates the absorption of nutrients, electrolytes and vitamins and acts as an effective barrier against the permeation of macromolecules, bacteria and luminal toxins.[71] Adverse effects of drugs on the small intestine are rarely considered in clinical practice, although the small bowel mucosa is often affected, as high drug concentrations occur there. This was most dramatically shown in 1983, when a novel osmotic-pump delivery system of indometacin (Osmosin) was withdrawn from the UK market because of reports of small bowel perforation and ulceration.[72]

Poor recognition of intestinal ADRs may be explained by the fact that there are often few symptoms of small intestinal disease until substantial damage has occurred. In addition, the small bowel is not readily accessible to clinical investigation.

NSAID enteropathy

NSAIDs damage the small intestine, causing small bowel inflammation (enteropathy), perforation, ulceration and stricture.[55,71,73–75] The overall incidence of NSAID-related injury to the GI tract distal to the duodenum is much less than that seen in the stomach and proximal duodenum. The prevalence of small intestinal inflammation in long-term NSAID users depends on the diagnostic technique used, and is 40–70%.[73] COX-2 inhibitors appear to have a lower incidence of this complication than do conventional NSAIDs. The vast majority of patients are asymptomatic. Clinical problems arise from the associated complications; these include blood loss of up to 10 mL/day; protein loss equivalent to 30–300 mL of serum per day; ulceration, and stricture formation. The strictures have a diaphragmatic appearance on endoscopy and may be multiple. They are thin (2–4 mm) and are due to submucosal fibrosis, without vascular change. Malabsorption of vitamin B_{12} and bile salts results in further nutritional problems. Problems, including blood and protein loss, may continue many months after treatment has been stopped. This condition is difficult to diagnose and is important to consider in patients with anaemia or malnutrition on NSAID therapy.

Other drug-induced ulceration of the small intestine, with risk of perforation, has also been described with slow-release potassium preparations, cocaine misuse (ischaemic disease due to vasospasm) and arsenic.

Paralytic ileus and pseudo-obstruction

Drug-induced intestinal obstruction or pseudo-intestinal obstruction are rare, but an important surgical differential diagnosis, as early recognition can prevent unnecessary surgical intervention.[76] The mechanisms by which this can occur include physical obstruction within the small bowel lumen (bezoars); bowel dysmotility due to drug effects on smooth muscle or autonomic nerve transmission; and obstruction from outside the gut wall as a result of vascular occlusion or peritoneal fibrosis.[76,77] Several patient groups may be at greater risk of these problems, such as those with a predisposing lesion (e.g. Crohn's disease, carcinoma) and patients with cystic fibrosis or autonomic neuropathy (diabetes). Neural control of the gut occurs via the sympathetic and parasympathetic nervous systems. Opioids, anticholinergics and calcium channel blockers are the most frequent drug groups involved, but secondary effects from electrolyte disturbance (e.g. hypokalaemia from diuretics) also need to be considered.

Atropine and related cholinergic muscarinic receptor antagonists, including tricyclic antidepressants, block parasympathetic transmission to the postganglionic muscarinic receptors. This results in reduced forward propulsion of intestinal contents. Phenothiazines also cause constipation and obstruction, and the problem can be made worse by anticholinergic drugs if they are required to treat the parkinsonian side effects of the antipsychotics. Clozapine has been reported to cause severe GI complications, including bowel obstruction, faecal impaction and paralytic ileus, and rarely death.[78–80] The mechanism is thought to relate to clozapine's anticholinergic effects and the risk is increased when it is given together with other anticholinergic medications. Patients with a history of colonic disease or previous bowel surgery may also be at greater risk.

Drug-induced neuropathy can also affect the nerve supply to the gut, producing a syndrome similar to paralytic ileus. This has been reported with vincristine. Table 6.11 shows some drugs that may cause intestinal obstruction and pseudo-obstruction.

The vascular supply of the bowel may be damaged in a number of ways. Mesenteric vein thrombosis has been associated with oral contraceptive use, but current low-dose formulations do not incur this risk.

Table 6.11 Some drugs that may cause intestinal obstruction and pseudo-obstruction

Acarbose	Opioids
Calcium channel blockers	Phenothiazines
Clozapine	Potassium salts
Colestyramine	Tricyclic antidepressants
Laxatives (bulk forming)	Vincristine
Loperamide	Vinorelbine

Other drug effects on the small bowel

Neomycin was previously used in the treatment of patients with hepatic encephalopathy to reduce bacterial colonisation of the intestine. In doses greater than 4 g daily it has a direct toxic effect on the enterocytes, causing villous atrophy resembling that seen in coeliac disease.[81] This results in reduced hydrolysis of disaccharidases and consequent carbohydrate malabsorption.

Colchicine is a notorious cause of nausea, vomiting, colicky abdominal pain and diarrhoea. The underlying mechanism is unclear, but appears to be local as symptoms are not seen after intravenous administration. These symptoms usually resolve within 24 hours of stopping the medicine.

Malabsorption

Malabsorption of medicines or nutrients can occur as a result of an interaction between these agents in the small bowel. The anion-exchange resins colestyramine and colestipol, and the faecal softener liquid paraffin, can interfere with the absorption of fat-soluble vitamins (A, D and K), calcium and other nutrients. Orlistat is an intestinal lipase inhibitor which has been shown to assist weight reduction by increasing faecal fat excretion. When fat excretion exceeds 20% of ingested fat, bulky, pale steatorrhoeic stools may become a problem. In addition, orlistat can interfere with the absorption of fat-soluble vitamins. Metformin can interfere with the absorption of vitamin B_{12} in a third of patients on long-term therapy, occasionally leading to megaloblastic anaemia.[82] Serum B_{12} levels should be checked annually in patients taking metformin. Cytotoxic medicines impair cell turnover in the small bowel lining and impair absorption. This is well documented, for example with high-dose methotrexate.[83]

Colon

Adverse drug reactions affecting colonic function are divided principally into (a) those affecting motility, and causing constipation or diarrhoea as an adverse effect, (b) those affecting the colonic contents, typically disturbing microflora, (c) those acting on the mucosa, causing colitis, and (d) those acting on the vascular supply to cause ischaemic colitis.

Diarrhoea

Diarrhoea is a common ADR that has been reported with many drugs.[84] Antimicrobials account for about 25% of drug-induced diarrhoea. The drugs most commonly implicated are shown in Table 6.12. The mechanism

Table 6.12 Some drugs that commonly cause diarrhoea

Acarbose	Laxatives
Antibiotics	Leflunomide
Biguanides	Magnesium-containing antacids
Bile salts	Misoprostol
Colchicine	Non-steroidal anti-inflammatory drugs
Cytotoxics (docetaxel, epirubicin, idarubicin, irinotecan, mitoxantrone)	(especially mefenamic acid) Olsalazine
Dipyridamole	Orlistat
Gold compounds	Ticlopidine
Iron preparations	

of these reactions is often multifactorial and sometimes remains unclear. Mechanisms involved include intraluminal osmotic change, increased secretion, impaired fluid absorption, motility change, overflow diarrhoea from constipation and colitis-induced diarrhoea. More than one of these mechanisms may be present simultaneously. In most cases of drug-induced diarrhoea there is no detectable organic lesion. Exceptions are antibiotic-associated pseudomembranous colitis and rare observations of enteropathy and colitis due to other drugs. Two main types of diarrhoea are seen: acute, which usually appears during the first few days of treatment, and chronic, lasting several weeks and which can appear a long time after the start of drug treatment. As the stomach's acidity is an important protective mechanism against enteropathogenic bacteria, treatment with proton pump inhibitors and H2A increase the risk of enteric infection.[85]

Antimicrobials

Diarrhoea occurs in up to 30% of individuals treated with antimicrobial agents.[85] Most cases can be classified into two categories: diarrhoea associated with *Clostridium difficile* infection, and cases in which no pathophysiological mechanism is identified. Most antimicrobial-induced diarrhoea is benign, appearing during the first few days of treatment and resolving after treatment stops. The cause is thought to be disruption of the normal intestinal microflora, which can lead to proliferation of pathogenic micro-organisms and impairment of the metabolic function of the microflora. Usually, changes in the composition of the gut microflora are of no clinical significance and the normal microflora is re-established shortly after antimicrobial treatment is complete. In some patients, however, modification of the microflora and the loss of normal colonisation resistance can lead to proliferation of opportunistic pathogens such as *C. difficile*, which is responsible for more than 20% of cases of antimicrobial-associated diarrhoea and almost all cases of pseudomembranous colitis. This organism can release specific toxins (A and B) which may cause mucosal damage and inflammation. Changes in the normal intestinal microflora can also lead to osmotic or secretory diarrhoea.

Pseudomembranous colitis

Pseudomembranous colitis is a rare but potentially severe complication of antimicrobial treatment and is characterised by the proliferation of *C. difficile* in the colon. Symptoms generally begin 5–10 days after the start of therapy, but both shorter and longer times to onset are possible. The acute colitis can be severe, with profuse watery diarrhoea (rarely with blood), abdominal pain, fever and bloating.[84,86] Endoscopy reveals raised plaques or membranes ('pseudomembranes') covering the colonic mucosa. The membranes consist of fragments of fibrin, leukocytes and epithelial cells. The diagnosis of *C. difficile* infection depends on the detection of its toxins in the stools. Outbreaks of *C. difficile* diarrhoea are common in hospitals and long-term care establishments.

   C. difficile-associated diarrhoea is more likely to occur with broad-spectrum antibiotics, such as amoxicillin, cephalosporins and clin-damycin, and those that achieve high concentrations in the intestinal lumen (e.g. agents that are poorly or incompletely absorbed or secreted into the bile) which lead to greater changes in gut commensals. For example, the third-generation cephalosporin ceftriaxone, which is mainly eliminated by biliary secretion, is associated with a 10–40% frequency of diarrhoea.[87]

   Other risk factors are the duration of antimicrobial therapy, multiple or repeated antibiotic regimens, severe underlying illness, advanced age, immunodeficiency, use of a nasogastric tube, intensive care and prolonged hospital stay. The dose of the antimicrobial and the route of administration are not risk factors, perhaps because doses used clinically are well above any threshold for affecting gut flora.

   C. difficile colitis may have a fatal outcome owing to both local complications (e.g. toxic megacolon, haemorrhage, perforation) and general complications (e.g. sepsis).

   Almost all antibiotics have been associated with pseudomembranous colitis. Antibiotic therapy should be stopped as soon as possible in a patient who develops severe diarrhoea. Patients with proven or suspected

C. *difficile* infection will require treatment with oral metronidazole or vancomycin. If an antimicrobial must be continued for the primary infection it should ideally be one that is less likely to cause C. *difficile* diarrhoea, such as a quinolone or a parenteral aminoglycoside. Because of the magnitude of the problem of antibiotic-associated colitis, care should be taken to ensure that an appropriate antibiotic is prescribed. Broad-spectrum antimicrobials should be reserved for severe infections.

Ischaemic colitis

Ischaemic colitis has been reported as a complication of treatment with various medicines. It commonly presents with sudden onset of severe abdominal pain, nausea, vomiting, diarrhoea and abdominal distension. Tachycardia, pyrexia, leukocytosis (raised white cell count) and bloody stools are often present. Other conditions associated with colonic ischaemia include atherosclerosis, arrhythmias, valvular heart disease and recent myocardial infarction. These increase the risk of drug-associated ischaemia. Examination of the colon may show erythematous, ulcerated, haemorrhagic mucosa. Medicines known to cause ischaemic colitis include ergotamine, oestrogens, amfetamines, digoxin and cocaine. Ergotamine, although now seldom used in migraine, can cause local ischaemia due to vasospasm.[88] Colitis has been described after oral administration and the suppositories can cause proctitis.

Ischaemic colitis has been reported in association with sumatriptan and with docetaxel and vinorelbine combination therapy.[89–91]

Other types of colitis

NSAIDs, particularly mefenamic acid, have been reported to cause or exacerbate colitis.[92,93] Loperamide, which controls diarrhoea by inhibiting GI peristalsis, has caused paralytic ileus that progressed to necrotising enterocolitis in both adults and children.[94–96] Thus, loperamide should not be used where ileus or abdominal distension are present, or in patients with acute pseudomembranous colitis associated with broad-spectrum antibiotics.

Gold compounds are known to cause diarrhoea. Occasionally, severe enterocolitis has also occurred, with rectal bleeding and vomiting, usually within the first 3 months of treatment. The colitis may remit once gold therapy is stopped, but septicaemia is a common complication.[97]

Table 6.13 Some drugs that may cause colitis

Amfetamines	Methysergide
Cocaine	Non-steroidal anti-inflammatory drugs
Digoxin	Oestrogens
Docetaxel	Salicylates
Ergotamine	Sulfasalazine
Gold compounds	Sumatriptan
Irinotecan	Vasopressin
Methotrexate	Vinorelbine
Methyldopa	

Proctocolitis was described in a patient taking isotretinoin; the symptoms resolved after medication withdrawal.

Severe colitis is a recognised complication of cancer chemotherapy and seems a particular problem with irinotecan, and during chemotherapy for colonic tumours.[98,99] Ulcerative colitis has been associated with simvastatin, and the rare condition of lymphocytic colitis with ticlopidine.[100,101] Some drugs that may cause colitis are shown in Table 6.13.

Other colonic adverse effects

Laxative abuse, possibly linked with an eating disorder, is a possible cause of chronic diarrhoea.[84,102] A rare complication is cathartic colon with severe diarrhoea and hypokalaemia. This has been linked with prolonged and surreptitious laxative consumption.

Gold therapy is associated with frequent diarrhoea in about 40–50% of patients, usually within the first 3 months of treatment.[97] The problem usually resolves on dosage reduction or with the use of antidiarrhoeal agents, but some patients may need to discontinue treatment. The laxative danthron is a mutagenic compound, and although the significance for human health is unclear its use is now limited to terminal illness as a precaution against bowel cancer promotion.[103]

Constipation

The fact that many medicines cause constipation is often overlooked. The drugs most frequently implicated include anticholinergic agents, opioids, iron salts and calcium antagonists, particularly verapamil. Common drug causes of constipation are shown in Table 6.14.

Table 6.14 Some drugs that commonly cause constipation

Anion exchange resins	Opioids
Anticholinergics	Peppermint oil
Antihistamines	Phenothiazines
Clozapine	Sucralfate
Diuretics	Tricyclic antidepressants
Iron preparations	Verapamil
Mebeverine	Vincristine
Monoamine oxidase inhibitors	

Pancreatitis

Pancreatitis is the acute or chronic inflammation of the pancreas due to autodigestion of pancreatic tissue by its own enzymes. Bile duct stones and alcohol abuse account for 80% of all cases of acute pancreatitis. Drug-induced pancreatitis is uncommon, as the cause of less than 2% of all cases.[104] Acute pancreatitis typically presents with sudden-onset upper abdominal pain and vomiting. Symptoms include tachycardia, fever, jaundice, and a rigid, tender abdomen. Serum amylase levels are normally over four times the upper limit of normal. There are no unique features that distinguish drug-induced pancreatitis from acute pancreatitis due to other causes.

The criteria that have been proposed to prove a drug was a cause of pancreatitis include:[105]

- Pancreatitis develops during treatment with the drug.
- Other likely causes of pancreatitis are not present.
- Pancreatitis resolves upon discontinuing the drug.
- Pancreatitis usually recurs upon readministration of the drug.

Given that pancreatitis is serious and may be fatal, the suspect medicine is only readministered if it is essential for the treatment of a serious illness.

The drugs associated with the highest incidence of acute pancreatitis are didanosine, sodium valproate, 5-aminosalicylates and oestrogens. Didanosine is reported to cause acute pancreatitis in between 3 and 23% of patients. This is associated with high dose and increased duration of therapy (i.e. longer than 10 weeks). The severity of AIDS and the concomitant use of pentamidine has also been associated with an increased incidence. Sodium-valproate-induced pancreatitis occurs in 50% of affected patients within the first 3 months of treatment and in 75% within the first year, but has not been reported to be related to dose. Sulfasalazine and other 5-aminosalicylates have been reported to cause pancreatitis.

Table 6.15 Some drugs that may cause pancreatitis

Didanosine	Sodium valproate
Furosemide and thiazide diuretics	Stibogluconate
Mesalazine	Sulfasalazine
Metronidazole	Sulfonamides
Oestrogens	Sulindac
Olsalazine	Tetracyclines
Pentamidine	

Positive crossover rechallenges have been seen between sulfasalazine and other 5-aminosalicylates and with use of rectal 5-aminosalicylate. Oestrogens appear to increase serum triglycerides in all patients. In patients with pre-existing hyperlipidaemia, severe hypertriglyceridaemia and pancreatitis can result.[104,106,107] Diuretics derived from thiazides, including furosemide, are also associated with an increased risk of pancreatitis.

Drugs implicated are listed in Table 6.15.

CASE STUDY 6.1

Mrs B is a 74-year-old woman with a history of coronary artery disease who has undergone coronary angioplasty and stenting. She is currently on clopidogrel, aspirin 75 mg daily, atorvastatin, isosorbide mononitrate, atenolol and diclofenac. The patient presents to the community pharmacist with indigestion, which has been a problem over the last few weeks.

What risk factors does this patient have for having a drug-induced gastric ADR?

This patient is currently taking two NSAIDs (aspirin and diclofenac) and is also on clopidogrel, all of which are known to cause gastrotoxicity. Her advanced age (>60 years) is an additional risk factor. Other possible risk factors to be clarified would include whether there is any history of previous GI problems, gastric or duodenal ulcer, concomitant corticosteroid use, smoking and alcohol use, and the presence of hepatorenal dysfunction.

What could be done to reduce the risk?

Ideally no more than one NSAID should be taken concurrently, and the combination of an NSAID with low-dose aspirin should only be used if absolutely

→

CASE STUDY 6.1 (continued)

necessary. If an elderly patient requires an analgesic for osteoarthritis then paracetamol should be used if possible. If an NSAID is considered essential, the use of a less gastrotoxic drug such as ibuprofen would be preferred. NSAIDs should be given at the lowest dose required to control the symptoms, together with a gastroprotectant such as misoprostol or a proton pump inhibitor. As Mrs B is taking both aspirin and clopidogrel, the use of any NSAID should be avoided.

Is indigestion likely to be a sign of gastrotoxicity?

Indigestion could be a symptom of gastro-oesophageal disease (e.g. reflux) or could be a sign of an ADR. Only 20% of patients who develop problems with NSAIDs report prior dyspepsia. If Mrs B reports having any blood-stained vomit or black tarry stools she should be referred to her doctor immediately.

What course of action should the community pharmacist take?

The community pharmacist should ensure that Mrs B has no signs of gastro-toxicity, such as black tarry stools or bloodstained vomit. Depending on the frequency and nature of the symptoms, and if the patient agrees, the pharmacist could contact her GP to discuss the issue. Alternatively, the pharmacist could advise the patient to make a routine appointment about the GI symptoms. There is an argument for advising the patient to stop taking the diclofenac as an interim measure. If antacids are purchased then the pharmacist should ensure Mrs B does not take them at the same time as her diclofenac, which is enteric coated.

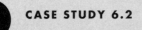

CASE STUDY 6.2

Mrs D is an 82-year-old woman with type 2 diabetes mellitus and osteoarthritis of the knees. Her regular medication consists of glipizide, metformin, diclofenac and omeprazole. She recently had a chest infection which was treated with a 7-day course of cefuroxime. Mrs D has now presented with watery diarrhoea.

→

CASE STUDY 6.2 (continued)

What would need to be eliminated as a cause of diarrhoea before considering her medicines?

It would be necessary to check for the presence of pathogens, ova and cysts, as well as checking for occult blood and considering the possibility of villous adenoma of the colon.

Which of her medicines could be a cause of the diarrhoea?

Diarrhoea has been reported as an ADR with all the medicines Mrs D is taking, although antimicrobials are the most commonly implicated. Diarrhoea normally starts during treatment but pseudomembranous colitis may occur during or after antimicrobial therapy. This would be diagnosed by the detection of *C. difficile* toxin in the stools.

NSAID-induced enteropathy may manifest as diarrhoea and can occur after more than 1 year's treatment. Diagnosis is difficult and is normally confirmed by the exclusion of other causes and endoscopy (strictures or small bowel obstruction may be seen).

Glipizide, metformin and omeprazole can all cause diarrhoea during treatment. If medication history reveals that diarrhoea started after the initiation of any new therapy this should alert the practitioner to the likely culprit. Use of omeprazole is known to increase the risk of bacterial food poisoning in younger patients (low gastric acidity is more common in the elderly but its relation to GI infection is less clear).

How should the *Clostridium difficile* diarrhoea be managed?

Patients with this condition require specific therapy for the infective organism, and appropriate management of fluid replacement. Isolation of such patients to prevent transmission to others is often indicated. Antibiotic treatment involves either metronidazole or vancomycin orally.

References

1. Smith CC, Bennett PM, Pearce HM, *et al*. Adverse drug reactions in a hospital general medical unit meriting notification to the Committee on Safety of Medicines. *Br J Clin Pharmacol* 1996; 42: 423–429.
2. Bates DW, Cullen DJ, Laird N, *et al*. Incidence of adverse drug events and potential adverse drug events. Implications for prevention. *JAMA* 1995; 274: 29–34.

3. Pirmohamed M, James S, Meakin S, *et al*. Adverse drug reactions as cause of admission to hospital: prospective analysis of 18 820 patients. *Br Med J* 2004; 329: 15–19.

4. Ackerman BH, Kasbekar N. Disturbances of taste and smell induced by drugs. *Pharmacotherapy* 1997; 17: 482–496.

5. Seymour RA. Oral and dental disorders. In: Davies DM, Ferner RE, de Glanville H, eds. *Davies's Textbook of Adverse Drug Reactions*, 5th edn. London: Chapman & Hall, 1999: Chapter 11.

6. Tomita H, Yoshikawa T. Drug-related taste disturbances. *Acta Otolaryngol* 2002; 546(Suppl): 116–121.

7. Alderman CP. Adverse effects of the angiotensin-converting enzyme inhibitors. *Ann Pharmacother* 1996; 30: 55–61.

8. Henkin RI. Drug-induced taste and smell disorders. Incidence, mechanisms, and management related primarily to treatment of sensory receptor dysfunction. *Drug Safety* 1994; 11: 318–377.

9. Galan D, Grymonpre R. Adverse oral effects of systemic drug use. *Can J Hosp Pharm* 1994; 47: 155–164.

10. Martinez-Mir I, Navano Badenes J, Palop Larrea V. Taste disturbance with acetazolamide. *Ann Pharmacother* 1997; 31: 373.

11. Adbollahi M, Radfar M. A review of drug-induced oral reactions. *J Contemp Dent Pract* 2002; 3: 10–31.

12. Golka K, Roth E, Huber J, *et al*. Reversible ageusia as an effect of clopidogrel treatment. *Lancet* 2000; 355: 465–466.

13. Taylor BA. Management of drug-induced gingival enlargement. *Aust Prescriber* 2003; 26: 11–13.

14. Brunet L, Miranda J, Farre M, *et al*. Gingival enlargement induced by drugs. *Drug Safety* 1996; 15: 219–231.

15. Meraw SJ, Sheridan PJ. Medically induced gingival hyperplasia. *Mayo Clin Proc* 1998; 73: 1196–1199.

16. Kleinegger CL, Hammond HL, Finkelstein MW. Oral mucosal hyperpigmentation secondary to antimalarial drug therapy. *Oral Surg Oral Med Oral Path Oral Radiol Endod* 2000; 90: 189–194.

17. Tanzi EL, Hecker MS. Minocycline-induced hyperpigmentation of the tongue. *Arch Dermatol* 2000; 136: 427–428.

18. Grisius MM. Salivary gland dysfunction: A review of systemic therapies. *Oral Surg Oral Med Oral Path Oral Radiol Endod* 2001; 92: 156–162.

19. Ettinger RL. Review: Xerostomia: A symptom which acts like a disease. *Age Aging* 1996; 25: 409–412.

20. Scully C. Drug effects on salivary glands: dry mouth. *Oral Dis* 2003; 9: 165–176.

21. LeSueur BW, Yiannias JA. Contact stomatitis. *Dermatol Clin* 2003; 21: 105–114.

22. Tack DA, Rogers III RS. Oral drug reactions. *Dermatol Ther* 2002; 15: 236–250.

23. Scully C, Gorsky M, Lozada-Nur F. Aphthous ulcerations. *Dermatol Ther* 2002; 15: 185–205.

24. Boyce HW. Jr. Drug-induced esophageal damage: diseases of medical progress. *Gastrointest Endosc* 1998; 47: 547–550.

25. O'Neill JL, Remington TL. Drug-induced esophageal injuries and dysphagia. *Ann Pharmacother* 2003; 37: 1675–1684.

26. Levine MS. Drug-induced disorders of the esophagus. *Abdom Imag* 1999; 24: 3–8.

27. Jaspersen D. Drug-induced oesophageal disorders. *Drug Safety* 2000; 22: 237–249.

28. Akhtar AJ. Oral medication-induced esophageal injury on elderly patients. *Am J Med Sci* 2003; 326: 133–135.

29. Hasler WL, Chey WD. Nausea and vomiting. *Gastroenterology* 2003; 125: 1860–1867.

30. Douthwaite AH, Lintott SAM. Gastroscopic observation of the effect of aspirin and certain other substances on the gut. *Lancet* 1938; 2: 1222–1225.

31. Vane JR. Inhibition of prostaglandin synthesis as a mechanism of action for aspirin-like drugs. *Nature* 1971; 231: 232–235.

32. Wallace JL. Nonsteroidal anti-inflammatory drugs and gastroenteropathy: the second hundred years. *Gastroenterology* 1997; 112: 1000–1016.

33. Anon. Rational use of NSAIDs for musculoskeletal disorders. *Drug Ther Bull* 1994; 32: 91–95.

34. Weil J, Langman MJS, Wainwright P, *et al*. Peptic ulcer bleeding: accessory risk factors and interactions with non-steroidal anti-inflammatory drugs. *Gut* 2000; 46: 27–31.

35. Singh G, Rosen Ramey DR. NSAID induced gastrointestinal complications: The ARAMIS Perspective – 1997. Arthritis, Rheumatism and Aging Medical Information System. *J Rheumatol* 1998; 25(Suppl 51): 8–16.

36. Langman MJ. Ulcer complications associated with anti-inflammatory drug use. What is the extent of the disease burden? *Pharmacoepidemiol Drug Safety* 2001; 10: 13–19.

37. Rees Willett L, Carson JL, Strom BL. Epidemiology of gastrointestinal damage associated with nonsteroidal anti-inflammatory drugs. *Drug Safety* 1994; 10: 170–181.

38. Tannenbaum H, Davis P, Russell AS, *et al*. An evidence-based approach to prescribing NSAIDs in musculoskeletal disease: a Canadian consensus. *Can Med Assoc J* 1996; 155: 77–88.

39. Langman MJS, Morgan L, Worrall A. Use of anti-inflammatory drugs by patients admitted with small or large bowel perforations and haemorrhage. *Br Med J* 1985; 290: 347–349.

40. Langman MJS, Weil J, Wainright P, *et al*. Risks of bleeding peptic ulcer associated with individual non-steroidal anti-inflammatory drugs. *Lancet* 1994; 343: 1075–1078.

41. Garcia Rodriguez LA, Jick H. Risk of upper gastrointestinal bleeding and perforation associated with individual non-steroidal anti-inflammatory drugs. *Lancet* 1994; 343: 769–772.

42. Gabriel SE, Jaakkimainen L, Bombardier C. Risk for serious gastrointestinal complications related to use of nonsteroidal anti-inflammatory drugs. A meta-analysis. *Ann Intern Med* 1991; 115: 787–796.

43. Armstrong CP, Blower AL. Non-steroidal anti-inflammatory drugs and life threatening complications of peptic ulceration. *Gut* 1987; 28: 527–532.

44. Steen KS, Lems WF, Aertsen J, *et al*. Incidence of clinically manifest ulcers and their complications in patients with rheumatoid arthritis. *Ann Rheum Dis* 2001; 60: 443–447.

45. Pilotto A, Franceschi M, Leandro G, *et al.* The risk of upper gastrointestinal bleeding in elderly users of aspirin and other non-steroidal anti-inflammatory drugs: the role of gastroprotective drugs. *Aging Clin Exp Res* 2003; 15: 494–499.
46. Wolfe MM, Lichtenstein DR, Singh G. Gastrointestinal toxicity of nonsteroidal anti-inflammatory drugs. *N Engl J Med* 1999; 340: 1888–1899.
47. Appleton I, Tomlinson A, Willoughby DA. Inducible cyclooxygenase (COX-2): a safer therapeutic target? *Br J Rheumatol* 1994; 33: 410–412.
48. Lipsky PE, Adamson SB, Crofford L, *et al.* The international Cox II study group. The classification of cyclooxygenase inhibitors. *J Rheumatol* 1998; 25: 2298–2303.
49. Schnitzer TJ, Burmester GR, Mysler E, *et al.* The TARGET study group. Comparison of lumiracoxib with naproxen and ibuprofen in the Therapeutic Arthritis Research and Gastrointestinal Event Trial (TARGET), reduction in ulcer complications: randomised controlled trial. *Lancet* 2004; 364: 639–640.
50. Langman MJ, Jensen DM, Watson DJ, *et al.* Adverse upper gastrointestinal effects of rofecoxib compared with NSAIDs. *JAMA* 1999; 282: 1929–1933.
51. Feldman M, McMahon AT. Do cyclooxygenase-2 inhibitors provide benefits similar to those of traditional nonsteroidal anti-inflammatory drugs, with less gastrointestinal toxicity? *Ann Intern Med* 2000; 132: 134–143.
52. Henry D, Dobson A, Turner C. Variability in the risk of major gastro-intestinal complications from nonaspirin non-steroidal anti-inflammatory drugs. *Gastroenterology* 1993; 105: 1078–1088.
53. Singh G, Triadafilopoulus G. Epidemiology of NSAID-induced GI complications. *J Rheumatol* 1999; 26(Suppl 26): 18–24.
54. Huang JQ, Sridhar S, Hunt RH. Role of *Helicobacter pylori* infection and non-steroidal anti-inflammatory drugs in peptic-ulcer disease: a meta-analysis. *Lancet* 2002; 359: 14–22.
55. Lanas A, Sekar MC, Hirschowitz BI. Objective evidence of aspirin use in both ulcer and nonulcer upper and lower gastrointestinal bleeding. *Gastroenterology* 1992; 103: 862–869.
56. Committee on Safety of Medicines. Relative safety of oral non-aspirin NSAIDs. *Curr Probl Pharmacovigilance* 1994; 20: 9–11.
57. Committee on Safety of Medicines. Non-steroidal anti-inflammatory drugs (NSAIDs) and gastrointestinal (GI) safety. *Curr Probl Pharmacovigilance* 2002; 28: 5.
58. Anon. Which prophylactic aspirin? *Drug Ther Bull* 1997; 35: 7–8.
59. Kelly JP, Kaufman DW, Jurgelon JM, *et al.* Risk of aspirin-associated major upper-gastrointestinal bleeding with enteric-coated or buffered product. *Lancet* 1996; 348: 1413–1416.
60. Chan FK, Graham DY. Review article: prevention of non-steroidal anti-inflammatory gastrointestinal complications – review and recommendations on risk assessment. *Aliment Pharmacol Ther* 2004; 19: 1051–1061.
61. Yeomans ND, Tulassay Z, Juhasz L, *et al.* A comparison of omeprazole with ranitidine for ulcers associated with nonsteroidal anti-inflammatory drugs. *N Engl J Med* 1998; 338: 719–726.
62. Silverstein FE, Graham DY, Senior JR, *et al.* Misoprostol reduces serious gastrointestinal complications in patients with rheumatoid arthritis receiving

nonsteroidal anti-inflammatory drugs: a randomized, double-blind, placebo-controlled trial. *Ann Intern Med* 1995; 123: 241–249.

63. Maiden N, Madhok R. Misoprostol in patients taking non-steroidal anti-inflammatory drugs. *Br Med J* 1995; 311: 1518–1519.

64. Desboeuf K, Lapeyre-Mestre M, Montastruc JL. Risk of gastrointestinal haemorrhage with calcium antagonists. *Br J Clin Pharmacol* 1998; 46: 87–89.

65. Kelly JP, L'aszio A, Kaufman DW, *et al*. Major upper gastrointestinal bleeding and the use of calcium channel blockers. *Lancet* 1999; 353: 559.

66. Smallery WE, Ray WA, Daugherty JR, *et al*. No association between calcium channel blocker use and confirmed bleeding peptic ulcer disease. *Am J Epidemiol* 1998; 148: 350–354.

67. Suissa S, Bourgault C, Barkun A, *et al*. Antihypertensive drugs and the risk of gastrointestinal bleeding. *Am J Med* 1998; 105: 230–235.

68. Piper JM, Ray WA, Daugherty JR, Griffin MR. Corticosteroid use and peptic ulcer disease: role of non-steroidal anti-inflammatory drugs. *Ann Intern Med* 1991; 114: 735–740.

69. Dalton SO, Johansen C, Mellemkjaer L, *et al*. Use of selective serotonin reuptake inhibitors and risk of upper gastrointestinal bleeding: a population based cohort study. *Arch Intern Med* 2003; 163: 59–64.

70. Chan FK, Ching JY, Hung LC, *et al*. Clopidogrel versus aspirin and esomeprazole to prevent recurrent ulcer bleeding. *N Engl J Med* 2005; 352: 238–244.

71. Tibble J, Smale S, Bjarnason I. Adverse effects of drugs on the small bowel. *Adv Drug React Bull* 1999; 198: 755–758.

72. Committee on Safety of Medicines. Osmosin (controlled release indomethacin). *Curr Probl* 1983; No 11.

73. Davies NM, Saleh JY, Skjodt NM. Detection and prevention of NSAID-induced enteropathy. *J Pharma Pharm Sci* 2000; 3: 137–155.

74. Lanza FL. A guideline for the treatment and prevention of NSAID-induced ulcers. *Am J Gastroenterol* 1998; 93: 2037–2046.

75. Bjorkman D. Nonsteroidal anti-inflammatory drug-associated toxicity of the liver, lower gastrointestinal tract, and esophagus. *Am J Med* 1998; 105: 17S–21S.

76. Iredale JP, George CF. Drugs causing gastrointestinal obstruction. *Adv Drug React Toxicol Rev* 1993; 12: 163–175.

77. Committee on Safety of Medicines. Bezoar formation with sucralfate (Antepsin). *Curr Probl Pharmacovigilance* 1999; 25: 1.

78. Schwartz BJ, Frisolone JA. A case report of clozapine-induced gastric outlet obstruction. *Am J Psychiatry* 1993; 150: 1563.

79. Erickson B. Clozapine-associated postoperative ileus: Case report and review of the literature. *Arch Gen Psychiatry* 1995; 52: 508–509.

80. Anon. Clozapine and gastrointestinal obstruction. *WHO Drug Inf* 1999; 13: 92.

81. Longstreth GF, Newcomer AD. Drug-induced malabsorption. *Mayo Clin Proc* 1975; 50: 284–293.

82. Adams JF, Clark JS, Ireland JT, *et al*. Malabsorption of vitamin B12 and intrinsic factor secretion during biguanide therapy. *Diabetologica* 1983; 24: 16–18.

83. Dagdemir A, Yildirim H, Aliyazicioglu Y, *et al*. Does vitamin A prevent high-dose-methotrexate-induced D-xylose malabsorption in children with cancer? *Support Care Cancer* 2004; 12: 263–267.

84. Chassany O, Michaux A, Bergmann JF. Drug-induced diarrhoea. *Drug Safety* 2000; 22: 53–72.

85. Bateman DN, Aziz, EE. Gastrointestinal disorders. In: Davies DM, Ferner RE, de Glanville H, eds. *Davies's Textbook of Adverse Drug Reactions*, 5th edn London: Chapman & Hall, 1991: 259–274.

86. Anon. Antibiotic-induced diarrhoea. *Drug Ther Bull* 1995; 33: 23–24.

87. Thompson JW, Jacobs RF. Adverse effects of newer cephalosporins. *Drug Safety* 1993; 9: 132–142.

88. Jost WH, Raulf F, Muller-Lobeck H. Anorectal ergotism: Induced by migraine therapy. *Acta Neurol Scand* 1991; 84: 73–74.

89. Knudsen JF, Friedman B, Goldwasser JE. Ischemic colitis and sumatriptan use. *Arch Intern Med* 1998; 158: 1946–1948.

90. Ibrahim NK, Sahin AA, Dubrow RA, et al. Colitis associated with docetaxel-based chemotherapy in patients with metastatic breast cancer. *Lancet* 2000; 355: 281–283.

91. de Matteis A, Nuzzo F, Rossi E, et al. Intestinal side-effects of docetaxel/vinorelbine combination. *Lancet* 2000; 355: 1098–1099.

92. Evans JMM, McMahon AD, Murray FE, et al. Non-steroidal anti-inflammatory drugs are associated with emergency admission to hospital for colitis due to inflammatory bowel disease. *Gut* 1997; 40: 619–622.

93. Cappell MS, Simon T. Colonic toxicity of administered medications and chemicals. *Am J Gastroenterol* 1993; 88: 1684–1699.

94. Olm M, Gonzalez FJ, Garcia-Valdecasas JC, et al. Necrotising enterocolitis with perforation in diarrhoeic patients treated with loperamide. *Eur J Clin Pharmacol* 1990; 40: 415–416.

95. Chow CB, Li SH, Leung NK. Loperamide associated necrotising enterocolitis. *Arch Pediatr Scand* 1986; 75: 1034–1036.

96. Motala C, Hill ID, Mann MD, Bowie MD. Effect of loperamide on stool output and duration of acute infectious diarrhoea in infants. *J Pediatr* 1990; 117: 467–471.

97. Marcuard SP, Ehrinpreis MN, Fitter WF. Gold-induced ulcerative proctitis: report and review of the literature. *J Rheumatol* 1987; 14: 142–144.

98. Sears S, McNally P, Bachinski MS, Avery R. Irinotecan (CPT-11) induced colitis: report of a case and review of Food and Drug Administration MED-WATCH reporting. *Gastrointest Endosc* 1999; 50: 841–844.

99. Dranitsaris G, Maroun J, Shah A. Severe chemotherapy-induced diarrhea in patients with colorectal cancer: a cost of illness analysis. *Support Care Cancer* 2004; Dec 22 Epub ahead of print.

100. Rea WE, Durrant DCS, Boldy DAR. Ulcerative colitis after statin treatment. *Postgrad Med J* 2002; 78: 286–287.

101. Fuerle GE, Bartz KO, Schmitt-Graff A. Lymphocytic colitis, induced by ticlopidine. *Gastroenterol* 1999; 37: 1105–1108.

102. Eastwood M. The dilemma of laxative abuse. *Lancet* 1995; 346: 1115.

103. Committee on Safety of Medicines. Danthron restricted to constipation in the terminally ill. *Curr Probl Pharmacovigilance* 2000; 26: 4.

104. Wilmink T, Frick TW. Drug-induced pancreatitis. *Drug Safety* 1996; 14: 406–423.

105. Mallory A, Kern F Jr. Drug-induced pancreatitis: a central review. *Gastroenterology* 1980; 78: 813–820.
106. Sakorafas GH, Tsiotou AG. Etiology and pathogenesis of acute pancreatitis: Current concepts. *J Clin Gastroenterol* 2000; 30: 343–356.
107. McArthur KE. Review article: drug-induced pancreatitis. *Aliment Pharmacol Ther* 1996; 10: 23–38.

Further reading

Bateman DN, Aziz EE. Gastrointestinal disorders. In: Davies DM, Ferner RE, de Glanville H, eds. *Davies's Textbook of Adverse Drug Reactions*, 5th edn London: Chapman & Hall, 1999: 259–274.

Chan FK, Graham DY. Review article: prevention of non-steroidal anti-inflammatory gastrointestinal complications – review and recommendations on risk assessment. *Aliment Pharmacol Ther* 2004; 19: 1051–1061.

Hasler WL, Chey WD. Nausea and vomiting. *Gastroenterology* 2003; 125: 1860–1867.

Henkin RI. Drug-induced taste and smell disorders. Incidence, mechanisms, and management related primarily to treatment of sensory receptor dysfunction. *Drug Safety* 1994; 11: 318–377.

Huang JQ, Sridhar S, Hunt RH. Role of *Helicobacter pylori* infection and non-steroidal anti-inflammatory drugs in peptic-ulcer disease: a meta-analysis. *Lancet* 2002; 359: 14–22.

McArthur KE. Review article: drug-induced pancreatitis. *Aliment Pharmacol Ther* 1996; 10: 23–38.

Seymour RA. Oral and dental disorders. In: Davies DM, Ferner RE, de Glanville H, eds. *Davies's Textbook of Adverse Drug Reactions*, 5th edn London: Chapman & Hall, 1999: Chapter 11.

Tibble J, Smale S, Bjarnason I. Adverse effects of drugs on the small bowel. *Adv Drug React Bull* 1999; 198: 755–758.

7

Hepatic disorders

Ewan Forrest

Introduction

Drug-induced hepatotoxicity accounts for approximately 2% of cases of inpatient jaundice, and the liver is involved in 3–10% of all adverse drug reactions (ADRs). Up to 50% of all cases of acute liver failure (which is associated with a 90% mortality rate) are thought to be drug related.[1–3] Furthermore, hepatotoxicity is the main cause of fatal ADRs and the most common reason for withdrawal of drugs from the market.[1] This chapter discusses the different types of hepatotoxic reaction that can be produced and the main drugs implicated.

The liver is central to the metabolism of virtually all foreign substances ingested. If these substances are potentially toxic, they can damage the liver either directly or as a consequence of the metabolic changes that occur in the organ. Most drugs have been implicated as a cause of liver injury, if all published case reports are taken into account. However, if only drugs where there is reasonable evidence of a causal relationship are considered, several hundred can be classed as hepatotoxic.[2] The spectrum of drug hepatotoxicity is wide, ranging from asymptomatic reversible alterations in liver function tests to fatal acute hepatic necrosis.

Classification and mechanisms

Adverse effects of drugs on the liver can be classified into two main types, namely predictable (type A) and unpredictable (type B). Predictable hepatic reactions are dose dependent and affect the majority of individuals who ingest a sufficient amount of the drug. Examples of dose-dependent hepatotoxins are paracetamol (acetaminophen), salicylates, tetracycline and methotrexate. Idiosyncratic or unpredictable liver reactions (type B) are generally less frequent, typically occurring in between 1 in every 1000 and 1 in every 100 000 patients.[1,4] Examples of drugs involved are chlorpromazine, halothane and isoniazid. Both types of reaction can cause similar patterns of liver damage, and several drugs can cause more than one type of damage. Drugs may have a direct hepatotoxic effect or may induce an immune reaction after biotransformation to peptides and other small molecules that bind to proteins in the liver, inducing antibody formation.[1] Direct effects lead to predictable, dose-dependent toxicity. Immune reactions are dose independent, occur rapidly (often within 1–5 days), and are associated with hypersensitivity phenomena such as fever, rash and eosinophilia.

The time between starting treatment and the appearance of liver injury (the latency period) varies greatly. The latency period for type A reactions generally ranges between days and weeks, whereas for type B reactions it may be months or even years.[2] Although drug-induced liver damage is relatively rare in comparison with some other types of ADR, healthcare professionals should have some knowledge of the problem. In particular, they should be familiar with the drugs most frequently implicated, the most susceptible patients, the types of damage that can occur, and the situations in which monitoring of liver function is advisable.

Signs and symptoms of liver disorders

There may be few clinical signs on physical examination of a patient with liver disease, other than fever and the general appearance of being unwell. The liver is often tender and may be slightly enlarged, and a skin rash may indicate a drug hypersensitivity reaction. Less frequent signs of hypersensitivity reactions include lymphadenopathy, splenomegaly and arthritis.[4]

Anorexia, nausea and vomiting are the usual presenting symptoms in patients with hepatitis. Abdominal discomfort is common, particularly in the right upper quadrant, whereas dark urine, pale stools and jaundice tend to become evident after the first few days of illness. The presence of pruritus indicates cholestasis, which may be due to intrahepatic damage to the small bile ductules or extrahepatic damage owing to possible obstruction of the common bile duct. In the absence of cholestasis, however, the presence of jaundice may indicate that the liver injury is severe. Fatalities from drug-induced hepatitis occur in between 5 and 30% of jaundiced patients, but are rare in those without jaundice.[4] Acute liver failure is recognised by the development of encephalopathy, which may be very subtle in its early stages. The longer the period from the onset of jaundice to the onset of encephalopathy, the worse the prognosis.

Risk factors

Pre-existing liver disease

Patients with liver disease may be at increased risk of ADRs because of a reduced drug-metabolising capacity of the affected liver.[5] The risk of terfenadine-induced ventricular arrhythmias, for example, is greater in patients with significant liver disease.[6] However, many enzyme systems are preserved, even in advanced liver disease, particularly those involved in conjugation reactions.[1] In severe liver disease the activity of the cytochrome P450 (CYP450) 2C19 isoenzyme is greatly decreased, whereas that of the 2D6 enzyme is intact. In general, patients with pre-existing liver disease such as alcoholic cirrhosis or chronic viral hepatitis are at no greater risk of idiosyncratic drug reactions. Examples of exceptions to this would be methotrexate and niacin.

Care should be taken with drug dosing in patients with cirrhosis, ascites or encephalopathy. For example, the prescription of analgesia for patients with liver disease is fraught with difficulties. Non-steroidal anti-inflammatory drugs (NSAIDs) are likely to precipitate worsening ascites and/or peripheral oedema, and renal dysfunction. Opioids may worsen encephalopathy both by a direct central nervous system depressant action and by causing constipation. In general terms paracetamol is safe for these patients as long as they do not have evidence of an active alcoholic hepatitis. As encephalopathy is more likely to be reversible than renal impairment, opioids may be preferred if more potent analgesia is required.

Gender

Women appear to be more susceptible to drug-induced liver disease than men.[1] For example, halothane-induced hepatitis occurs more often in women,[7] and the rate of isoniazid hepatotoxicity appears to be higher in women.[8] Men, however, may be more susceptible to cholestatic reactions (e.g. co-amoxiclav, azathioprine).

Age

Older patients have a higher incidence of drug-induced liver disease and reactions tend to be more severe.[9] In general, drug-induced liver disease is rare in children, except in those receiving sodium valproate. Children under the age of 2 years on multiple enzyme-inducing antiepileptics and with developmental delay seem to be particularly susceptible to idiosyncratic hepatotoxicity with sodium valproate.[10] The mechanism is not fully understood, but is thought to involve a toxic metabolite.[11]

The other drug causing hepatotoxicity specifically in children is aspirin. The use of salicylates in children with a viral infection results in a greater risk of developing Reye's syndrome. The condition is characterised by coma, hypoglycaemia, seizures and hepatic steatosis leading to fulminant liver failure. Once the association with aspirin was confirmed by epidemiological studies,[12,13] aspirin became contraindicated in children under 12 years except for use in juvenile arthritis. The mechanism of the toxicity remains unknown. More recent data suggest that cases of aspirin-induced Reye's syndrome in children still occur.[14] In the UK aspirin is no longer recommended in young people under 16 years of age unless on the advice of a doctor.[15] Healthcare professionals should ensure that children are not inadvertently treated with aspirin.

Children appear to be less susceptible than adults to the hepatotoxic effects of paracetamol in overdose; severe or fatal reactions are rare in this age group.[16] This may be because children have an enhanced capacity for sulphate conjugation and a relative immaturity of microsomal enzymes catalysing formation of the active metabolite.[17,18]

Genetic factors

Genetic factors are increasingly recognised as potentially important determinants of drug-induced liver disease. The composition of the CYP450 isoenzymes in the liver is genetically determined, and the relative concentrations of these can determine the extent to which an individual may produce toxic metabolites or have reduced protective mechanisms when exposed to a particular drug.[19] Genetic variation in these isoenzymes alone is unlikely to cause severe toxicity, given that severe liver toxicity occurs so infrequently. The potential for drugs to complex with proteins leading to antigen development depends on human leukocyte antigen (HLA) configurations that have been genetically defined (see Chapter 3). For example, a specific HLA haplotype believed to be associated with hepatitis induced by the administration of amoxicillin-clavulanate was found in 57% of patients with the illness but in only 12% of unaffected persons.[1]

Epidemiological studies have not led to a definitive conclusion on whether acetylator status is an important determinant of isoniazid-induced liver damage. Rapid acetylators of isoniazid were originally believed to be more susceptible to hepatotoxicity, but further studies have refuted this and some have suggested that the risk is in fact higher in slow acetylators.[4]

Enzyme inducers

Enhancement of drug-metabolising enzymes via the induction of CYP450 isoenzymes may lead to an increased risk of liver damage when an individual is subsequently exposed to drugs that can produce toxic metabolites. For example, the incidence of hepatotoxicity due to sodium valproate is increased in patients on enzyme-inducing antiepileptics,[10] and the hepatotoxicity of statins may be precipitated by the addition of diltiazem.[20]

Alcohol

Chronic ethanol consumption induces the CYP450 system and, as a result, can potentiate toxicity induced by certain drugs. Doses of paracetamol smaller than those that are usually hepatotoxic may cause liver damage in chronic alcohol abusers. In addition, toxicity caused by isoniazid and methotrexate is more likely in alcoholics.[4] There has been a report of a polyunsaturated fatty acid preparation causing acute hepatitis in an alcohol abuser.[21]

Multidrug regimens

There are some circumstances in which combinations of medicines are associated with an increased risk of toxic reactions. In these cases one drug commonly causes induction of CYP450, which then increases the quantity of the toxic metabolite formed by the other drug. For example, the risk of hepatotoxicity with isoniazid is substantially greater when rifampicin is given concomitantly.[22]

Other diseases

Certain pre-existing conditions can increase the risk of drug-induced hepatic injury. For example, patients with insulin-dependent diabetes mellitus are at increased risk of hepatic fibrosis caused by methotrexate. The risk of liver injury caused by tetracycline is increased in patients with renal failure.[23]

Nutritional status

Obesity increases the risk of liver injury caused by methotrexate and halothane. Fasting patients are more likely to be predisposed to hepatotoxicity caused by paracetamol as hepatic glutathione, which is needed for normal paracetamol metabolism, is depleted.[23]

Diagnosis of drug-induced liver damage

To assess the likelihood that a particular drug or compound is responsible for causing liver disease, several factors must be considered. These include drug exposure, time to onset of abnormalities, time to resolution of abnormalities, clinical features, exclusion of other causes of liver disease, liver function tests (LFTs) and biopsy results. A clinical diagnostic scale has been described which takes into account many of these factors.[24] This practical score correlates well with international consensus classification of drug-induced hepatotoxicity.

Routine LFTs involve measurement of total bilirubin, alanine transaminase and alkaline phosphatase. Impairment of the synthetic function of the liver is detected by total protein, albumin and prothrombin time. The gamma-glutamylpeptidase level may also be elevated in drug-induced liver disease. Conjugated bilirubin may be measured to establish whether there is biliary obstruction. Liver biopsy and histological evaluation are useful in the diagnosis of acute hepatocellular dysfunction where a drug-induced cause is suspected.

Drug exposure

It is essential that a detailed and thorough medication history is obtained from any patient in whom liver disease is suspected. This history should include all medicines (current and past), with specific questions about the use of over-the-counter medicines, herbal remedies, oral contraceptives and any drugs of abuse. Some medicines, including digoxin and theophylline, are seldom implicated as causes of liver injury, whereas drugs such as NSAIDs and some antibiotics (e.g. flucloxacillin) are commonly implicated.[3] Liver injury induced by complementary therapies has become more common as the use of these medications has increased. Various compounds, including kava, black cohosh, germander, chaparral leaf and many others, have been associated with hepatotoxicity.

Onset of abnormalities

The most effective way to identify the drug causing a reaction is to consider carefully when drugs were ingested in relation to the onset of signs and symptoms. Healthcare professionals should be particularly suspicious of any potentially hepatotoxic drug begun during the 3 months before the onset of symptoms.[3] There is usually a latent period between the first administration of a drug and the onset of an adverse reaction in the liver. The interval may vary from a few hours (in the case of a drug causing potent dose-dependent hepatotoxicity) to several weeks (for most forms of drug-induced acute hepatitis or cholestasis), to more than 6 months (in cases of chronic liver disease). Although there is some variability, the latent period for many drugs is sufficiently reproducible to be of some diagnostic value.

Resolution of abnormalities

A striking improvement in symptoms of liver impairment when a drug is discontinued strongly suggests that it may be implicated as a hepatotoxin. Time to resolution of abnormalities will depend very much on the individual drug and the type of disease it has induced. The recovery period can be many months. Confirmation of drug-induced hepatotoxicity can sometimes be sought by rechallenge with the suspected drug, but as this is potentially dangerous for the patient it is usually unacceptable in practice.[3] In some cases, such as when a patient with tuberculosis develops abnormal liver function while taking isoniazid or rifampicin, therapy is often reintroduced sequentially, with careful monitoring, as the potential benefits of therapy generally outweigh the risks associated with not giving the most effective antituberculous regimen.[25] If the patient develops further liver abnormalities, an alternative drug may then need to be substituted.

Clinical features

The clinical features that guide causality assessment in drug-induced hepatotoxicity include an evaluation of the signs and symptoms at diagnosis, the systemic features of the reaction, and the availability of a specific diagnostic test. If drug-induced hepatotoxicity is suspected and the liver injury is accompanied by fever, rash and eosinophilia, for example, it is possible that the patient is suffering from an immunologically mediated (type B) ADR.[4]

There are very few specific diagnostic tests that can confirm drug-induced liver disease other than routine determinations of liver function.

One possible exception relates to halothane hepatotoxicity, which involves both direct hepatotoxicity and immune mechanisms. The major metabolite of halothane is trifluoroacetic acid (TFA). TFA–liver protein complexes are formed in all individuals exposed to halothane, yet only those who develop severe halothane hepatitis have antibodies to them.[26,27]

Exclusion of other possible causes

It is essential to exclude other possible causes of liver disease, in case the hepatic changes are unrelated to drug exposure. Viral and autoimmune causes of hepatitis and intrahepatic cholestasis can be identified by serological tests, and in cases of jaundice the common bile duct can be investigated radiologically to exclude physical obstruction by gallstones, other masses or strictures.

Liver function tests

Abnormalities in liver function tests (LFTs) may indicate the presence of liver disease, although some are crude and non-specific. In general, markers of liver damage (such as serum gamma-glutamyl transferase, alanine transaminase, aspartate transaminase, alkaline phosphatase or the conjugated bilirubin concentration) are defined as abnormal when they are increased to more than twice the upper limit of the normal reference range.[28] Elevations in LFTs are common with certain drugs, but only in a minority of cases does significant hepatic injury follow.[17] For example, serum transaminases rise in up to 40% of patients taking isoniazid, but symptomatic hepatotoxicity occurs in fewer than 5%.[25]

Patterns of changes in LFTs may distinguish the type of liver disease present, which in turn may help to determine whether a particular drug is implicated. Marked increases in LFTs, together with signs and symptoms associated with liver disease (nausea, vomiting, abdominal pain, ascites, pruritus, jaundice), suggest that liver injury has occurred. Predominant elevations of transaminases (alanine transaminase and aspartate transaminase) suggest hepatitis. Cholestasis is indicated by predominant elevations of alkaline phosphatase and gamma-glutamyl transferase. Both types of reaction may be associated with a raised serum bilirubin, resulting in jaundice. A combination of cholestasis and hepatitis is not uncommon in ADRs (cholestatic hepatitis). These blood tests may indicate the nature of hepatotoxicity, but true liver function is better indicated by measurement of the prothrombin time.

When potentially hepatotoxic drugs are prescribed, it is important to measure LFTs before the start of treatment so that baseline values are available to compare with subsequent measurements. Monitoring LFTs in the first few weeks of therapy with drugs known to cause hepatic damage by metabolic idiosyncrasy (e.g. isoniazid, pyrazinamide) can give early warning of an impending severe reaction.

Liver biopsy

Data on the histological and ultrastructural features of hepatic lesions may be necessary to confirm a suspected diagnosis. This is generally achieved by taking a needle biopsy of the liver through the abdomen under local anaesthetic. Certain drugs cause characteristic lesions: for example, amiodarone therapy can lead to infiltration of the hepatocytes with phospholipid droplets.[29] Liver biopsy is not a risk-free procedure, and should only be performed in cases when there is serious doubt regarding the diagnosis. In patients prescribed low-dose methotrexate for psoriasis or rheumatoid arthritis, regular liver biopsy is unlikely to be beneficial[30,31] but may be appropriate where the cumulative methotrexate dose is high and if liver damage is suspected.[31,32]

Types of drug-induced liver disease

Tables 7.1–7.6 illustrate the diversity of drugs that have the potential to have adverse effects on the liver. They are not exhaustive summaries of all the medicines implicated in liver injury, but select those most frequently documented in the literature.

Dose-dependent hepatocellular damage

A number of hepatotoxic ADRs are dose dependent. These include cyclophosphamide and heavy metal (for example mercury) toxicity. However, the most important clinical dose-dependent hepatotoxic drug is paracetamol.

Paracetamol is generally safe when taken in the recommended therapeutic dose of 1–4 g daily, but in excessive doses it is hepatotoxic. It is the most common cause of drug-induced liver disease, leading to about 200 deaths each year in the UK.[33] In therapeutic doses, paracetamol is mainly metabolised by conjugation to the glucuronide and sulphate compounds, which are then excreted in the urine. A small proportion (5–10%) is oxidised by mixed-function oxidase enzymes to form the highly reactive

Table 7.1 Some drugs that may cause acute hepatocellular necrosis and hepatitis

Allopurinol
Angiotensin-converting enzyme (ACE) inhibitors
Aspirin
Carbamazepine
Chinese herbs (Jin Bu Huan)
Cocaine
Co-trimoxazole
Cyclophosphamide
Cyproterone
Dantrolene
Didanosine
'Ecstasy' (MDMA; methylenedioxymethamfetamine)
Halothane
Isoniazid
Ketoconazole
Labetalol
Leflunomide
Methyldopa
Minocycline
Monoamine oxidase inhibitors (MAOIs)
Nitrofurantoin
Non-steroidal anti-inflammatory drugs (NSAIDs), e.g. indometacin, diclofenac
Paracetamol
Pennyroyal (herbal)
Phenytoin
Rifampicin
Sodium valproate
Sulfasalazine
Sulfonamides
Tricyclic antidepressants
Troglitazone

N-acetyl-p-benzoquinoneimine (NAPQI). In overdose, the conjugation pathway becomes saturated and a greater proportion of paracetamol is oxidised. As a result, liver glutathione stores become depleted and the liver is unable to deactivate the toxic metabolite NAPQI. This compound can bind directly to liver cells, leading to necrosis.

Replenishment of glutathione stores is of value in paracetamol poisoning. Intravenous acetylcysteine and oral methionine are effective antidotes, provided they are administered within 8–10 hours of ingestion of the overdose.[34] For this reason, all patients should be referred to hospital immediately if there is a suspicion that they have taken an overdose of paracetamol.

After an overdose of paracetamol patients usually remain asymptomatic for the first 24 hours, although anorexia, nausea and vomiting are sometimes present. The absence of symptoms can lead to a delay in seeking medical advice, and thus increase the risk of potentially fatal liver failure. Liver damage is not usually detectable by routine LFTs until at least 18 hours after ingestion of the drug. Hepatic tenderness and abdominal pain are seldom seen before the second day after ingestion. Maximum liver damage, as assessed by plasma alanine transaminase (ALT) or aspartate aminotransferase (AST) activities or prothrombin time, occurs 72–96 hours after ingestion. Hepatic failure (manifest by jaundice and encephalopathy) may then develop between the third and fifth days; the rate of clinical deterioration reflects the severity of the overdose. Hepatic coma, metabolic acidosis, high peak prothrombin time and renal failure are all indicators of poor outcome. Death can occur between 4 and 18 days after the overdose, usually from cerebral oedema, sepsis and multi-organ failure. The overall mortality from paracetamol poisoning in untreated patients is about 5%.

Any patient who ingests more than 150 mg/kg bodyweight of paracetamol, or more than 12 g in total, should be considered at risk of severe liver damage. Patients who present 12 hours or more after ingestion are at greater risk of serious liver damage, as the antidotes are less effective after this time. Patients taking enzyme-inducing drugs, those with eating disorders, and chronic alcohol abusers are at greater risk of hepatotoxic damage. In patients with a high alcohol intake paracetamol doses of 2–6 g have been associated with fatal hepatotoxicity. Treatment with acetylcysteine or methionine should be initiated at lower plasma paracetamol concentrations in these high-risk patients.

Points to remember about paracetamol include the following:

- There is evidence that the public has a poor knowledge of paracetamol's toxicity in overdose. There is a tendency to misjudge the potentially lethal dose.
- Accidental deaths have occurred after self-medication with multiple paracetamol-containing preparations at the same time.
- Healthcare professionals have an active role to play in educating the public about the dangers of paracetamol overdose. Patients should be counselled about the importance of not exceeding the maximum daily dose of 4 g.
- Any patient who reports having taken a paracetamol overdose, either accidentally or deliberately, should be advised to seek medical advice immediately.

Immunologically mediated hepatocellular damage

Hepatocellular damage from dose-independent reactions can present with a wide spectrum of changes, from mild asymptomatic elevations in serum transaminases to a severe hepatic illness with jaundice. Minor abnormalities in LFTs are sometimes self-limiting and resolve with continued drug administration, whereas in other cases they progress to symptomatic hepatitis. Hepatitis from some drugs often occurs in the context of a hypersensitivity reaction, with prominent skin rashes, arthralgia and eosinophilia, whereas for other agents such features are rarely, if ever, seen.

Granulomatous hepatitis is characterised by proliferative inflammatory lesions and is often the result of an immunoallergic reaction. Resolution of the clinical, laboratory and histological abnormalities usually occurs promptly after discontinuation of the responsible drug.

Idiosyncratic metabolic hepatocellular damage

This type of liver disease is frequently thought to be due to metabolic idiosyncrasy. Halothane, for example, can produce severe hepatocellular necrosis leading to fulminant hepatic failure. Halothane hepatitis has a low incidence (estimated at between 1 in 22 000 and 1 in 35 000 halothane anaesthetics) but a high mortality. Severe hepatic damage is more common in patients who have been exposed to halothane on more than one occasion, particularly if the interval between exposures is short.[17,23] For this reason it is recommended that repeat exposure within 3 months should be avoided.[35,36] In practice, the use of halothane has been superseded by newer and safer anaesthetic agents.

A hepatotoxic ADR of a drug may be reflective of reactivity to that class of drug, such as statins. However, in others the reaction may be more individual. For example, troglitazone was associated with severe

Table 7.2 Some drugs causing granulomatous hepatitis

Allopurinol	Phenylbutazone
Carbamazepine	Phenytoin
Chlorpromazine	Procainamide
Diltiazem	Quinidine
Gold	Quinine
Hydralazine	Sulfasalazine
Methyldopa	Sulfonamides
Nitrofurantoin	Sulfonylureas
Penicillin	Tacrine

hepatotoxicity, although the rest of the thiazolidinediones do not appear to have such problems.[37]

Steatosis and steatohepatitis

Steatosis or fatty liver can be characterised into two categories, an acute microvesicular (small droplet) form and a subacute or chronic macrovesicular (large droplet) form. Microvesicular steatosis is part of the spectrum of metabolic idiocyncratic hepatotoxicity and can be caused by drugs such as tetracycline, sodium valproate and L-asparaginase. Blood glucose may be low and blood ammonia levels high, and the clinical picture may resemble Reye's syndrome. Macrovesicular fatty liver that resembles alcoholic-related liver damage, usually termed non-alcoholic fatty liver disease or, in its more aggressive form, non-alcoholic steatohepatitis. Simple steatosis may be caused by corticosteroids and methotrexate.[4,23] Steatohepatitis differs from diffuse fatty change as there is evidence of hepatocellular damage. Amiodarone can complex with phospholipids, causing chronic steatohepatitis. This may progress to cirrhosis.

Non-alcoholic fatty liver disease may occur without a drug reaction. Patients at risk are those with diabetes mellitus, obesity and hyperlipidaemia.[38] This can lead to confusion, as the LFTs of patients with hyperlipidaemia may be abnormal owing to either hyperlipidaemia related non-alcoholic fatty liver disease or to a reaction to lipid-lowering statin therapy. In this regard it is very useful to know the patient's LFTs before commencing statin therapy. There is no evidence to suggest that patients with non-alcoholic fatty liver disease are at greater risk of statin hepatotoxicity.

Chronic hepatitis (Table 7.3)

Drug-induced chronic hepatitis has mixed characteristics, with features of both acute and chronic hepatic injury. Serum transaminases are usually raised and serum albumin low. The disease is defined as 'chronic' when present for more than 3 months, as determined by histological and laboratory results. The histology resembles that of autoimmune chronic active hepatitis and is associated with circulating antibodies. The condition usually resolves on drug withdrawal.

Cholestasis (Tables 7.4 and 7.5)

Partial or complete obstruction of the common bile duct, with resulting retention of bile acids, leads to the condition known as cholestasis. This may occur with or without associated hepatitis and bile duct injury or destruction. Long-standing obstruction of the bile outflow from the liver can cause inflammation, scarring, and eventually cirrhosis. Cholestasis without hepatitis is associated with a raised bilirubin and a normal or

Table 7.3 Some drugs causing chronic hepatitis

Cimetidine
Dantrolene
Diclofenac
Etretinate
Herbal medicines (e.g. germander, chaparral)
Isoniazid
Minocycline
Nitrofurantoin
Paracetamol
Phenytoin
Sulfonamides
Tricyclic antidepressants

Table 7.4 Some drugs causing cholestasis with hepatitis

ACE inhibitors	Nitrofurantoin
Azathioprine	NSAIDs, e.g. sulindac
Carbimazole	Penicillamine
Chlorpropamide	Phenindione
Cimetidine	Phenothiazines, e.g. chlorpromazine
Clavulanic acid	Phenytoin
Co-trimoxazole	Ranitidine
Dextropropoxyphene	Sulfonamides
Erythromycin	Sulphonylureas
Flucloxacillin	Ticlopidine
Flutamide	Tricylic antidepressants
Fusidic acid	Thiouracil
Gold salts	Troglitazone
Ketoconazole	

Table 7.5 Some drugs causing cholestasis without hepatitis

Ciclosporin	Oral contraceptives
Flucloxacillin	Tamoxifen
Glibenclamide	Warfarin
Griseofulvin	

minimally raised ALT level. No inflammation or hepatocellular necrosis is seen. In contrast, in cholestasis associated with hepatitis the laboratory picture is normally one of elevated levels of alkaline phosphatase, ALT and conjugated bilirubin.

Chlorpromazine is a common cause of cholestasis, with an estimated incidence of 0.5–1% in patients taking the drug for more than 2 weeks. The median latent period is 2–3 weeks, with symptoms usually resolving within 4 weeks of discontinuation in the majority of cases. Abnormal LFTs without jaundice are much more common and may be seen in a quarter or more of patients treated with phenothiazines.[17]

Chronic cholestasis

A syndrome that clinically and histologically resembles primary biliary cirrhosis (PBC) occurs in association with a number of drugs, all of which have been shown to produce acute cholestasis. Histologically there is disappearance of small intrahepatic bile ducts (vanishing bile duct syndrome). The syndrome may be manifested as chronic cholestatic jaundice with its attendant complications, or just as persistently abnormal LFTs (predominantly alkaline phosphatase) with no symptoms or signs. Even when the offending agent is stopped there is usually chronic cholestasis, often with jaundice, and high alkaline phosphatase and gamma-glutamyl-transpeptidase activities for several years.[39] In some cases abnormalities may be permanent. Some drugs reported to cause chronic cholestasis are shown in Table 7.6.

Fibrosis and cirrhosis

Fibrosis may occur without cirrhosis and is partially reversible, whereas cirrhosis is characterised by dense fibrosis and hepatocellular regeneration, which is irreversible. In fibrosis, serum transaminases may be only transiently raised and are not good predictors of hepatic damage.

Table 7.6 Some drugs causing chronic cholestasis

Anabolic and contraceptive steroids	Erythromycin
Carbamazepine	Flucloxacillin
Chlorpromazine	Phenytoin
Co-amoxiclav	Prochlorperazine
Co-trimoxazole	Sulfonamides

Microscopy shows deposition of fibrous tissue. Cirrhosis results from continued injury to hepatocytes, which may occur in chronic cholestasis, steatohepatitis and chronic active hepatitis, although it may also develop despite discontinuation of a causal drug.[40] Methotrexate and vitamin A have both been implicated in causing a gradual progression to cirrhosis without any symptoms or abnormalities in LFTs.

Methotrexate-induced liver damage is dose related. The high incidence of hepatic fibrosis and cirrhosis reported in early studies reflected the use of high daily doses of the drug. There is also good evidence that daily dosing is more hepatotoxic than giving the same cumulative amount in weekly doses. With the doses currently used in psoriasis and rheumatoid arthritis the incidence of liver damage is minimal. Other factors that increase susceptibility to liver injury from methotrexate include underlying liver disease, alcohol abuse, and the combination of obesity and diabetes mellitus. The incidence of liver toxicity also seems to be higher in patients with psoriasis than in those with rheumatoid arthritis. This is probably related both to dose and the higher prevalence of alcohol abuse in psoriasis patients. Regular monitoring of LFTs is required in patients taking methotrexate.

Vascular disorders

A variety of drugs can cause veno-occlusive disease and Budd–Chiari syndrome. Veno-occlusive disease is characterised by non-thrombotic concentric narrowing of the central hepatic veins by connective tissue. Severe centrilobular congestion and necrosis reflect the venous blockage. Presentation may be acute with right upper quadrant pain, ascites, and, in the most severe cases, hepatic failure. In those who survive this progresses to cirrhosis. Alternatively, cirrhosis may develop insidiously over a number of years and present with its complications, including hepatocellular carcinoma. Veno-occlusive disease may be caused by azathioprine, dactinomycin, dacarbazine and high-dose busulfan or cyclophosphamide. High-dose chemotherapy with busulfan or cyclophosphamide for bone marrow transplantation is complicated by veno-occlusive disease of the liver in about 25% of cases.[41] The risk of this complication may be reduced by careful dose adjustment and heparin prophylaxis. Herbal remedies containing pyrrolizidine alkaloids, for example comfrey and heliotropium, have also been reported to cause veno-occlusive disease.[42]

Budd–Chiari syndrome is characterised by the obstruction of large hepatic veins, and has been reported in association with oral contraceptives and cytotoxic agents.[43,44]

Hepatic tumours

Hepatocellular adenoma and carcinoma, although rare, have been associated with the use of steroidal compounds such as the oral contraceptives, danazol and anabolic steroids.[4,17]

Management of patients with drug-induced hepatic disease

Stopping the administration of a suspected hepatotoxic drug is the most important action in the management of drug-induced liver disease. In some circumstances attempts to remove a drug from the body can be made, i.e. with dose-dependent acute hepatotoxins such as paracetamol or heavy metal poisoning, where the unabsorbed drug may be removed by emptying the stomach. If available, a suitable antidote, such as acetylcysteine or methionine, may be used as a cytoprotectant in the management of paracetamol overdose.

There are conflicting views on the value of using corticosteroids as anti-inflammatory agents to treat drug-induced liver disease. It is generally considered reasonable to give corticosteroids to patients with a hepatocellular drug-induced injury if improvement is not apparent within 3 months of discontinuing the drug, or possibly as early as 6 weeks where deterioration persists after the causative agent has been stopped.[23]

Patients with a predominantly cholestatic reaction may be treated with ursodeoxycholic acid, but evidence with regard to its effectiveness is lacking.

Additional, supportive therapy may be needed, ranging from the symptomatic management of pruritus with systemic antihistamines or colestyramine, to liver transplantation for cases where acute hepatic failure has developed.

Liver dysfunction of any kind is classed as a serious reaction, so any suspicion that a drug has had an adverse effect on the liver should be reported to the appropriate regulatory authority.

Prevention of drug-induced hepatic damage

Regular monitoring of LFTs should be carried out for all patients treated with certain drugs that are common causes of hepatotoxicity (Table 7.7). Baseline LFTs should be carried out before treatment starts. There is uncertainty about the level of abnormality at which drugs should be discontinued. In general, an increase in any one parameter to two to three times the baseline measurement may indicate drug-induced hepatotoxicity, and

Table 7.7 Some drugs for which regular monitoring of liver function tests is recommended

Drug	LFT monitoring recommended (in UK)
Amiodarone	Monitor LFTs (particularly transaminases) at baseline and then every 6 months
Cyproterone	Check baseline LFTs and then recheck if symptoms develop
Dantrolene	Check baseline LFTs and repeat 6 weeks after starting therapy
Leflunomide	Check baseline LFTs and repeat periodically thereafter
Methotrexate	Check baseline LFTs, then every 2–3 months
Methyldopa	Check baseline LFTs, then at intervals during first 6–12 weeks of treatment
Nevirapine	Check baseline LFTs then every 2 weeks during first 2 months of treatment, at the third month and then on a 3–6-monthly basis
Rifampicin	In patients with pre-existing liver disease or if pretreatment LFTs abnormal, LFTs should be checked weekly for the first 2 weeks then at 2–4-week intervals
Rosiglitazone	Check baseline LFTs then repeat every 2 months for the first 12 months, and periodically thereafter
Sodium valproate	Check baseline LFTs and repeat periodically during first 6 months of therapy
Statins	Check baseline LFTs and check periodically after that (e.g. every 6–12 months)
Sulfasalazine	As for methotrexate

the drug should be withdrawn. However, where drugs are commonly known to cause elevations in certain liver enzymes then the threshold for discontinuing the drug may be higher.

Patient education is essential in the prevention of drug-induced hepatotoxicity. Many drug reactions can develop within days, so monitoring of LFTs is not a complete safeguard against toxicity. Patients who do not realise that drug-induced injury is possible, and those who continue to take a drug despite initial signs of toxicity, are at highest risk of fatal reactions. For example, patients taking antituberculous medication should be encouraged to report to their doctor any gastrointestinal symptoms that may indicate drug-induced hepatitis, such as anorexia, nausea, vomiting or abdominal pain.

One area where healthcare professionals can have a valuable educational role is with over-the-counter preparations, which members of the public widely assume to be safer than drugs available only on prescription. Health food products ('nutraceuticals') and herbal remedies may also be judged to be innocuous, but toxic reactions, including liver damage, may occur.[42]

Finally, the latency period of many hepatotoxic reactions may lead to diagnostic difficulties when patients present with the non-specific signs of actual or impending hepatic damage. Ensuring adequate monitoring of patients, and providing information to prescribers about drugs that are potentially hepatotoxic, is therefore an essential educational role.

 CASE STUDY 7.1

Mr A is a 46-year-old man with a history of type 2 diabetes mellitus diagnosed 2 years ago. He is found at a screening clinic to have significant hypercholesterolaemia and reckoned to be at high risk of cardiac events in the future. It is decided to prescribe a statin to treat this. Although he has no symptoms he has his LFTs checked prior to commencing treatment. These are as follows, with normal level in brackets:

Albumin 35 g/L (normal 35–55)
Aspartate transaminase (AST) 56 units/L (<35)
Alanine transaminase (ALT) 89 units/L (<50)
Alkaline phosphatase 253 units/L (70–290)
Bilirubin 15 µmol/L (3–17)

What is the likely cause of the abnormal LFTs?

The most likely cause of these minor abnormalities is non-alcoholic fatty liver disease related to his diabetes and hyperlipidaemia. However, it would be important to exclude other potential causes of liver disease, such as chronic viral hepatitis, autoimmune liver disease or metabolic liver diseases (such as haemochromatosis). The fatty change is often noted on ultrasound examination of the liver.

Should the statin be prescribed?

Despite the LFTs being abnormal, there is no reason to withhold the statin, and he is prescribed simvastatin, titrated to 60 mg. Subsequent LFTs do not change significantly. However, 1 year later he develops significant hypertension. This does not respond optimally to angiotensin-converting enzyme inhibitor treatment, and it is decided to start diltiazem in addition. Two weeks later he complains

→

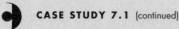

CASE STUDY 7.1 (continued)

of muscle aches and then develops nausea and upper abdominal discomfort. Further blood results are as follows:

Albumin 34 g/L (normal 35–55)
Aspartate transaminase (AST) 985 units/L (<35)
Alanine transaminase (ALT) 638 units/L (<50)
Alkaline phosphatase 347 units/L (70–290)
Bilirubin 34 μmol/L (3–17)
Creatine kinase (CK) 2529 units/L (<150)

What type of liver dysfunction is indicated by these results?

This is a predominantly hepatitic abnormality. There is no significant jaundice or elevation of the alkaline phosphatase to indicate cholestasis. The creatine kinase is also elevated, which reflects muscle damage. Aspartate transaminase is also derived from muscle, and so is disproportionately elevated relative to the alanine transaminase.

What do you think is the cause of the hepatotoxicity?

The combination of the muscle injury (myositis) and hepatitis is highly suggestive of statin-induced hepatotoxicity. It is probable that the injudicious use of diltiazem has precipitated the statin toxicity, as diltiazem inhibits the cytochrome P450 metabolism of some statins. The risk of serious myopathy is increased when high doses of simvastatin are combined with diltiazem. The Committee on Safety of Medicines has recently advised that the dose of simvastatin should not exceed 40 mg daily in patients taking diltiazem.[45]

How should his hyperlipidaemia be treated in the future?

Once the acute episode is settled, the statin could be restarted without the coadministration of diltiazem. Alternatively, another statin could be prescribed. The LFTs should of course be closely monitored.

CASE STUDY 7.2

Mrs B is a 71-year-old woman who recently suffered a myocardial infarction. At the time of discharge she was prescribed aspirin, atenolol, enalapril and

→

◗ CASE STUDY 7.2 (continued)

simvastatin. Three months later she presented to her doctor with a 4-week history of lethargy and increasing nausea. For the previous 4 days she has noted yellowing of her eyes and darkening of her urine. In the last 2 days she has suffered from widespread itch, which has prevented her from sleeping.

What form of liver disease is suggested by this presentation?

General malaise, tiredness and gastrointestinal symptoms of nausea and vomiting are common signs of drug-induced liver disease. Pruritus in particular is associated with liver dysfunction of cholestatic origin, although the mechanism for this is unclear.

What are the other possible causes, and how what questions would you ask?

It is important to obtain details of time of symptom onset in relation to drug ingestion. Onset of illness associated with statins is usually within 1–6 weeks of starting the drug, but may occur later. The onset of angiotensin-converting enzyme inhibitor hepatotoxicity is often delayed up to months after starting treatment. Although it may be likely that this is a drug reaction, a full clinical history should still be taken to exclude other causes of potential illness. The patient may have a history of liver disease, which might confuse the picture, and this should be clarified. It is possible that congestive heart failure could cause liver dysfunction after a myocardial infarction, and so signs such as the presence of peripheral oedema should be sought.

The patient was admitted to hospital. LFTs on admission were as follows:

Albumin 37 g/L (normal 35–55)
Aspartate transaminase (AST) 172 units/L (<35)
Alanine transaminase (ALT) 211 units/L (<50)
Alkaline phosphatase 1975 units/L (70–290)
Bilirubin 172 μmol/L (3–17)

What type of liver dysfunction is indicated by these results?

The LFTs reveal a mixed cholestatic and hepatic picture of injury. The cholestasis appears to predominate, suggesting that this is a cholestatic hepatitis. The albumin is in the normal reference range, which indicates that the liver injury is acute rather than chronic. LFTs can only provide a crude guide to the type of liver disease, and changes do not always accurately indicate the extent of liver damage.

→

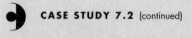

CASE STUDY 7.2 (continued)

How would you treat her symptoms?

Pruritus is a common and debilitating effect of cholestatic injury, and will probably be the main symptomatic complaint. Once the patient has been assessed, treatment with antihistamines, colestyramine and/or topical therapy with menthol in aqueous cream may be considered. In general, sedating antihistamines, such as chlorphenamine, are used because of their longer-term safety record and because lack of sleep is a debilitating feature of pruritus. However, they should only be used in patients with stable liver disease. Non-sedating antihistamines, such as loratadine and cetirizine, may also be of some benefit. Resolution of the underlying condition will provide the most effective relief from the pruritus.

What changes to treatment would you recommend?

This case indicates the difficulties faced with an ADR in the context of polypharmacy. There are two potential culprit drugs: simvastatin and enalapril. The cholestatic hepatitis favours the enalapril as a cause, as opposed to the more 'pure' hepatitis of statin toxicity. Both agents should be discontinued. After resolution of the liver abnormalities, the least likely cause of the hepatotoxicity may be restarted with careful monitoring of the LFTs. There may be cross-reactivity with other angiotensin-converting enzyme inhibitors, so if this is enalapril hepatotoxicity then an alternative class of drug, such as angiotensin-II receptor antagonists, may need to be used.

References

1. Lee WM. Medical progress: Drug-induced hepatotoxicity. *N Engl J Med* 2003; 349: 474–485.
2. Dossing M, Sonne J. Drug-induced hepatic disorders. Incidence, management and avoidance. *Drug Safety* 1993; 9: 441–449.
3. Farrell GC. Drug-induced hepatic injury. *J Gastroenterol Hepatol* 1997; 12: S242–250.
4. Farrell GC. *Drug-induced Liver Disease*. Melbourne: Churchill Livingstone, 1994.
5. Bass NM, Williams RL. Guide to drug dosage in hepatic disease. *Clin Pharmacokinet* 1988; 15: 396–420.
6. Committee on Safety of Medicines. Ventricular arrhythmias due to terfenadine and astemizole. *Curr Probl* 1992; November.

7. Benjamin SB, Goodman ZD, Ishak KG, *et al.* The morphologic spectrum of halothane-induced hepatic injury: analysis of 77 cases. *Hepatology* 1985; 5: 1163–1171.

8. Nolan C, Goldberg SV, Buskin SE. Hepatotoxicity associated with isoniazid preventive therapy. *JAMA* 1999; 281: 1014–1018.

9. James OFW. Drugs and the aging liver. *J Hepatol* 1985; 1: 431–435.

10. Pirmohamed M, Kitteringham NR, Park BK. The role of active metabolites in drug toxicity. *Drug Safety* 1994; 11: 114–144.

11. Anderson GD, Acheampong AA, Wilensky AJ, *et al.* Effect of valproate dose on formation of hepatotoxic metabolites. *Epilepsia* 1992; 33: 736.

12. Starko KM, Ray GC, Dominguez LB, Stromberg WL, Woodall DF. Reye's syndrome and salicylate use. *Pediatrics* 1980; 66: 859–864.

13. Hall SM, Plaster PA, Glasgow JFT, *et al.* Admission antipyretics in Reye's syndrome. *Arch Dis Child* 1988; 63: 857–866.

14. Poss WB, Vernon DD, Dean JM. A re-emergence of Reye's syndrome. *Arch Pediatr Adolesc Med* 1994; 148: 879–882.

15. Committee on Safety of Medicines. New advice on aspirin in under 16s. *Curr Probl Pharmacovigilance* 2002; 28: 7.

16. Penna A, Buchanan N. Paracetamol poisoning in children and hepatotoxicity. *Br J Clin Pharmacol* 1991; 32: 143–149.

17. Davis M. Drugs and abnormal liver function tests. *Adv Drug React Bull* 1989; 139: 520–523.

18. Choonara I, Gill A, Nunn A. Drug toxicity and surveillance in children. *Br J Clin Pharmacol* 1996; 42: 407–410.

19. Finlayson NDC. Drugs and the liver. *Medicine Int* 1994; 22: 455–458.

20. Kanathur N, Mathai MG, Byrd RP Jr, Fields CL, Roy TM. Simvastatin-diltiazem drug interaction resulting in rhabdomyolysis and hepatitis. *Tennessee Med* 2001; 94: 339–341.

21. Grattagliano I, Palmieri VO, Palasciano G. Hepatotoxicity of polyunsaturated fatty acids in alcohol abuser. *J Hepatol* 2002; 37: 291–292.

22. Steele MA, Burke RF, Des Prez RM. Toxic hepatitis with isoniazid and rifampicin. A meta-analysis. *Chest* 1991; 99: 465–471.

23. Lee WM. Drug-induced hepatotoxicity. *N Engl J Med* 1995; 333: 1118–1127.

24. Aithal GP, Rawlins MD, Day CP. Clinical diagnostic scale: a useful tool in the evaluation of suspected hepatotoxic adverse drug reactions. *J Hepatol* 2000; 33: 949–952.

25. Ormerod LP, Skinner C, Wales J. Hepatotoxicity of antituberculous drugs. *Thorax* 1996; 51: 111–113.

26. Kenna JG, Neuberger J, Williams R. Evidence for expression in human liver of halothane-induced neoantigens recognised by antibodies in sera from patients with halothane hepatitis. *Hepatology* 1988; 8: 1635–1641.

27. Howard Fee JP, Thompson GH. Comparative tolerability profiles of the inhaled anaesthetics. *Drug Safety* 1997; 16: 157–170.

28. Danan G, Benichou C. Causality assessment of adverse reactions to drugs. I. A novel method based on the conclusions of international consensus meetings: application to drug-induced liver injuries. *J Clin Epidemiol* 1993; 46: 1323–1330.

29. Richer M, Robert S. Fatal hepatotoxicity following oral administration of amiodarone. *Ann Pharmacother* 1995; 29: 582–586.

30. Neuberger J. Selected side-effects: 16. Methotrexate and liver disorders. *Prescribers J* 1995; 35: 158–163.
31. Aithal GP, Haugk B, Das S, *et al.* Monitoring methotrexate-induced hepatic fibrosis in patients with psoriasis: are serial liver biopsies justified? *Aliment Pharmacol Ther* 2004; 19: 391–399.
32. American College of Rheumatology Ad Hoc Committee on Clinical Guidelines. Guidelines for monitoring drug therapy in rheumatoid arthritis. *Arthritis Rheum* 1996; 39: 723–731.
33. Fagan E, Wannan G. Reducing paracetamol overdoses. *Br Med J* 1996; 313: 1417–1418.
34. Vale JA, Proudfoot AT. Paracetamol (acetaminophen) poisoning. *Lancet* 1995; 346: 547–552.
35. Committee on Safety of Medicines. Halothane hepatotoxicity. *Curr Probl Pharmacovigilance* 1986; September.
36. Committee on Safety of Medicines. Reminder: Halothane hepatotoxicity. *Curr Probl Pharmacovigilance* 1997; May.
37. Tolman KG, Chandramouli J. Hepatotoxicity of the thiazolidinediones. *Clin Liver Dis* 2003; 7: 369–379.
38. Ludwig J, McGill DB, Lindor KD. Review: Nonalcoholic steatohepatitis. *J Gastroenterol Hepatol* 1997; 12: 398–403.
39. McCarthy M, Wilkinson ML. Hepatology. *Br Med J* 1999; 318: 1256–1259.
40. Cadman B. Drug induced liver disease. *Hosp Pharm* 1996; 3: 31–35.
41. Styler MJ, Crilley P, Biggs J, *et al.* Hepatic dysfunction following busulfan and cyclophosphamide myeloablation: a retrospective multicentre analysis. *Bone Marrow Transplant* 1996; 18: 171–176.
42. Pittler MH, Ernst E. Hepatotoxic events associated with herbal medicinal products. *Aliment Pharmacol Ther* 2003; 18: 451–471.
43. Maddrey WC. Hepatic vein thrombosis (Budd–Chiari syndrome): possible association with the use of oral contraceptives. *Semin Liver Dis* 1987; 7: 32–39.
44. Valla D, Benhamou JP. Drug-induced vascular and sinusoidal lesions of the liver. *Baillieres Clin Gastroenterol* 1988; 2: 481–500.
45. Committee on Safety of Medicines. Statins and cytochrome P450 interactions. *Curr Probl Pharmacovigilance* 2004; 30: 1–2.

Further reading

Danan G, Benichou C. Causality assessment of adverse reactions to drugs. I. A novel method based on the conclusions of international consensus meetings: application to drug-induced liver injuries. *J Clin Epidemiol* 1993; 46: 1323–1330.
Farrell GC. *Drug-Induced Liver Disease.* Melbourne: Churchill Livingstone, 1994.
Kirchain WR, Gill MA. Drug-induced liver disease. In: DiPiro JT, Talbert RL, Yee GC, *et al.*, eds. *Pharmacotherapy: A Pathophysiologic Approach*, 5th edn. New York: McGraw-Hill, 2002.
Lee WM. Drug-induced hepatotoxicity. *N Engl J Med* 2003; 349: 474–485.
Rashid M, Goldin R, Wright M. Drugs and the liver. *Hosp Med* 2004; 65: 456–461.

8

Renal disorders

Sharon Hems and Aileen Currie

Introduction

Drug-induced renal impairment is an important clinical problem. Studies suggest that up to 30% of cases of acute renal failure are secondary to medication and chemicals, and that 2–5% of hospitalised patients develop drug-induced acute renal impairment.[1-3] In one analysis, medicines contributed to 29% of all cases of acute renal failure in hospital patients, with antibiotics, non-steroidal anti-inflammatory drugs (NSAIDs), angiotensin-converting enzyme (ACE) inhibitors and diuretics most commonly implicated.[3] Hospital-acquired acute renal failure is often due to a combination of factors, such as the use of aminoglycosides in patients with sepsis, or the use of radiocontrast media in patients on ACE inhibitors. Herbal medicines also have the potential to cause renal impairment, notably nephropathy associated with the use of Chinese herbal medicines containing aristolochia.[4]

The kidneys together weigh less than 500 g but receive 25% of cardiac output. They have an essential role in the elimination of many substances, control of fluid and electrolyte balance, and hormonal homoeostasis. They are particularly susceptible to the toxic effects of medicines. Such toxicity may occur through a variety of mechanisms, including direct and indirect biochemical effects as well as immunological effects. The spectrum of drug-induced renal disease is wide: many drugs can cause several types of defect. For example, NSAIDs can cause functional renal insufficiency, interstitial nephritis, glomerulonephritis, oedema, hyponatraemia and hyperkalaemia.

Loss of renal function is often reversible on discontinuation of therapy, but may occasionally lead to end-stage renal failure. Renal dysfunction of any kind is considered a serious reaction and, if suspected to be due to a medicine, should always be reported to the appropriate regulatory authority.

Risk factors

Patients at particular risk of nephrotoxicity include those with pre-existing renal impairment, dehydration, sodium-retaining states such as cirrhosis or heart failure, and specific clinical conditions such as diabetes. Patients receiving multiple nephrotoxic agents and seriously ill patients with sepsis, shock, or failure of multiple body systems are also at increased risk. The elderly appear to be more susceptible to renal toxicity than younger people, possibly because of reduced renal reserve.

Diagnosis of drug-induced renal dysfunction

Several criteria are important in determining whether renal dysfunction has occurred. There is a fall in glomerular filtration rate (GFR), manifest as a rise in blood urea or creatinine. A change in the volume of urine output may also be significant: output may be reduced to less than 400 mL/day (oliguria), or it may be increased (polyuria). Healthy adults may excrete up to 200 mg of protein daily in urine. Heavy proteinuria is usually due to an abnormally permeable glomerular membrane, and suggests glomerular disease.[5] Other causes of proteinuria include reduced tubular reabsorption due to tubular damage, or overflow of proteins present in the plasma at high concentrations.

Routine dipstick testing of the urine for blood, protein and sugar is carried out in all patients suspected of having renal disease. Microscopy of urine may reveal 'casts', which are cylindrical bodies moulded in the shape of the distal tubular lumen.[6] Casts are composed of glycoprotein, cells, cell debris and other proteins. The characteristics of the casts may be helpful: pigmented granular casts are typically found in acute tubular necrosis, white cell casts in interstitial nephritis, and red cell casts in glomerulonephritis.

Imaging techniques such as ultrasonography may be useful in the diagnosis of obstruction or the estimation of renal size. Renal biopsy is of value where a knowledge of the histology will influence management. Tissue should be examined by conventional histochemical staining, electron microscopy and immunofluorescence.

Acute renal failure

In acute renal failure (ARF), kidney function deteriorates rapidly over days or weeks. It is a medical emergency characterised by a rapid rise in serum creatinine and usually accompanied by oliguria, although this is less common in drug-induced ARF.[6] Symptoms are often non-specific and renal failure is commonly diagnosed after incidental observation of elevated creatinine or urea. Hyperkalaemia, hypocalcaemia or hyperphosphataemia may also be present.[7,8]

In the later stages of failure, an accumulation of excess urea and other substances in the blood leads to uraemia and associated symptoms. These include nausea, vomiting, gastrointestinal haemorrhage, muscle cramps, predisposition to infection and decreased consciousness. The overall mortality due to ARF depends on the cause, but averages about 50%; septicaemia is the most common cause of death.

As shown in Figure 8.1, ARF is generally categorised as prerenal, intrarenal or postrenal.

Prerenal failure

Prerenal failure is precipitated by a fall in renal perfusion.[9] Usually renal function returns to normal once the offending drug is withdrawn and perfusion restored. However, if it persists, acute tubular necrosis may develop (see Intrarenal Failure, below). Renal perfusion may decline for a number of reasons, such as volume depletion secondary to excessive use of diuretics or laxatives.[10] Volume depletion may manifest as fatigue, hypotension and muscle cramps. Patients especially at risk include the elderly, those with renal impairment and those receiving other nephrotoxic agents.[11]

Intrarenal failure

This condition arises from changes to the renal infrastructure. It can be subdivided into effects on the GFR, acute interstitial nephritis, acute tubular necrosis and glomerulonephritis.

Effects on the glomerular filtration rate

The GFR is largely controlled by the relative tone of the afferent and efferent arterioles. In the afferent arteriole, tone is mainly mediated by vasodilatory prostaglandins, whereas in the efferent arteriole the renin–angiotensin–aldosterone system is mainly involved. When renal perfusion falls, activation of these systems will help to control the filtration pressure across an individual glomerulus.[1] Angiotensin (AT)-II does this via vasoconstriction of the efferent glomerular arteriole, whereas prostaglandins stimulate vasodilation of the afferent glomerular arteriole.

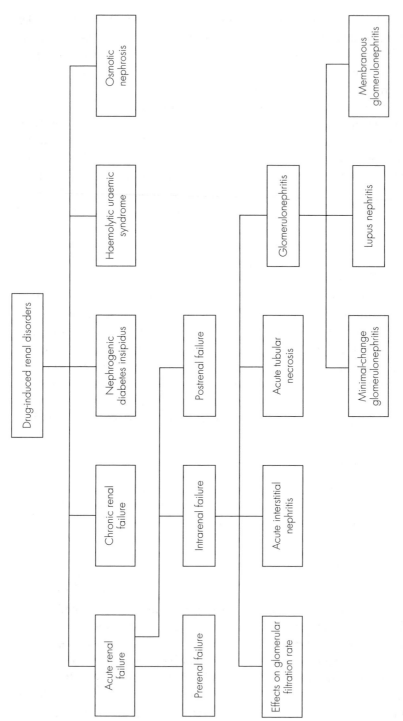

Figure 8.1 Classification of drug-induced renal disorders.

ACE inhibitors and angiotensin-II receptor antagonists   ACE inhibitors prevent the conversion of angiotensin-I to angiotensin-II in the renin–angiotensin–aldosterone system. Angiotensin-II is a potent vasoconstrictor of the systemic and the renal vascular bed. Consequently, ACE inhibitors produce systemic and renal vasodilation, resulting in decreased blood pressure and increased renal blood flow. As renal vasodilation is mainly mediated by the efferent arteriole, filtration pressure is reduced by ACE inhibition. The lower filtration pressure does not automatically lead to a reduction in GFR, but this may occur in some situations.[12] Patients at risk include those with renal artery stenosis, particularly bilateral stenoses, those with severe cardiac failure and those receiving NSAIDs or diuretics. The overall incidence of ARF in patients taking ACE inhibitors is less than 1%. However, it increases to 25% in those with bilateral renal disease; it is therefore essential to monitor renal function regularly both before and during therapy in at-risk patients.

Several angiotensin-II receptors have been identified, but the haemodynamic effects of angiotensin-II appear to be mediated mainly via AT1 receptor stimulation.[13] Most clinical data suggests that angiotensin-II receptor antagonists, which inhibit binding of angiotensin II to the AT1 receptor, exert the same systemic and renal haemodynamic effects as ACE inhibitors. These agents should therefore be used with the same precautions as ACE inhibitors.

NSAIDs   NSAIDs vary in their selectivity for inhibiting different types of cyclooxygenase. Conventional NSAIDs inhibit both isoforms of cyclooxygenase (COX-1 and COX-2), an enzyme that converts arachidonic acid to prostaglandins. Where renal blood flow is decreased, vasodilatory prostaglandins E_2, D_2 and I_2 (prostacyclin) protect against renal ischaemia by antagonising vasoconstrictor substances. In some circumstances, when renal blood flow is already compromised, as in congestive cardiac failure or cirrhosis, the inhibition of prostaglandin production by NSAID therapy can precipitate an acute fall in GFR. Mild cases are manifest only as increased serum creatinine or hypertension due to salt and water retention, but ARF can occur. NSAIDs have been associated with 7% of all cases of ARF and 36% of drug-related cases.[14] Functional renal insufficiency is the most common adverse renal effect of NSAIDs. Patients who are volume depleted or those with pre-existing renal impairment are also particularly susceptible.[15]

Until recently COX-1 was believed to be responsible for the synthesis of renal prostaglandins.[16] It was therefore thought that selective COX-2 inhibitors, such as celecoxib and rofecoxib, would not produce the renal adverse effects associated with conventional NSAIDs. However, studies suggest that COX-2 may be important in regulating renal perfusion and glomerular haemodynamics. The GFR has been shown to fall in young and elderly sodium-depleted individuals receiving selective COX-2 inhibitors. Selective COX-2 inhibitors have also been associated with ARF in elderly patients with comorbid conditions such as chronic renal insufficiency, cardiomyopathy or diabetic nephropathy. Further investigation is needed to determine the frequency of nephrotoxicity with COX-2 inhibitors, and whether there are differences between the individual agents.[17] Clinical experience indicates, however, that conventional NSAIDs and selective COX-2 inhibitors exert similar effects on renal haemodynamics and homoeostasis. Therefore, the same precautions should be applied to selective COX-2 inhibitors as to NSAIDs when used in patients at risk of nephrotoxic events.[18,19]

Acute interstitial nephritis

Acute interstitial nephritis (AIN) is a hypersensitivity reaction characterised by interstitial inflammation and tubular damage. It is found in 15% of all biopsy specimens performed for investigation of ARF, and is often drug induced.[20] ARF normally occurs within 2 weeks of drug exposure.[21] The signs and symptoms are fever, skin rash, arthralgias, gross haematuria, blood eosinophilia and a variable degree of ARF. However, studies suggest that the classic triad of fever, rash and eosinophilia occurs in fewer than 30% of cases.[1,22,23] Mild proteinuria and microscopic haematuria are always present, with urinary white and red cell casts. Proteinuria within the nephrotic range is almost exclusively found in NSAID-related acute interstitial nephritis. The renal failure is often non-oliguric and dialysis is required in about a third of patients. Most patients recover fully following withdrawal of the nephrotoxin, but in over a third of cases renal failure continues to deteriorate after the causative drug has been withdrawn.[20] The recovery of renal function may take several months, and is dependent on how long renal failure had been present before the discovery of AIN. Although evidence for their use is limited, corticosteroids may be prescribed to shorten recovery time if spontaneous recovery does not occur within 10 days of drug withdrawal.[24] Steroids should be discontinued if no response is obtained after up to 4 weeks of treatment. Many medicines have been implicated in AIN, of which the most common are beta-lactam antibiotics and NSAIDs (Table 8.1).

Table 8.1 Some drugs associated with acute interstitial nephritis

Allopurinol	Non-steroidal
Azathioprine	anti-inflammatory drugs
Captopril	Omeprazole
Cephalosporins	Penicillins
Cimetidine	Phenobarbital
Co-trimoxazole	Phenytoin
Erythromycin	Pyrazinamide
Fluoroquinolones	Rifampicin
Furosemide	Sulfonamides
Isoniazid	Thiazides
Methyldopa	Vancomycin
Minocycline	

Beta-lactam antibiotics   Beta-lactams give the most characteristic picture of drug-induced AIN.[23] Many cases of methicillin-induced AIN were reported during the 1970s. The incidence of renal dysfunction ranged between 12 and 20% of patients treated. Symptoms of AIN appeared between 2 and 60 days after the start of treatment. Fever often occurred, and about half of affected adults had an increased blood urea. Macroscopic haematuria, skin rash, blood eosinophilia and eosinophiluria were present in one-third of patients. More than 90% of affected patients recovered. Other penicillin derivatives linked to AIN are ampicillin, amoxicillin, benzylpenicillin and piperacillin, although the problem is comparatively rare with these agents. Renal and extrarenal symptoms may recur if the patient is rechallenged with the same or chemically related drugs. All beta-lactam antibiotics are best avoided in anyone who has developed AIN during treatment with a penicillin or cephalosporin. Cephalosporins are a rare cause of AIN.

NSAIDs   NSAIDs are a recognised cause of AIN, but the clinical picture is different from that seen with beta-lactam antibiotics. There may be no symptoms or signs of hypersensitivity, and renal insufficiency has a progressive onset, discovered several months or years after the start of treatment. Extrarenal signs are rare. More than 80% of patients with NSAID-induced AIN develop a nephrotic syndrome; with beta-lactams this occurs in less than 1% of patients.[25] In biopsies the glomeruli show minimal change. Minimal-change nephrotic syndrome without AIN has also been reported with many NSAIDs (see Minimal-Change Glomerulonephritis, p. 229). AIN has been reported with celecoxib and rofecoxib, and demonstrates the need for caution with the use of COX-2 inhibitors in high-risk patients.[26–28]

Allopurinol AIN has also been described in association with the allopurinol hypersensitivity syndrome, where additional symptoms include rash, hepatotoxicity, fever, eosinophilia and leukocytosis.[29,30] The syndrome usually develops within 6 weeks of starting therapy, although this is variable, and overall mortality is about 25%. Fortunately, the syndrome is rare, although it has been described in patients with renal impairment in whom the drug dose has not been reduced appropriately. This results in accumulation of allopurinol and its metabolite (oxipurinol), and a hypersensitivity reaction to the metabolite develops.[30]

Rifampicin Rifampicin-induced AIN usually occurs following intermittent therapy, and is a dose-dependent effect.[24] It is thought that anti-rifampicin antibodies, still detectable weeks to months after rifampicin withdrawal, stimulate an immunological reaction when the drug is reintroduced.[24,31] Initial symptoms often include an influenza-like illness (fever, malaise, chills, myalgia, headache), typically following 3–6 months of intermittent therapy.[32] These symptoms generally develop within 2 hours of rifampicin administration and resolve within 8 hours. Intermittent rifampicin therapy should therefore be avoided and patients previously exposed to rifampicin should be closely monitored on re-exposure.

Aristolochia Chinese-herb nephropathy, first identified in 1992, is characterised by rapidly progressive fibrosing interstitial nephritis.[33] In Belgium, in 1993, over 70 cases of renal failure were reported due to the presence of aristolochia in a slimming regimen that contained Chinese herbs. Aristolochia species contain aristolochic acids, which are genotoxic carcinogens and associated with interstitial nephropathy. It was banned in the UK in 1999 following a review of safety information, including two cases of end-stage renal failure in patients using Chinese herbal medicines for eczema.[4,34]

Aminosalicylates Interstitial nephritis has been reported more frequently with mesalazine than with sulfasalazine, the incidence ranging from 1 in 150 and 0 in 500 patients treated, to renal impairment with increased serum creatinine in 0.2% of 2940 patients.[35] Renal impairment has been associated with higher mesalazine doses, and tubular proteinuria has occurred in up to one-third of patients treated with doses over 3 g daily.

In patients receiving mesalazine it has been suggested that serum urea and creatinine levels should be monitored every 4 weeks for the first 3 months, then every 3 months up to 1 year and annually thereafter. Where renal impairment has occurred, the available evidence suggests that renal function returns to normal if drug therapy is withdrawn early, with 85% of cases of renal impairment resolving where treatment was stopped within 10 months.

Acute tubular necrosis

Acute tubular necrosis (ATN) is the most common drug-induced renal disease. The most important causes are aminoglycosides, amphotericin, cisplatin, ciclosporin and radiocontrast agents (Table 8.2).[10] These drugs produce a direct toxic effect on the renal tubule, resulting in necrosis of the tubular cells. However, ATN may also result from persistent renal hypoperfusion, which causes ischaemic tubular cell damage and necrosis.[1,7]

Acyclic nucleoside phosphonates The acyclic nucleoside phosphonates cidofovir and adefovir have been associated with significant nephrotoxicity, ranging from isolated proximal tubular defects and Fanconi-like syndrome to severe ATN requiring renal replacement therapy.[36,37] Cidofovir is a nucleotide analogue of cytosine that forms cidofovir-phosphocholine (an analogue of cytidine 5-diphosphocholine) in cells. It is thought that cidofovir-phosphocholine interferes with the synthesis and/or degradation of membrane phospholipids, producing proximal tubular injury and, in severe cases, cell necrosis. Adefovir is a nucleotide analogue of adenine that undergoes mono- and diphosphorylation in cells. It then interferes with a number of adenosine triphosphate (ATP)-related processes: ATP synthesis, ATP-dependent processes, and/or transport of adenine nucleotides.[37] Co-treatment with probenecid and prior hydration with intravenous fluids can minimise the nephrotoxicity of these agents.

Table 8.2 Some drugs associated with acute tubular necrosis

Amphotericin	Gentamicin
Ciclosporin	Methotrexate
Ciprofloxacin	Radiocontrast agents
Cisplatin	Rifampicin

Tenofovir disoproxil fumarate (DF) is structurally similar to cidofovir and adefovir but was thought to be minimally nephrotoxic.[37] However, two cases of ARF and tubular injury have recently been reported. Tenofovir should therefore be avoided, or used with caution at a significantly reduced dose and monitoring, in patients with chronic renal disease.

Aminoglycoside antibiotics Aminoglycoside antibiotics cause transient renal failure in 10–30% of patients and are the cause of half of all cases of drug-induced ARF in hospitals.[38] Clinical features include mild elevation of creatinine accompanied by normal urine output (non-oliguric renal failure). Serum creatinine levels typically increase after 3–5 days of treatment, but occasionally ARF may only become apparent after treatment is stopped.

The major site of aminoglycoside damage is the proximal renal tubule. The exact mechanism of nephrotoxicity is unclear, but accumulation of drug and phospholipids within lysosomes is involved. The lysosomes become overloaded with phospholipid, destabilise and rupture, releasing acid hydrolases and high concentrations of aminoglycoside into the cytoplasm, where they disrupt cell structure and function.[39] The toxic potential of individual aminoglycosides is directly related to their capacity to disrupt lysosomal membrane function. It has been suggested that the aminoglycosides may be ranked in decreasing order of nephrotoxicity as follows: gentamicin > tobramycin > amikacin > netilmicin, although the differences may only be marginal.

It is essential that plasma drug concentrations and renal function are monitored throughout aminoglycoside therapy and doses adjusted as appropriate. Gentamicin is the most frequently implicated, with 6–26% of recipients developing renal impairment within 10 days of treatment.[40] Development of renal failure is dependent on the dose and duration of therapy, as well as the presence of risk factors such as renal or hepatic disease, or concurrent administration of other nephrotoxic agents[41,42] (Table 8.3). Renal function usually recovers completely when aminoglycosides are withdrawn, although this may take several weeks.

The approach to aminoglycoside dosing has moved towards the use of larger doses given less frequently. It is believed that once-daily dosing will lead to reduced tissue accumulation and so decrease the incidence of nephrotoxicity. However, there is no agreed way of monitoring aminoglycoside concentrations to ensure optimum efficacy and safety with once-daily dosing.[43]

Amphotericin Parenteral amphotericin still has an important role in the management of systemic fungal infections, but dose-dependent

Table 8.3 Risk factors for aminoglycoside nephrotoxicity

Choice of aminoglycoside	High total dose of aminoglycoside
Concurrent liver disease	Hypotension
Concurrent use of other nephrotoxic drugs	Volume depletion
High peak or trough serum concentrations	

nephrotoxicity occurs to some degree in almost all patients receiving the drug.[44] Toxicity may be manifest as a decrease in renal blood flow and GFR with increased serum creatinine, distal renal tubular acidosis, and renal tubular potassium, sodium and magnesium wasting into urine. Toxicity may occur with doses as low as 300 mg, and the prevalence is about 80% with cumulative doses approaching 4 g. Risk factors include high mean daily doses, diuretic use and volume depletion, and abnormal baseline renal function.[45,46] The risk of nephrotoxicity may be minimised by volume repletion and administration with an intravenous saline load. Preparations of amphotericin in which the drug is encapsulated in, or available as a complex with, liposomes are less toxic.[47] If nephrotoxicity occurs, the drug should be stopped. Renal tubular dysfunction and glomerular filtration will improve in most patients, although in some cases damage may be irreversible.

Radiocontrast media   The incidence of nephrotoxicity associated with radiocontrast agents varies from 0.6% in patients with normal renal function and to as high as 50% in high-risk patients. The pathogenesis of contrast nephropathy includes both direct tubular nephropathy and renal ischaemia. Pre-existing renal impairment is the major risk factor, present in 60% of cases, but other factors may be implicated, such as congestive heart failure, myeloma and dehydration.[8] Renal failure usually develops within 24 hours of administration of the radiocontrast agent, with serum creatinine concentrations reaching a maximum within 4 days, followed by gradual recovery within 10 days.

Contrast nephropathy can be prevented by using alternative imaging procedures in high-risk patients. If contrast media must be used, the smallest adequate dose, preferably of a low-osmolality agent, should be administered. In addition, it has been recommended that patients at risk should receive intravenous fluids (0.9% or 0.45% saline) before and after administration of these agents to protect against ARF.[48–51] In patients able to take oral fluids, hydration can be achieved through ingestion of fluid before and after the procedure. Allowing at least 48 hours to elapse between procedures in which contrast material is used allows the kidneys to recover. Recent trials using acetylcysteine have shown it to be protective against contrast-agent-induced nephrotoxicity. It is believed that it may help prevent direct oxidative tissue damage, through its ability to scavenge oxygen free radicals. Although not all studies have shown a protective effect, several randomised placebo-controlled trials have found that administration of acetylcysteine prevented a significant rise in creatinine in patients with underlying renal insufficiency who received low doses of contrast agent.[51] A recent review concluded that acetylcysteine may be recommended to prevent ARF in at-risk patients receiving radiocontrast media.[52] It should be administered orally (600 mg twice daily on the day before and the day of the procedure). In addition, adequate hydration should be maintained before and after contrast administration.

Glomerulonephritis

Glomerulonephritis is a disorder in which there is immunologically mediated damage to the glomeruli of both kidneys. There are several forms of glomerulonephritis, including membranous, minimal-change glomerulonephritis and lupus nephritis.[9] Drug-induced glomerulonephritis may present as proteinuria which, if prolonged and severe (usually >3.5 g/day), leads to oedema and hypoalbuminaemia; this is known as nephrotic syndrome.[9,52]

Membranous glomerulonephritis In membranous glomerulonephritis, antigens stimulate the production of antibodies and then combine with them to form an immune complex. The immune complex deposits in the kidney to produce thickening of the capillary basement membrane. This form of glomerulonephritis has been described in association with gold and penicillamine therapy.[6] Genetic factors appear to be important in conferring susceptibility.

With gold therapy, proteinuria has been described in 2–19% of patients.[53] Onset is usually within the first 6 months of treatment, but appears to be unrelated to the daily or cumulative dose. It is more common with parenteral than with oral gold therapy. Usually renal function remains normal and proteinuria resolves 6–12 months following drug withdrawal.[21,53] However, about 10–30% of affected patients develop nephrotic syndrome, usually with membranous glomerulonephritis as the underlying pathology.[53,54] To minimise the risk of complications, urinalysis must be carried out regularly during gold therapy and treatment discontinued if severe proteinuria develops.

Penicillamine causes proteinuria in up to 30% of patients, usually within the first 12 months. The incidence is dose related. The problem usually resolves within 6–12 months after drug withdrawal.[1,52] However, as proteinuria often remits with continued treatment, therapy may be continued as long as renal function remains normal, oedema is absent, and urinary protein excretion does not exceed 2 g/24 hours.

Membranous glomerulonephritis is found in 12% of patients treated with penicillamine and 85% of those with penicillamine-induced nephrotic syndrome.[52,55] Urinalysis should be conducted regularly throughout therapy.

Minimal-change glomerulonephritis In minimal-change glomerulonephritis, light microscopy of biopsy tissue shows normal glomeruli but electron microscopy reveals abnormal epithelial cells.[6] It is most commonly observed with NSAIDs, especially in patients with renal failure and elderly patients on diuretics.[1,52] The nephrotic syndrome develops following 2 weeks to 2 years of therapy, and usually disappears following drug withdrawal, although this may take several weeks.[24] Steroids may assist recovery, but progression to chronic renal failure has been described despite their administration.

Lupus nephritis More than 50 drugs have been associated with a syndrome resembling the autoimmune disease systemic lupus erythematosus (SLE).[55] In the US, about 10% of cases of SLE are estimated to be drug related, and symptoms resemble those of the spontaneously occurring disease: antinuclear antibodies are present, and there may be fever, arthralgia, rashes, pleurisy, pleural effusions and pericarditis. Renal involvement in drug-induced SLE (lupus nephritis) is rare (about 5%), and the disease usually resolves following drug withdrawal.[1,55,56]

Lupus erythematosus was recognised with hydralazine in the 1950s, and has been reported in 10–20% of patients, of whom 2–20% have renal involvement.[2,57] The risk is increased in women, patients who are slow acetylators or possess the HLA-DR4 genotype, and following prolonged therapy, particularly if doses exceed 100 mg daily.[2] Acetylator status should be determined if the dose is to be increased beyond 100 mg daily. Initial symptoms of lupus nephritis may include microhaematuria, proteinuria, and positive titres of antinuclear factors, and regular urinalysis is therefore important during long-term therapy.

Procainamide is the commonest cause of drug-induced SLE, with antinuclear antibodies appearing in 50–100% of patients, of whom

5–30% develop signs and symptoms of SLE.[57] Usually the lupus-like syndrome appears after 2–6 months of therapy, more commonly in slow acetylators. There have been several reports of lupus nephritis associated with procainamide, but this appears to occur less frequently than with hydralazine.[56,57]

Postrenal failure

Postrenal failure results from urinary tract obstruction. It may develop during chemotherapy, when the breakdown of tumour cells leads to over-production of uric acid, which precipitates and blocks the renal tubules. This can be prevented by prior administration of allopurinol, which inhibits uric acid production, and by ensuring adequate hydration and alkalinisation of the urine.

Obstruction may also occur from precipitation of the drug itself. For example, aciclovir crystals may precipitate in the renal collecting tubules following intravenous administration, because of the drug's low solubility.[55,58] The incidence of aciclovir-associated renal failure has been reported as 12–48%. Risk factors include bolus administration, pre-existing renal impairment, hypovolaemia and high dosage. Crystal nephropathy often develops within 24–48 hours of aciclovir administration and usually resolves following drug withdrawal and volume resuscitation.[37] With high-dose intravenous aciclovir, adequate hydration and slow infusion are essential to prevent crystallisation. Similarly, methotrexate or its metabolites may precipitate in the renal tubules when administered in high doses. Adequate hydration and alkalinisation of the urine is recommended to avoid this problem.

Renal calculi

Drug-induced calculi represent 1–2% of all renal calculi. The drugs implicated include poorly soluble drugs with high urine excretion that favours crystallisation in the urine; and drugs that provoke urinary calculi as a result of their metabolic effects, such as calcium/vitamin D supplements, furosemide and aluminium-containing preparations.[59]

For many years sulfonamides have been known to cause obstructive nephropathy because of the formation of crystals, which obstruct the urinary tract, leading to haematuria, renal colic and anuria.[60] The risk of nephrotoxicity depends on the solubility of the sulfonamide, the dose, the presence of pre-existing renal impairment, dehydration or low urinary pH. Older agents such as sulfadiazine and sulfapyridine are more likely to cause these problems than newer, more soluble sulfonamides such as sulfamethoxazole. Sulfamethoxazole is frequently associated with crystalluria, but this is rarely responsible for obstructive uropathy.[59] Obstructive nephropathy has been reported in patients with HIV infection treated with high doses of sulfonamides for *Pneumocystis carinii* pneumonia infection or toxoplasma encephalitis.[61]

The protease inhibitor indinavir is now the leading cause of drug-induced nephrolithiasis (kidney stone formation). The initial prescribing information for indinavir mentioned its potential to cause urinary calculi. However, it soon became clear that the incidence was higher than at first thought, with as many as 40% of treated patients affected.[59] The clinical presentation of indinavir-associated nephrolithiasis includes renal colic, flank or loin pain, or dysuria.[37] Indinavir renal stones result from precipitation and crystallisation of the drug (as indinavir monohydrate) in the collecting tubule owing to its low solubility at physiologic pH.[62] Approximately 20% of patients receiving indinavir will develop crystalluria that is usually asymptomatic, whereas the incidence of nephrolithiasis has been reported as 3.6–12.4%.[63–65] It has been suggested that crystalluria precedes nephrolithiasis. Usually symptoms resolve with increased fluid intake and analgesia, although there is a risk of recurrence. Indinavir stones may be passed spontaneously or removed by urologic procedures to control pain or relieve urinary obstruction.[37] The majority of cases of renal failure associated with indinavir have been mild and reversible, although more severe renal failure due to obstructing indinavir calculi and chronic kidney disease have also been described. Patients on indinavir therapy should be advised to drink at least 2–3 L of fluid daily to maintain high urinary flow rates and prevent crystal deposition in the kidneys. The dose should be reduced in severe hepatic impairment. Usually nephrotoxicity reverses when indinavir is withdrawn.

Rhabdomyolysis

In rhabdomyolysis acute muscle damage occurs, causing the release of cell contents such as myoglobin, enzymes and electrolytes into the circulation.[66] Several mechanisms have been suggested to explain the ensuing ARF, such as impaired renal vascular flow, or tubular obstruction by myoglobin casts or urate crystals.[67] At urinary pH less than 5.6, myoglobin is converted to ferrihaem, which may act as a direct tubular cell toxin or may precipitate and obstruct the tubules. Alternatively, it may be that by scavenging vasodilatory nitric oxide, myoglobin produces intrarenal vasoconstriction and ARF.

Table 8.4 Some drugs associated with rhabdomyolysis

Amphotericin	Lithium
Barbiturates	Monoamine oxidase inhibitors
Benzodiazepines	Opioids
Cimetidine	Phenothiazines
Colchicine	Retinoids
Co-trimoxazole	Statins
Fibrates	Theophylline

It has been estimated that about 30% of patients with rhabdomyolysis develop ARF.[66] Drugs have been implicated in about 80% of cases of rhabdomyolysis, with alcohol accounting for at least 20% (Table 8.4).[67] The risk of rhabdomyolysis in association with lipid-lowering agents (fibrates and statins) is recognised.[68] The incidence of rhabdomyolysis with statin monotherapy is 0.04–0.2%, with case reports describing occurrence following 2 weeks to 5 years of therapy.[69] Presenting symptoms include muscle pain, weakness, tenderness or cramps. The risk of statin-induced myopathy is increased in patients with renal impairment, untreated hypothyroidism, alcohol abuse, and age >70 years. The risk is also increased by concomitant use of other lipid-lowering agents, e.g. fibrates or nicotinic acid, or drugs that can increase plasma levels of statins through cytochrome P450 interactions, e.g. macrolide antibiotics, ciclosporin, azole antifungals and protease inhibitors. Patients receiving any statin should be asked to report muscle pain, weakness or cramp to the prescriber immediately, especially if accompanied by malaise, fever or dark urine. Patients experiencing any of these symptoms should stop therapy and have their creatine kinase (CK) level measured. If the CK level is significantly elevated (>5 times upper limit of normal) or if symptoms are severe, statin therapy should be withheld.

Retroperitoneal fibrosis

Bromocriptine, pergolide, methysergide and other ergot derivatives and beta-blockers have been implicated in retroperitoneal fibrosis.[70,71] This is characterised by fibrosis over the posterior abdominal wall and retroperitoneum.[6] The ureters become embedded in the fibrous tissue, resulting in an obstructive uropathy. Symptoms of retroperitoneal fibrosis may include malaise, fatigue, back pain, weight loss, abdominal pain, flank pain and dysuria.[70] Because of the hazards, continuous therapy with methysergide should not exceed 6 months without a drug-free period of at least 1 month. Although retroperitoneal fibrosis usually recedes following drug withdrawal, it may progress and require corticosteroid therapy or surgery.[55]

Ergot-derived dopamine receptor agonists (bromocriptine, cabergoline, lisuride, pergolide) may cause pulmonary, retroperitoneal and pericardial fibrotic reactions.[72] Of these ergot-derivatives, pergolide appears to be associated with a higher reporting rate of such reactions. Progression of fibrosis can be prevented by early diagnosis and withdrawal of treatment. Patients should be monitored for dyspnoea, persistent cough, chest pain, cardiac failure, and abdominal pain or tenderness. Before starting treatment it may be appropriate to perform baseline investigations such as erythrocyte sedimentation rate, serum creatinine and chest X-ray. Lung function tests may also be helpful if long-term treatment is anticipated.

Chronic renal failure

Chronic renal failure (CRF) is defined as a gradual deterioration in renal function developing over months or years. Typical signs and symptoms are shown in Table 8.5.[5] Analgesic nephropathy is the commonest drug cause. Long-term abuse or use of analgesics for chronic pain disorders, such as rheumatoid arthritis, can lead to chronic interstitial nephritis and renal papillary necrosis.[15] The problem was identified in the early 1950s and phenacetin was the first drug to be incriminated. However, the problem has not resolved with phenacetin's withdrawal. Studies have shown that analgesic nephropathy is usually associated with combinations of paracetamol with salicylates, codeine or caffeine. The mechanism involved is not clear, but is thought to involve the generation of reactive metabolites. Stopping analgesic use generally results in stabilisation or improvement of renal function, whereas continued use leads to progressive renal damage.[2]

Abuse of compound analgesics is more common in women and has been attributed to the presence of addictive substances, such as caffeine.

Table 8.5 Signs and symptoms associated with chronic renal failure

Anaemia	Oedema
Breathlessness	Paraesthesia
Drowsiness	Polyuria
Electrolyte disturbances (e.g. hyperkalaemia, hypocalcaemia)	Pruritus
	Renal bone disease
Hypertension	Restless legs syndrome
Malaise	Seizures
Muscle cramps	Tiredness
Nausea/vomiting	

In contrast, abuse of single-component analgesics (paracetamol, aspirin, codeine, NSAIDs) and nephropathy secondary to their chronic use, is rare.[10,73] Paracetamol has been implicated more often than NSAIDs or aspirin. The low doses of aspirin used for its antiplatelet effect are unlikely to affect the kidneys in this way.[74]

The prevalence of analgesic nephropathy varies widely throughout the world. Surveys have shown that the percentage of patients with end-stage renal disease (ESRD) associated with analgesic abuse is as high as 36% in Belgium and as low as 0.07–0.4% in the UK.[75] In Australia, in the 1970s, a quarter of all patients commencing dialysis had developed renal failure secondary to analgesic nephropathy.[10] In Australia, Sweden and Canada, the withdrawal of over-the-counter sales of compound analgesics significantly reduced the incidence of analgesic nephropathy.[15] This led to an ad hoc committee of the US National Kidney Foundation recommending that compound analgesics should be available only on prescription, and that all NSAIDs and compound analgesics should be clearly labelled with a warning about the risk of nephrotoxicity.

Nephrogenic diabetes insipidus

In nephrogenic diabetes insipidus the renal tubules are partially or totally resistant to the effects of antidiuretic hormone (ADH, vasopressin), resulting in polyuria and polydipsia.[76] Unlike central diabetes insipidus, it does not respond to desmopressin. It has been described in association with lithium, which reduces the responsiveness of the kidney to ADH. This impairs the kidney's ability to concentrate urine, causing polyuria in up to one-third of patients. Polyuria often occurs shortly after commencing lithium therapy, with symptoms such as polydipsia, extreme thirst and dry mouth. Urine volumes of about 3–4 L in 24 hours may be produced and indometacin may be prescribed to control polyuria.[77] Nephrogenic, lithium-induced diabetes insipidus is diagnosed when diuresis increases above these values. The decline in urine concentrating ability is probably progressive over the first 10 years of therapy.[78] However, although initially functional and reversible, renal dysfunction may become structural and irreversible with long-term treatment.[79] The elderly are particularly at risk for nephrogenic diabetes insipidus, and coadministration of other drugs, such as tricyclic antidepressants, may also sensitise patients to nephrogenic polyuria. Recommendations to reduce the risk of renal dysfunction include monitoring serum lithium levels to achieve optimal efficacy at the lowest possible concentration. In addition, serum creatinine levels should be monitored regularly during therapy.

Demeclocycline also produces a reversible, dose-dependent nephrogenic diabetes insipidus. In this case, however, the 'adverse effect' has been put to therapeutic use in the management of hyponatraemia caused by the syndrome of inappropriate antidiuretic hormone secretion (SIADH).

Haemolytic uraemic syndrome

The haemolytic uraemic syndrome (HUS) is associated with the production of microthrombi in the renal arterioles and glomeruli, with symptoms including haemolytic anaemia, thrombocytopenia and ARF.[9,80] It usually affects young children following gastrointestinal infection with shiga toxin-producing *Escherichia coli*. However, 'atypical' HUS, which may occur due to a number of factors, including drugs, accounts for 11% of patients with HUS. Thrombotic thrombocytopenic purpura (TTP) may also be caused by shiga toxin-producing *E. coli*, but usually affects adults. Approximately 40% of patients with TTP will present with renal impairment, thrombocytopenia, microangiopathic haemolytic anaemia, neurological abnormalities and fever, and 75% will have anaemia, thrombocytopenia and neurological abnormalities. The clinical features of TTP and HUS are similar, and they are therefore sometimes described as a single disorder (TTP-HUS) in adults. HUS has been associated with ciclosporin, oral contraceptives and, in children, metronidazole.[55] A number of chemotherapeutic agents (gemcitabine, cisplatin, bleomycin, mitomycin) have also been associated with this syndrome.[81] The incidence of HUS following mitomycin is 2–15%, but it occurs much less frequently with other chemotherapeutic agents. Chemotherapy-associated HUS has a case-fatality rate of 50–70%. Glucocorticoids and plasma infusion may be used initially, but plasma exchange is the mainstay of treatment.

The first reports of quinine-induced HUS appeared in 1991.[82] Unlike HUS due to other drugs, with quinine the problem is immune mediated. Quinine-dependent antibodies directed against red cells, granulocytes and platelets have been demonstrated.[83] Treatment with corticosteroids and plasma exchange has been suggested. The prognosis is often favourable, with many reports documenting normal renal function at follow-up. However, a more recent case series reported that three of 17 patients (18%) diagnosed with TTP/HUS died during initial hospitalisation. Eight of 14 patients who survived the initial episode developed CRF.[84] Because quinine is widely consumed, either as a treatment for muscle cramps or in drinks such as tonic water and bitter lemon, careful questioning of the patient is vital in order to identify quinine as a possible cause of HUS.

Table 8.6 Some drugs for which regular renal function monitoring is recommended

Aminoglycoside antibiotics (systemic)	Cisplatin
Amphotericin	Cyclophosphamide
Angiotensin-converting enzyme inhibitors	Gold (injectable and oral)
Angiotensin-II receptor antagonists	Methotrexate
Carboplatin	Penicillamine
Chlorambucil	Tacrolimus
Ciclosporin	Vancomycin

Osmotic nephrosis

Intravenous immunoglobulin (IVIG) has been associated with osmotic nephropathy in older patients and those with pre-existing renal disease.[37] Osmotic nephrosis is recognised by proximal tubular cell swelling and vacuolisation, together with tubular luminal occlusion from swollen tubular cells. ARF developed after approximately 3 days of therapy with IVIG, and was usually oliguric. The duration of renal impairment was about 2 weeks, and renal replacement therapy was required in one-third of patients. In 84% of cases ARF was reversible and renal function returned to baseline following withdrawal of IVIG therapy. Sandoglobulin, which contains sucrose as the stablilising agent, was the brand of IVIG used in more than 80% of cases and it has been suggested that this plays a role in the development of ARF. It seems likely that renal injury in the majority of patients treated with IVIG is caused by the uptake of sucrose into proximal tubular cells, which can lead to narrowing and occlusion of the tubular lumina. A reduction in nephrotoxicity may be achieved by avoiding IVIG, which uses sucrose as a stabiliser, and sucrose-containing IVIG preparations should be used cautiously in patients with pre-existing renal impairment and older age. Limiting the dose of IVIG or increasing the dosing interval may also benefit these patients.

Conclusion

Many drugs can cause renal failure, from mild reversible to severe irreversible. Some drugs for which renal function monitoring is recommended are shown in Table 8.6. There is a wide spectrum of renal lesions, and many drugs can produce more than one type. A knowledge and understanding of the pathogenesis assists early diagnosis and prevents unnecessary interventions.

CASE STUDY 8.1

Mr BC is a 70-year-old man admitted to an orthopaedic ward with a fractured neck of femur. He has a past medical history of asthma and hypertension. His current medication consists of:

Salbutamol MDI inhaler 100 µg/puff, 2 puffs when required for shortness of breath
Beclometasone MDI inhaler 100 µg/puff, 2 puffs twice daily
Bendroflumethiazide 2.5 mg in the morning
Aspirin 75 mg daily
Simvastatin 40 mg at night.

After surgery, Mr BC is commenced on diclofenac 50 mg three times a day when required for pain relief. Three days later (Friday), he develops a wound infection and is started on intravenous gentamicin 80 mg three times daily. On Monday, urea, electrolytes and serum gentamicin concentrations are measured. They are reported as:

Sodium 134 mmol/L
Potassium 5 mmol/L
Bicarbonate 22 mmol/L
Urea 15 mmol/L
Creatinine 210 µmol/L
Gentamicin trough concentration 4 mg/L (target <2 mg/L)
Gentamicin peak concentration 17 mg/L (target 5–10 mg/L)
Patient's body weight 60 kg.

Mr BC is reviewed by the renal team and the diclofenac and gentamicin are discontinued. His renal function slowly recovers.

What may have caused the renal impairment?

Mr BC may have developed interstitial nephritis secondary to gentamicin. Gentamicin exerts a nephrotoxic effect as a result of the accumulation of drug and phospholipids within lysosomes. These become overloaded and rupture, releasing acid hydrolases and high concentrations of aminoglycoside into the cytoplasm, causing disruption of the cell structure and function. This produces damage within the proximal renal tubule. Aminoglycosides in general account for a high proportion of hospital-acquired ARF, with gentamicin being the most nephrotoxic.

Risk factors are:

- Dose and duration of treatment
- Concomitant renal or hepatic disease

→

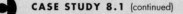

CASE STUDY 8.1 (continued)

- Other nephrotoxins, e.g. diclofenac
- Hypotension
- Volume depletion
- Elderly (reduced renal reserve)
- Various disease states, for example heart failure, cirrhosis, diabetes, sepsis
- Renal ischaemia.

How should gentamicin be monitored?

Baseline urea and electrolytes should be checked before commencing gentamicin to ensure that the patient does not have renal impairment. Gentamicin concentrations should be measured when steady state is achieved, after 24 hours of therapy. The dose or frequency should be adjusted according to serum gentamicin and creatinine concentrations. The peak gentamicin concentration should be measured 60 minutes after the dose, and the trough concentration just before the dose is given.

It has been reported that 25% of courses of gentamicin are complicated by ARF, even when appropriate levels are maintained.

What other gentamicin dose schedules are available?

Theoretically gentamicin should be less nephrotoxic when given as a single daily dose of 3–7 mg/kg (ideal body weight) instead of 3–5 mg/kg daily in three divided doses, as the transport mechanism for gentamicin into the renal cortex is saturable. Single daily dosing has the advantage of a simpler blood sampling routine: the concentration is measured after 6–14 hours and analysed against the Hartford nomogram to determine how often the dose should be given. In contrast, when administered as 3–5 mg/kg daily in three divided doses, both peak and trough concentrations are required.

In renal units, gentamicin is normally administered as 2–3 mg/kg after haemodialysis, or every 48 hours if the patient is on peritoneal dialysis or has severe renal impairment. The dose is then adjusted according to serum gentamicin concentrations. In haemodialysis patients a predialysis trough concentration of less than 4 mg/L is acceptable, as approximately 50% of the drug is removed by haemodialysis, although in peritoneal dialysis the gentamicin trough concentration should still be less than 2 mg/L. A lower peak concentration (approximately 5 mg/L) is aimed for, as gentamicin concentrations tend to remain relatively constant until the next dialysis session.

⟩ **CASE STUDY 8.2**

Mrs AD is a 70-year-old woman with a 10-year history of hypertension. Her current medication is:

Bendroflumethiazide 2.5 mg daily
Enalapril 10 mg daily
Aspirin 75 mg in the morning
Paracetamol 1 g every 6 hours when required for pain relief.

Mrs AD presents at the GP's surgery with a history of cough, breathlessness, and feeling quite wheezy. She has not eaten or drunk much over the last few days. She is diagnosed as having a chest infection and prescribed co-amoxiclav 375 mg three times a day for 7 days. Three days later, she presents with nausea, diarrhoea, vomiting and fatigue. Urea and electrolytes (previously normal) are measured and reported as:

Sodium 145 mmol/L
Potassium 5.9 mmol/L
Bicarbonate 21 mmol/L
Urea 21.3 mmol/L
Creatinine 393 μmol/L.

Mrs AD is admitted to the renal unit. Intravenous fluids are administered, and bendroflumethiazide and enalapril discontinued. Her renal function improves over a 3-week period.

What could be the cause of her renal impairment?

Mrs AD's renal impairment was probably primarily caused by volume depletion as a result of reduced fluid intake and increased output due to vomiting and diarrhoea. This leads to prerenal failure and may result in ATN if not corrected. Mrs AD is also at risk of intrarenal toxicity due to enalapril. This occurs because volume depletion results in a reduction in renal blood flow; angiotensin-II and renin are then produced via a compensatory mechanism to cause constriction of the efferent glomerular arteriole and therefore maintain GFR. However, ACE inhibitors prevent the compensatory vasoconstrictive effects of angiotensin-II and renin. Vasodilation therefore occurs at the efferent glomerular arterioles, leading to a decrease in filtration pressure, which then causes a reduction in GFR in susceptible people, for example those with renal artery stenosis. In the case of Mrs AD, hypovolaemia may have precipitated renal dysfunction. Once the causative factors have been removed, and renal blood flow and glomerular filtration pressure improved, her renal function should return to baseline levels.

→

> ◗ **CASE STUDY 8.2** (continued)
>
> Another potential cause of renal impairment in Mrs AD is a hypersensitivity reaction and subsequent AIN due to co-amoxiclav. This results in a reduction in GFR and significant proteinuria, macroscopic or microscopic haematuria, fever, arthralgia and abnormal liver function tests. More than 70 medicines have been associated with AIN, and drugs account for 4–8% of cases of ARF. The infection itself may also be implicated, as bacterial toxins can produce an inflammatory-mediated reaction leading to ATN. However, Mrs AD's renal impairment is more likely to have been due to hypovolaemia increasing her susceptibility to enalapril-induced ARF. Her age may also have contributed: older patients are at increased risk of drug-induced nephrotoxicity, as GFR decreases with increasing age.
>
> **How could ARF have been avoided?**
>
> Mrs AD should have been told to omit the ACE inhibitor and diuretic for a few days while she was not drinking and had diarrhoea and vomiting. She should also have been advised to return to the GP's surgery in a few days for the situation to be reviewed and to contact the GP immediately if she did not tolerate co-amoxiclav.
>
> **Would you restart the ACE inhibitor?**
>
> Yes. Enalapril can be restarted once renal function has improved. Although enalapril may have contributed to her renal impairment, it is unlikely to have been the primary cause as she has taken this for many years without any problem. However, initially urea and electrolytes should be measured regularly to ensure that her renal function does not deteriorate.

References

1. Hoitsma AJ, Wetzels JFM, Koene RAP. Drug-induced nephrotoxicity. Aetiology, clinical features and management. *Drug Safety* 1991; 6: 131–147.
2. Cove-Smith R. Drugs and the kidney. *Medicine* 1995; 23: 165–173.
3. Davidman M, Olson P, Kohen J, *et al*. Iatrogenic renal disease. *Arch Intern Med* 1991; 151: 1809–1812.
4. Committee on Safety of Medicines. Renal failure associated with Chinese herbal medicines. *Curr Probl Pharmacovigilance* 1999; 25: 18.
5. Gaskin G. Signs and symptoms of renal disease. *Medicine* 1999; 27: 1–4.
6. Cattell WR, Baker LRI, Greenwood RN. Renal disease. In: Kumar PJ, Clark ML, eds. *Clinical Medicine*, 3rd edn. London: Bailliere Tindall, 1998: Chapter 9.

7. Harper A. Acute renal failure. In: Walker R, Edwards C, eds. *Clinical Pharmacy and Therapeutics*. London: Churchill Livingstone, 1994: Chapter 14.

8. Swan SK, Bennett WM. Nephrotoxic acute renal failure. In: Lazarus JM, Brenner BM, eds. *Acute Renal Failure*, 3rd edn. London: Churchill Livingstone, 1993.

9. Becker GJ, Whitworth JA, Kincaid-Smith P. *Clinical Nephrology in Medical Practice*. Oxford: Blackwell Scientific, 1992.

10. Wang A, Lai KN. Drug-induced renal diseases. *Adv Drug React Bull* 1994; 168: 635–638.

11. Burnett JC. Acute renal failure associated with cardiac failure and hypovolaemia. In: Lazarus JM, Brenner BM, eds. *Acute Renal Failure*, 3rd edn. London: Churchill Livingstone, 1993: Chapter 7.

12. Navis G, Faber HJ, de Zeeuw D, *et al*. ACE inhibitors and the kidney. *Drug Safety* 1996; 15: 200–211.

13. Thuran JM, Schrier RW. Comparative effects of angiotensin-converting enzyme inhibitors and angiotensin receptor blockers on blood pressure and the kidney. *Am J Med* 2003; 114: 588–598.

14. Porile JL, Bakris GL, Garella S. Acute interstitial nephritis with glomerulopathy due to nonsteroidal anti-inflammatory agents: a review of its clinical spectrum and effects of steroid therapy. *J Clin Pharmacol* 1990; 30: 468–475.

15. Henrich W, Agodoa L, Barrett B, *et al*. Analgesics and the kidney: Summary and recommendations to the scientific advisory board of the National Kidney Foundation from an Ad Hoc Committee of the National Kidney Foundation. *Am J Kidney Dis* 1996; 27: 162–165.

16. Morales E, Mucksavage JJ. Cyclooxygenase-2 inhibitor-associated acute renal failure: case report with rofecoxib and review of the literature. *Pharmacotherapy* 2002; 22: 1317–1321.

17. Gambaro G, Perazella MA. Adverse renal effects of anti-inflammatory agents: evaluation of selective and nonselective cyclooxygenase inhibitors. *J Intern Med* 2003; 253: 643–652.

18. Brater DC. Renal effects of cyclooxygenase-2-selective inhibitors. *J Pain Symptom Manage* 2002; 23: S15–S20.

19. DeMaria AN, Weir MR. Coxibs – beyond the GI tract: renal and cardiovascular issues. *J Pain Symptom Manage* 2003; 25S: S41–S49.

20. Myers RP, McLaughlin K, Hollomby DJ. Acute interstitial nephritis due to omeprazole. *Am J Gastroenterol* 2001; 96: 3428–3431.

21. Mathew TH. Drug-induced renal disease. *Med J Aust* 1992; 156: 724–729.

22. Hussain N, MacKinnon M, Akbari A. Zopiclone-induced acute interstitial nephritis. *Am J Kidney Dis* 2003; 41: E17.

23. Davison AE, Stewart Cameron AE, Grunfeld JP, *et al*. *Oxford Textbook of Clinical Nephrology*. Oxford: Oxford University Press, 1997.

24. Murray KM, Keane WR. Review of drug-induced acute interstitial nephritis. *Pharmacotherapy* 1992; 12: 462–467.

25. Grunfeld JP, Kleinknecht D, Droz D. Acute interstitial nephritis. In: Schrier RW, Gottschalk CW, eds. *Diseases of the Kidney*, 5th edn. Vol. 2. Boston: Little Brown, 1993: 1331–1353.

26. Alper AB, Meleg-Smith S, Krane NK. Nephrotic syndrome and interstitial nephritis associated with celecoxib. *Am J Kidney Dis* 2002; 40: 1086–1090.

27. Henao J, Hisamuddin I, Nzerue CM, Vasandani G, Hewan-Lowe K. Celecoxib-induced acute interstitial nephritis. *Am J Kidney Dis* 2002; 39: 1313–1317.

28. Markowitz GS, Falkowitz DC, Isom R, *et al.* Membranous glomerulopathy and acute interstitial nephritis following treatment with celecoxib. *Clin Nephrol* 2003; 59: 137–142.

29. Elasy T, Kaminsky D, Tracy M, *et al.* Allopurinol hypersensitivity syndrome revisited. *West J Med* 1995; 162: 360–361.

30. Arellano F, Sacristan J. Allopurinol hypersensitivity syndrome: A review. *Ann Pharmacother* 1993; 27: 337–343.

31. Bennett WM, Elzinga LW, Porter GA. Tubulointerstitial disease and toxic nephropathy. In: Brenner BM, ed. *Brenner & Rector's The Kidney*, 4th edn. London: WB Saunders, 1991: Chapter 29.

32. Levine M, Collin K, Kassen BO. Acute hemolysis and renal failure following discontinuous use of rifampin. *Ann Pharmacother* 1991; 25: 743–744.

33. Yang C, Lin C, Chang S, Hsu H. Rapidly progressive fibrosing interstitial nephritis associated with Chinese herbal drugs. *Am J Kidney Dis* 2000; 35: 313–318.

34. Lord GM, Tagore R, Cook T, Gower P, Pusey CD. Nephropathy caused by Chinese herbs in the UK. *Lancet* 1999; 354: 481–482.

35. Ransford RAJ, Langman MJS. Sulphasalazine and mesalazine: serious adverse reactions re-evaluated on the basis of suspected adverse reaction reports to the Committee on Safety of Medicines. *Gut* 2002; 51: 536–539.

36. Coca S, Perazella MA. Acute renal failure associated with tenofovir: evidence of drug-induced nephrotoxicity. *Am J Med Sci* 2002; 324: 342–344.

37. Perazella MA. Drug-induced renal failure: update on new medications and unique mechanisms of nephrotoxicity. *Am J Med Sci* 2003; 325: 349–362.

38. Bennett WM, Porter GA. Nephrotoxicity of common drugs used by urologists. *Urol Clin North Am* 1990; 17: 145–156.

39. Begg EJ, Barclay ML. Aminoglycosides – 50 years on. *Br J Clin Pharmacol* 1995; 39: 597–603.

40. Humes HD. Aminoglycoside nephrotoxicity. *Kidney Int* 1988; 33: 900–911.

41. Appel GB. Aminoglycoside nephrotoxicity. *Am J Med* 1990; 88(Suppl 3C): 16–20.

42. Swan SK. Aminoglycoside nephrotoxicity. *Semin Nephrol* 1997; 17: 27–33.

43. Anon. Aminoglycosides once daily? *Drug Ther Bull* 1997; 35: 36–37.

44. Hoeprich PD. Clinical use of amphotericin B and derivatives: Lore, mystique, and fact. *Clin Infect Dis* 1992; 14(Suppl 1): S114–S119.

45. Fisher MA, Talbot GH, Maislin G, *et al.* Risk factors for amphotericin B-associated nephrotoxicity. *Am J Med* 1989; 87: 547–552.

46. Sabra R, Branch RA. Amphotericin B nephrotoxicity. *Drug Safety* 1990; 5: 94–108.

47. Barrett JP, Vardulaki KA, Conlon C, *et al.* A systematic review of the antifungal effectiveness and tolerability of amphotericin B formulations. *Clin Ther* 2003; 25: 1295–1320.

48. Barrett BJ, Parfrey PS. Prevention of nephrotoxicity induced by radiocontrast agents. *N Engl J Med* 1994; 331: 1449–1450.

49. Barrett BJ. Contrast nephrotoxicity. *J Am Soc Nephrol* 1994; 5: 125–137.

50. Oliveira DBG. Prophylaxis against contrast-induced nephropathy. *Lancet* 1999; 353: 1638–1639.

51. Guru V, Fremes SE. The role of *N*-acetylcysteine in preventing radiographic contrast-induced nephropathy. *Clin Nephrol* 2004; 62: 77–83.

52. Cox CD, Tsikouris JP. Preventing contrast nephropathy: what is the best strategy? A review of the literature. *J Clin Pharmacol* 2004; 44: 327–337.

53. Collins AJ. Gold treatment for rheumatoid arthritis: reassurance on proteinuria. *Br Med J* 1987; 295: 739–740.

54. Hall CL, Fothergill NJ, Blackwell MM, *et al*. The natural course of gold nephropathy: long term study of 21 patients. *Br Med J* 1987; 295: 745–748.

55. Cassidy MJD, Kerr DNS. Renal disorders. In: Davies DM, ed. *Textbook of Adverse Drug Reactions*, 4th edn. Oxford: Oxford University Press, 1991: Chapter 12.

56. McLaughlin K, Gholoum B, Guiraudon C, *et al*. Rapid development of drug-induced lupus nephritis in the absence of extrarenal disease in a patient receiving procainamide. *Am J Kidney Dis* 1998; 32: 698–702.

57. Stratton MA. Drug-induced systemic lupus erythematosus. *Clin Pharmacol* 1985; 4: 657–663.

58. Krieble BF, Rudy DW, Glick MR, Clayman MD. Case-report: Acyclovir neurotoxicity and nephrotoxicity – the role for hemodialysis. *Am J Med Sci* 1993; 305: 36–39.

59. Daudon M, Jungers P. Drug-induced renal calculi: epidemiology, prevention and management. *Drugs* 2004; 64: 245–275.

60. Cribb AE, Lee BL, Trepanier LA, *et al*. Adverse reactions to sulphonamide and sulphonamide – trimethoprim antimicrobials: clinical syndromes and pathogenesis. *Adv Drug React Toxicol Rev* 1996; 15: 9–50.

61. Simon DI, Brosius FC, Rothstein DM. Sulfadiazine crystalluria revisited. The treatment of toxoplasma encephalitis in patients with acquired immunodeficiency syndrome. *Arch Intern Med* 1990; 150: 2379–2384.

62. Herman JS, Ives NJ, Nelson M, Gazzard BG, Easterbrook PJ. Incidence and risk factors for the development of indinavir-associated renal complications. *J Antimicrob Chemother* 2001; 48: 355–360.

63. Famularo G, Di Toro S, Moretti S, De Simone C. Symptomatic crystalluria associated with indinavir. *Ann Pharmacother* 2000; 34: 1414–1418.

64. Jaradat M, Phillips C, Yum Moo-Nahm, Cushing H, Moe S. Acute tubulo-interstitial nephritis attributable to indinavir therapy. *Am J Kidney Dis* 2000; 35: E16.

65. Reilly RF, Tray K, Perazella MA. Indinavir nephropathy revisited: a pattern of insidious renal failure with identifiable risk factors. *Am J Kidney Dis* 2001; 38: E23.

66. Molnar ZL, Shearer ES. Rhabdomyolysis on the intensive care unit – an under-diagnosed condition. *Care Critically Ill* 1996; 12: 165–168.

67. Prendergast BD, George CF. Drug-induced rhabdomyolysis – mechanisms and management. *Postgrad Med J* 1993; 69: 333–336.

68. Committee on Safety of Medicines. HMG-CoA reductase inhibitors (statins) and myopathy. *Curr Probl Pharmacovigilance* 2002; 28: 8–9.

69. Modi JR, Cratty MS. Fluvastatin-induced rhabdomyolysis. *Ann Pharmacother* 2002; 36: 1870–1874.

70. Lim C, Devane CL. Retroperitoneal fibrosis and migraine therapy. *Drug Intell Clin Pharm* 1988; 22: 405–406.

71. Hely MA, Morris JGL, Lawrence S, *et al*. Retroperitoneal fibrosis, skin and pleuropulmonary changes associated with bromocriptine therapy. *Aust NZ J Med* 1991; 21: 82–84.

72. Committee on Safety of Medicines. Fibrotic reactions with pergolide and other ergot-derived dopamine receptor agonists. *Curr Probl Pharmacovigilance* 2002; 28: 3.

73. Elseviers MM, de Broe ME. Combination analgesic involvement in the patho-genesis of analgesic nephropathy: the European perspective. *Am J Kidney Dis* 1996; 28(Suppl 1): S48–S55.
74. Patrono C. Aspirin as an antiplatelet agent. *N Engl J Med* 1994; 330: 1287–1294.
75. McGoldrick MD, Bailie GR. Non-narcotic analgesics: prevalence and estimated economic impact of toxicities. *Ann Pharmacother* 1997; 31: 221–227.
76. Burke C, Fulda GJ, Castellano J. Lithium-induced nephrogenic diabetes insipidus treated with intravenous ketorolac. *Crit Care Med* 1995; 23: 1924–1927.
77. Anon. Adverse drug reactions to lithium. *Adv Drug React Bull* 2001; 206: 788.
78. Gitlin M. Lithium and the kidney. *Drug Safety* 1999; 20: 231–243.
79. Waller D. Lithium-induced polyuria. *Prescribers J* 1997; 37: 24–28.
80. Abuelo JG. Diagnosing vascular causes of renal failure. *Ann Intern Med* 1995; 123: 601–614.
81. Walter RB, Joerger M, Pestalozzi BC. Gemcitabine-associated haemolytic–uremic syndrome. *Am J Kidney Dis* 2002; 40: E16.
82. McDonald SP, Shanahan EM, Thomas AC, *et al.* Quinine-induced hemolytic uremic syndrome. *Clin Nephrol* 1997; 47: 397–400.
83. Anon. Quinine and haemolytic uraemic syndrome. *Aust Adv Drug React Bull* 1996; 15: 2.
84. Kojouri K, Vesely SK, George JN. Quinine-associated thrombotic thrombocy-topenic purpura–hemolytic uremic syndrome: frequency, clinical features, and long-term outcomes. *Ann Intern Med* 2001; 135: 1047–1051.

Further reading

Cove-Smith R. Drugs and the kidney. *Medicine* 1995; 23: 165–173.
Critchley JAJH, Chan TYK, Cumming AD. Renal diseases. In: Speight TM, Holford NHG, eds. *Avery's Drug Treatment*, 4th edn. New Zealand: Adis International Limited, 1997: Chapter 24.
Gaskin G. Signs and symptoms of renal disease. *Medicine* 1999; 27: 1–4.
Perazella MA. Drug-induced renal failure: update on new medications and unique mechanisms of nephrotoxicity. *Am J Med Sci* 2003; 325: 349–362.

9

Endocrine and metabolic disorders

Janice Watt

Introduction

Endocrine glands secrete hormones that evoke a specific response in other parts of the body. Examples include the thyroid, parathyroid, adrenal and pituitary glands. Endocrine disease affects a wide range of body systems; the majority is idiopathic, has an autoimmune cause, or is secondary to an endocrine tumour (most commonly of the pituitary, thyroid or parathyroid). Autoimmune diseases are characterised by the presence of specific antibodies in the serum that may be present for many years before symptoms occur. Autoimmune disease has been observed involving every endocrine organ.[1] A wide range of drugs affects the functions of the endocrine glands. Drugs may act on the synthesis and release of endocrine hormones, or may interfere with the tests used to identify endocrine disease. Some knowledge of medicines that interfere with tests for endocrine disease is particularly important, as if this is not considered, misdiagnosis may result in inappropriate treatment. This chapter gives an overview of drugs that affect the endocrine system, highlighting those commonly implicated. Note that osteoporosis and subfertility, although endocrine disorders by definition, are covered in Chapter 11 (Musculoskeletal disorders) and Chapter 16 (Sexual dysfunction and infertility), respectively.

Drugs affecting thyroid function

Thyroid hormone is synthesised from dietary iodine. The recommended daily intake of iodine should be at least 140 µg. There is an autoregulatory mechanism within the thyroid gland that protects against iodine deficiency and excess. Iodine is reduced to iodide in the gastrointestinal tract and, following its absorption, is 'organified' (i.e. combines with

Table 9.1 Some drugs that can affect thyroid function

Drugs associated with hyperthyroidism
Amiodarone
Lithium
Interferon alfa
Radiographic contrast media (transient)
Drugs associated with hypothyroidism
Amiodarone
Lithium
Interferon alfa

tyrosyl residues of thyroglobulin) to form monoiodotyrosines and di-iodotyrosines. Release of thyroid-stimulating hormone (TSH) from the pituitary results in these compounds being coupled to form thyroxine (T_4) and tri-iodothyronine (T_3), which are then released from the thyroid. T_3 and T_4 are transported throughout the body via carrier proteins, including thyroxine-binding globulin (TBG). Most thyroid disease is secondary to autoimmune processes, but some medicines cause thyroid dysfunction by interacting with aspects of thyroid hormone synthesis and release (Table 9.1).

Iodine and the thyroid gland

Iodine has complex effects on the thyroid gland and thyroid status and is recognised as causing both hypothyroidism and thyrotoxicosis (hyperthyroidism).[2] However, in iodine-replete areas, such as the UK and US, the effects of iodine and iodine-containing preparations on thyroid function are seldom clinically relevant.

Amiodarone

Amiodarone contains 37% by weight of iodine; a daily dose of 200–400 mg provides 6–12 mg of free iodine, which is about 100 times that consumed in an average diet.[3] Thyroid hormone dynamics change in almost all patients receiving amiodarone. This results in the following typical abnormal thyroid function tests in most patients: elevated T_4 (free and total), elevated TSH (may also be normal or low) and decreased T_3 (free and total). Abnormal thyroid function tests, without clinical signs of thyroid dysfunction, occur more often as the duration of treatment increases and the drug accumulates. Alternative reference values for thyroid function tests in patients receiving amiodarone have been devised.[4] Amiodarone may cause clinical hypothyroidism or thyrotoxicosis months to years after starting therapy. The effect of the drug depends on whether it has been given in the context of previous iodine deficiency or in the presence of overt or subclinical thyroid disease. In the first few weeks following initiation of amiodarone, the excess iodide load commonly inhibits thyroid hormone synthesis and release (Wolff–Chaikoff effect).[5] The normal thyroid is usually able to overcome this effect and thyroid hormone levels return to normal. However, if this does not happen hypothyroidism may result. Hypothyroidism secondary to amiodarone has been reported in 1–32% of patients on long-term therapy.[6] It is most prevalent in populations with high dietary iodine intake, such as the US, and is most common in females with pre-existing thyroid autoantibodies. Such women are about 14 times more likely than men without antibodies to present with hypothyroidism secondary to amiodarone.[6]

Symptoms of hypothyroidism include fatigue, intolerance of cold, mental and physical sluggishness and dry skin. Management involves either stopping the drug or, if this is not possible, thyroxine replacement therapy. Levothyroxine should be started at a dose of 25–50 μg and increased at 4–6-week intervals to maintain thyroid hormone levels at the upper end of the reference range.

In some circumstances amiodarone may cause hyperthyroidism (thyrotoxicosis), which in some cases has been fatal. Two subtypes of amiodarone-induced thyrotoxicosis (AIT) have been proposed.[4] Type I occurs when the thyroid gland has a pre-existing abnormality (i.e. in patients with subclinical thyroid disorders). It is caused by iodine-induced excessive thyroid hormone synthesis and release, and occurs more commonly in iodine-deficient areas. Type II AIT is a destructive thyroiditis that results in the release of preformed thyroid hormones from the damaged thyroid gland. It is more common in iodine-replete areas. Mixed forms of AIT may also occur. The reported incidence of clinically significant hyperthyroidism ranges between 1 and 23%.[6]

Patients with thyrotoxicosis secondary to amiodarone may present with unexplained weight loss, muscle weakness, goitre and tremor. They may also have an exacerbation of their pre-existing cardiac arrhythmia. Some classic symptoms (e.g. hyperactivity, heat intolerance and sweating) may be masked by the pharmacological properties of the drug. Symptoms are generally accompanied by a raised serum T_4, a decreased serum T_3 and a suppressed TSH concentration or an absent TSH response to thyrotropin-releasing hormone (TRH). If thyrotoxicosis occurs, amiodarone should be stopped wherever possible. However, owing to its long elimination half-life, it may take 8 months or more for the problem to resolve. In patients with serious cardiac arrhythmias it may not be possible to stop amiodarone. In these cases, antithyroid therapy, such as carbimazole or propylthiouracil, and a beta-blocker may be given, although higher than usual doses may be necessary.[2,6] Antithyroid therapy is less useful in patients with type II AIT. In these patients corticosteroids (e.g. prednisolone 40–60 mg daily) may also be useful.[4] Radioactive iodine is not usually a suitable treatment because high systemic iodine concentrations prevent the uptake of radioactive iodine into the thyroid.[6] Thyroid surgery may be considered.[4]

Lithium

Lithium may also cause hypothyroidism or thyrotoxicosis. As with amiodarone, women with pre-existing thyroid autoantibodies are predominantly affected. Lithium-induced hypothyroidism is thought to involve inhibition of iodotyrosine and iodothyronine biosynthesis and inhibition of thyroid hormone release from the gland. As many as 30% of patients treated are thought to develop subclinical hypothyroidism. However, long-term studies indicate that although T_3 and T_4 tend to fall in the first few months of treatment, they return to pretreatment levels within 12 months and can exceed pretreatment values afterwards.[7] Conversely, TSH tends to rise in the first few months but gradually returns to pretreatment levels after more than 12 months. Only about 2% of patients develop clinical features of hypothyroidism requiring thyroxine replacement.

Thyrotoxicosis due to lithium is rare. In most cases, symptoms develop several years after starting the drug and occasionally appear after it is stopped.[8] The mechanism is unclear, but in more than 50% of patients there is evidence of autoimmune thyroid disease. Several theories have been proposed, including overcompensation in response to abnormalities in iodine pharmacokinetics induced by lithium. When lithium treatment is stopped rebound hyperthyroidism may occur, because thyroid hormone synthesis is no longer inhibited. Management involves either withdrawing lithium therapy or giving carbimazole.[9]

Interferons

Hypothyroidism and thyrotoxicosis have been reported in patients receiving long-term treatment with recombinant interferon alfa.[10] The incidence is thought to be about 7% and 4%, respectively, and is highest in patients with chronic hepatitis C. Patients with thyroid autoantibodies are at greatest risk of thyroid disease, but the exact mechanism is unclear. There is some evidence that interferon alfa may inhibit iodide organification in the thyroid, thus inhibiting thyroid hormone biosynthesis. Thyroid dysfunction has also been reported during clinical trials with pegylated interferon alfa preparations, and rarely with interferon beta-1b.

Medicines that may interfere with thyroid function tests

Many drugs affect thyroid function tests through alterations in the synthesis, transport and metabolism of thyroid hormones, as well as via influences on thyroid-stimulating hormone synthesis and secretion.[11] T_4 and T_3 are transported in the bloodstream by three carrier proteins; only 0.03% of total T_4 and 0.3% of total T_3 circulate in the free or unbound form, but it is this small fraction that is biologically active. The thyroid function tests used most widely are total plasma T_4 and T_3, plasma basal TSH and free T_4.

Often drugs have only a minor effect on thyroid function tests, so that results remain within the normal reference range. However, results outside the reference range can arise in the absence of any clinical evidence of thyroid dysfunction. It is important to be aware of the potential influence of medication so that inappropriate investigations and therapy can be avoided. Some medicines that can interfere with thyroid function tests are shown in Table 9.2. Oestrogens, in combined oral contraceptives or hormone replacement therapy, result in a dose-dependent increase in TBG concentrations.[12] Serum T_4 concentrations are increased, but the proportions of active free T_4 and TSH are usually unaltered and clinical hyperthyroidism is absent. TBG serum concentrations may also be increased in long-term heroin or methadone users or patients receiving fluorouracil. Conversely, androgens, including danazol and anabolic steroids, and glucocorticoids decrease TBG concentrations.[12]

Table 9.2 Some drugs that can interfere with thyroid function tests

Amiodarone	Corticosteroids
Anabolic steroids	Danazol
Aspirin	Heparin
Beta-blockers	Non-steroidal anti-inflammatory drugs
Carbamazepine	Oestrogens
Contrast media	Phenytoin

Phenytoin, carbamazepine and rifampicin increase the metabolism and elimination of thyroid hormones, probably because of their ability to induce hepatic enzymes. This results in a fall in serum T_3 and T_4 concentrations, but patients remain euthyroid and TSH is normal or only slightly raised.[11]

Because of their high iodine content, radiographic contrast media may cause an increase in circulating T_4, which reaches a maximum 3–4 days after administration and returns to normal within 14 days. Care should be taken when interpreting thyroid function tests carried out within 2 weeks of exposure. However, clinical hyperthyroidism requiring treatment has been reported rarely.[13]

Heparin causes a rapid increase in the serum T_4 concentration, which peaks 15 minutes after injection but returns to normal after 60 minutes. For this reason, where possible, thyroid function tests should be postponed until after heparin therapy is stopped.[3] Corticosteroids are known to inhibit TSH release and small decreases in T_3 and T_4 may occur, although concentrations rarely fall outside normal limits.[11]

Drugs affecting adrenal function

Glucocorticoids

Cortisol production is stimulated by adrenocorticotrophic hormone (ACTH) produced by the pituitary gland. Cortisol in turn influences both corticotropin-releasing factor (CRF) production in the hypothalamus and ACTH release by the pituitary, via negative feedback. When steroids are given even for a few days, the feedback system is interrupted and suppression of the hypothalamic–pituitary–adrenal (HPA) system occurs.

Cushing's syndrome occurs when there is adrenal hyperfunction due to chronic glucocorticoid excess. Administration of pharmacological doses of corticosteroids causes iatrogenic Cushing's syndrome. This usually occurs within 2 weeks of starting therapy at daily doses in excess of hydrocortisone 50 mg (or equivalent). However, there is great variability in patient response and some may exhibit symptoms at much lower doses. Symptoms are usually absent with doses of less than 20 mg hydrocortisone.[14] Typical signs include 'moon face' and 'buffalo hump', weight gain, psychiatric symptoms and skin thinning.

Prolonged administration of corticosteroids in excess of physiological doses (i.e. >7.5 mg prednisolone daily or equivalent) results in suppression of the HPA axis. In the absence of ACTH release, the adrenals become atrophied and can no longer synthesise and release glucocorticoids.[14]

If corticosteroid therapy is stopped abruptly, a withdrawal syndrome may occur. Typically, patients experience headache, dizziness, joint pain, weakness and emotional changes, but symptoms may be much more severe, particularly after long-term therapy, and fatalities have been reported.

It is essential that patients treated with corticosteroids are counselled about the potential consequences of stopping treatment abruptly and that they carry a steroid warning card. Steroids should always be given for the shortest length of time at the lowest dose that is clinically necessary. Once-daily dosing in the morning and, if disease control will allow, alternate-day dosing may reduce suppression of the HPA axis.[15] Patients receiving long-term inhaled steroids in excess of 1.5 mg beclometasone dipropionate daily (or its equivalent) and those using high-potency topical preparations may also show signs of HPA suppression.[16] Increasing potency, prolonged application of large quantities, young age and occlusion of the skin at the site of application are all risk factors for HPA suppression with topical corticosteroids.[17] Suppression of the HPA axis results in the adrenals responding inadequately to physiological stress. An increased dose of systemic corticosteroid must therefore be given during serious illness or surgery.[18]

Patients stopping systemic corticosteroids after long-term treatment must have therapy withdrawn gradually. The British Thoracic Society asthma management guidelines advise that therapy may be stopped abruptly if the patient has been treated for less than 3 weeks and is receiving regular inhaled steroids.[19] Patients at greatest risk of HPA suppression are those who have been treated for more than 3 weeks, have had repeated courses of systemic corticosteroids, received more than 40 mg prednisolone or the equivalent, received a short course of steroids within 1 year of stopping long-term steroids, and those with underlying adrenocortical insufficiency. A reducing course of corticosteroids should be considered in all of these patients.[20] In patients treated with corticosteroids for 18 months or more the HPA axis may take up to 1 year to recover.[15] When tailing off corticosteroids in patients on chronic high-dose therapy a short Synacthen test may be useful in assessing the recovery of the HPA axis once a dose of 5 mg prednisolone is reached.[21]

Metyrapone/aminoglutethimide

Metyrapone and aminoglutethimide are both used in the treatment of Cushing's syndrome. They act by blocking corticosteroid biosynthesis, and therefore when used in excess can result in hypoadrenalism.[7]

Ketoconazole

Ketoconazole is a potent inhibitor of adrenal glucocorticoid synthesis. It acts at two enzyme steps in the adrenal steroid biosynthesis pathway: 11β-hydroxylase, and conversion of cholesterol to pregnenolone. The effect seems to be dose related, but adrenal insufficiency has been reported with oral doses as low as 200 mg twice daily after 2 days' treatment.[22,23] Signs and symptoms include lethargy, anorexia, weight loss, hyponatraemia and hyperkalaemia. Patients may be treated by withdrawing the drug or by corticosteroid replacement therapy. Because of its effects on steroid biosynthesis, attempts have been made to use ketoconazole in the treatment of Cushing's syndrome in patients unresponsive to conventional therapy.[22]

Rifampicin

Rifampicin has been reported to precipitate acute adrenal insufficiency in patients with pre-existing hypoadrenalism.[24] This is thought to be due to an increase in glucocorticoid metabolism secondary to microsomal enzyme induction. It is recommended that such patients should have their steroid replacement dose doubled or tripled on starting rifampicin.

Aldosterone synthesis

Aldosterone is the most potent mineralocorticoid secreted by the adrenal cortex; it increases sodium and water retention and potassium and hydrogen secretion by the kidney. Aldosterone production is regulated mainly by changes in blood volume, mediated through the renin–angiotensin system (RAS), which interacts with the sympathetic nervous system and prostaglandins. Other factors controlling its secretion include changes in potassium and ACTH. Some drugs that can cause hyperaldosteronism are shown in Table 9.3.

Angiotensin-converting enzyme (ACE) converts angiotensin-I to angiotensin-II which, as well as being a potent vasoconstrictor, is the primary stimulator of aldosterone. ACE inhibitors can produce

Table 9.3 Some drugs that may cause hyperaldosteronism

Carbenoxolone	Oral contraceptives
Lithium	Spironolactone
Loop diuretics	Thiazides

hyperreninaemic hypoaldosteronism, which manifests as hyperkalaemia with a hyperchloraemic metabolic acidosis. Angiotensin-II receptor antagonists can also lead to a reduction in aldosterone. Non-steroidal anti-inflammatory drugs inhibit renin secretion and hence aldosterone release, which can lead to a syndrome of hyporeninaemic hypoaldosteronism.[25,26] Even at low doses, standard or low molecular weight heparins can produce hypoaldosteronism. Aldosterone suppression occurs within a few days of initiation of therapy, is reversible, and is independent of either anticoagulant effect or route of administration.[27,28] A clinically significant increase in the serum potassium level may occur in about 7% of patients. Some patient groups appear to be more susceptible to the suppression of aldosterone secretion, such as those with diabetes mellitus, chronic renal impairment, pre-existing acidosis, raised plasma potassium, or those taking potassium-sparing medication.[29] Plasma potassium should be measured in at-risk patients before starting heparin and monitored regularly thereafter, particularly if heparin is to be continued for more than 7 days.

Drugs affecting gonadotrophin release and gonadal function

Glucocorticoids

Release of gonadotrophin-releasing hormones (GnRH or LnRH) from the hypothalamus stimulates follicle-stimulating hormone (FSH) and luteinising hormone (LH) release from the pituitary. FSH and LH stimulate spermatogenesis and testosterone production in males, and maturation of the follicle and the production of oestrogen and progestogen in females. High doses of corticosteroids inhibit pituitary gonadotrophin release and result in ovarian and testicular dysfunction.[14]

Ketoconazole

Ketoconazole directly inhibits testicular steroidogenesis by inhibiting the 17 α-hydroxylase enzyme at doses as low as 400 mg daily.[30] This is probably the mechanism by which ketoconazole causes gynaecomastia.

Danazol

Testosterone is transported in the body via sex-hormone-binding globulin. Danazol decreases the ability of testosterone to bind to this protein, resulting in an increase in the free, active form of testosterone in the plasma.[7] This may explain the virilisation and hirsutism observed in patients treated with danazol, although the drug also has weak androgenic properties.

Gynaecomastia

Gynaecomastia is the abnormal accumulation of tissue in the male breast. It can occur physiologically in three phases of life: in the neonatal period, following exposure to maternal oestrogens; at puberty (in up to two-thirds of adolescent males); and in old age, owing to a reduction in endogenous testosterone levels.[31] About 50% of cases of gynaecomastia have a physiological cause and about 10–20% are secondary to drug therapy.[32]

Drug-induced gynaecomastia may be very embarrassing and distressing for the patient but is rarely a cause for alarm. A wide variety of drugs have been implicated, and for most the mechanism for the adverse effect is unknown. Two recognised mechanisms are (1) increased serum

Table 9.4 Some drugs that can cause gynaecomastia

Drugs with oestrogenic activity
Clomifene
Digitalis glycosides
Oestrogens
Spironolactone

Drugs reducing testosterone synthesis or effects
Alcohol
Alkylating agents, e.g. vinblastine
Cimetidine
Cyproterone
Flutamide
Ketoconazole
Phenytoin
Spironolactone

Drugs where the mechanism is uncertain
Antipsychotics, e.g. chlorpromazine
Calcium channel blockers, e.g. verapamil, nifedipine
Isoniazid
Marijuana
Methadone
Methyldopa
Protease inhibitors
Stavudine
Tricyclic antidepressants

oestrogen concentration or enhanced activity, and (2) blockade of the synthesis or effect of testosterone.[31] Table 9.4 lists drugs that have been reported to cause gynaecomastia and the proposed underlying mechanism. Drug-induced gynaecomastia usually develops soon after drug therapy is initiated and resolves when the drug is stopped.[33]

Hyperprolactinaemia

Prolactin is a hormone synthesised and released from the anterior pituitary. It has a major role in preparing the breast for lactation and maintenance of lactation. The release of prolactin from the pituitary is inhibited by dopamine from the hypothalamus and stimulated by the release of serotonin. Excess prolactin release (hyperprolactinaemia) may cause galactorrhoea, amenorrhoea, impotence or infertility. Galactorrhoea can be defined as the persistent discharge of milk or a milk-like substance from the breast in the absence of parturition, or at least 6 months postpartum in mothers who are not breastfeeding.[34]

Drugs that have been implicated in the development of hyperprolactinaemia (Table 9.5) usually act in one of three ways. They may interfere with the production and release of dopamine from the hypothalamus. For example, reserpine and methyldopa deplete catecholamine stores in the hypothalamus, reducing the amount of dopamine available for release. Drugs may also cause hyperprolactinaemia by blocking dopamine receptors. Antipsychotic agents, including the phenothiazines and the butyrophenones, are thought to cause hyperprolactinaemia and galactorrhoea in this way.[34,35] The atypical antipsychotics used in schizophrenia (e.g. clozapine, olanzapine and quetiapine) have a prolactin-sparing effect and are less likely to cause this problem. However, at higher doses the atypical antipsychotic risperidone can cause an increase in serum prolactin similar to the major tranquillisers.[36] Hyperprolactinaemia may

Table 9.5 Some drugs that may cause hyperprolactinaemia

Antihypertensives, e.g. reserpine, methyldopa, verapamil
Antipsychotics, e.g. haloperidol, chlorpromazine
Antidepressants (tricyclic and SSRI)
Antiulcer drugs, e.g. cimetidine, ranitidine
Analgesics, e.g. methadone, morphine
Benzodiazepines
Oestrogens

SSRI, selective serotonin reuptake inhibitor.

also be caused by drugs that interfere with serotonin reuptake or the sensitivity of postsynaptic serotonin receptors. Tricyclic antidepressants and selective serotonin reuptake inhibitors (SSRIs) probably cause hyperprolactinaemia in this way.

Cimetidine and ranitidine may also cause hyperprolactinaemia, and therefore it is likely that histamine also affects prolactin secretion. Other drugs reported to cause hyperprolactinaemia and galactorrhoea include oestrogens, morphine, methadone, benzodiazepines and verapamil. However, the exact mechanism for these adverse effects is unclear.[34] Drug-induced hyperprolactinaemia and galactorrhoea usually resolve within weeks of stopping the causative drug. However, for antipsychotics administered as an intramuscular depot injection, prolactin levels may remain raised for 6 months after the last dose.[37]

Syndrome of inappropriate secretion of antidiuretic hormone

Antidiuretic hormone (ADH, vasopressin) is released from the posterior pituitary, primarily in response to changes in osmotic pressure. When the plasma osmolality increases, e.g. during dehydration, ADH is released. ADH then acts on vasopressin-2 (V2) receptors in the collecting duct of the renal tubule, resulting in an increase in the reabsorption of water and the formation of more concentrated urine. Syndrome of inappropriate secretion of antidiuretic hormone (SIADH) occurs when ADH is released from the pituitary under inappropriate circumstances, i.e. when the plasma osmolality is normal or low. This causes the extracellular fluid to become more dilute and to increase in volume.

Many of the symptoms of SIADH are secondary to hyponatraemia (serum sodium <135 mmol/L). Early symptoms include weakness, lethargy and weight gain. Headache, anorexia, nausea and vomiting may also be present. If the condition remains untreated, worsening hyponatraemia may result in confusion, convulsions, coma and death. The three main causes of SIADH are:[38]

- Release of ADH from sites other than the pituitary, e.g. malignancies such as small cell lung carcinoma;
- Abnormal secretion of ADH due to central nervous system disorders such as a cerebrovascular accident;
- Drugs, which may cause SIADH by enhancing the release of ADH or by increasing the responsiveness of the kidney to ADH release.

Psychotropics

SIADH has been associated with various centrally acting antipsychotic drugs, including phenothiazines, and with tricyclic antidepressants, SSRIs, venlafaxine and reboxetine.[39–41] Diagnosis is complicated by the observation that patients with untreated psychiatric disease may drink large quantities of water, but polydipsia alone does not usually result in clinical hyponatraemia.[39] The mechanism is thought to involve increased secretion or potentiation of the effects of ADH. Hyponatraemia secondary to these drugs usually occurs soon after the drug is started, although in some cases symptoms may occur after several years.

Carbamazepine

SIADH secondary to carbamazepine is well known and the incidence may be as high as 22% in patients with epilepsy or trigeminal neuralgia.[39] Carbamazepine enhances the release of ADH from the pituitary.

Cytotoxic agents

Cyclophosphamide, cisplatin, high-dose melphalan, vincristine, vinblastine and vinorelbine have all been reported to cause SIADH.[38,42] The mechanism is unclear. With vincristine it has been suggested that the neurotoxic effect causes the osmoreceptors that control ADH to respond inappropriately.[36]

Hypoglycaemic agents

Chlorpropamide and tolbutamide may cause hyponatraemia secondary to SIADH. The effect is more common with high doses, but symptoms have been observed at doses as low as 125 mg chlorpropamide and 500 mg tolbutamide.[43] The incidence of SIADH appears to be higher with chlorpropamide than with tolbutamide.

Chlorpropamide probably enhances the release of ADH from the pituitary and increases the sensitivity of the cyclic AMP–adenylate cyclase system in the ADH-sensitive cells of the kidney.

Angiotensin-converting enzyme (ACE) inhibitors

In most patients treated with ACE inhibitors serum sodium remains normal, but severe hyponatraemia has been reported.[44] The exact mechanism is unclear. ACE inhibitors block the conversion of angiotensin-I to angiotensin-II in the peripheral circulation, but not in the brain. It is possible that conversion of increased concentrations of angiotensin-I to angiotensin-II in the brain stimulate thirst and ADH release, leading to hyponatraemia. Assessing the precise role of ACE inhibitors in causing hyponatraemia is complicated by the fact that many patients are also taking diuretics.

Treatment of SIADH

The mainstay of treatment of drug-induced SIADH is to remove the cause. It is also essential to restrict fluid intake to 500–1000 mL/day. This will result in a gradual increase in plasma sodium concentration and osmolality and an improvement in symptoms. In patients with severe life-threatening symptoms it may be necessary to administer hypertonic sodium chloride solution at a rate that increases the serum sodium by 1–2 mmol/L/h, in addition to restricting fluid intake, until the serum sodium concentration exceeds 125 mmol/L. Some authors have recommended the administration of a 3% sodium chloride solution for this purpose. Over-rapid correction of hyponatraemia, particularly in patients with hyponatraemia of more than 2 days' duration, can result in 'osmotic demyelinisation syndrome' (bulbar palsy, paralysis of all limbs, coma and death), and therefore hypertonic sodium chloride solution should only be administered to patients with life-threatening symptoms. Osmotic demyelinisation syndrome does not usually occur in patients with acute-onset severe hyponatraemia if the rate of correction of hyponatraemia does not exceed 24 mmol/L over 48 hours.[45]

In chronic SIADH, where other methods have proved ineffective, demeclocycline 900–1200 mg daily has been used successfully. Demeclocycline inhibits the renal effects of ADH. An initial response is usually observed within 1–2 weeks, after which the dose should be gradually reduced to the lowest possible at which the serum sodium concentration remains normal.[46] It has been suggested that patients being initiated on drugs known to cause SIADH, particularly antipsychotics and carbamazepine, should have their serum sodium concentration measured before treatment is started, and again after 1–4 weeks.[39]

Hyperglycaemia and diabetes

Blood glucose is regulated in the body by a number of mechanisms. Insulin lowers blood glucose by suppressing hepatic glucose production and lipolysis. It also enhances glucose uptake for utilisation or storage in the liver, muscle or adipose tissue. In contrast, blood glucose may be increased by glucagon, adrenaline (epinephrine), cortisol and growth hormone. The effects of these hormones are closely intertwined. Glucagon stimulates hepatic gluconeogenesis and glyconeogenesis. Noradrenaline (norepinephrine) and adrenaline act by enhancing glucagon secretion and stimulating lipolysis. Cortisol promotes gluconeogenesis and increases the synthesis and release of adrenaline from the adrenal medulla, and growth hormone exerts both insulin-like and insulin antagonist effects.

Because under normal circumstances insulin and other hormones are released in response to increased blood glucose concentrations, drug-induced hyperglycaemia only usually occurs in patients with diabetes mellitus or those with latent disorders of glucose handling.

Corticosteroids

Hyperglycaemia secondary to corticosteroid treatment is well recognised. In one large case–control study of 11 855 patients newly commenced on an oral hypoglycaemic agent or insulin, the relative risk of hyperglycaemia (requiring treatment) secondary to corticosteroids was 2.2.[47] The risk increased with average daily dose. When expressed as hydrocortisone equivalents the relative risk was 1.77 for 1–39 mg/day, 3.02 for 40–79 mg/day, 5.82 for 80–119 mg/day, and 10.34 for more than 120 mg hydrocortisone per day. At equivalent doses methylprednisolone appears to be more likely to cause hyperglycaemia than hydrocortisone. Deflazacort, an oxazoline derivative of prednisolone, has been shown in small studies to cause less derangement in blood glucose, but further studies are needed to confirm this.[14]

Diuretics

Glucose intolerance has been reported in 3% of patients treated with diuretics. It is more common with long-acting diuretics and relatively rare with loop diuretics, although an isolated case of non-ketotic hyperglycaemia in diabetics has been reported. Hyperglycaemia with thiazide diuretics is dose related and seems to occur most commonly in the first 4–8 weeks of treatment.[48] As the hypotensive effects of thiazides are not related to dose, the lowest possible dose should be given and susceptible patients monitored closely for the first few months of treatment. Hypokalaemia may contribute to hyperglycaemia, as potassium depletion causes inhibition of insulin secretion. Insulin resistance is another possible mechanism.

Antipsychotics

The association between atypical antipsychotics, in particular clozapine, olanzapine, quetiapine and risperidone, and glucose intolerance is becoming increasingly well recognised.[49] Early studies also suggested an association between conventional antipsychotics and altered glucose–insulin homoeostasis, but this appears to be less common. The mechanism is not yet known, but atypical antipsychotics may exert direct effects on glucose–insulin homoeostasis and lipid metabolism, causing hyperinsulinaemia and hyperlipidaemia which lead to insulin resistance.[50] Risk factors for glucose intolerance may include male gender, increasing body weight and underlying diabetes. Schizophrenia has also been linked to the development of hyperglycaemia and diabetes mellitus. The adverse effect appears to be more common with clozapine and olanzapine and less common with risperidone. Most cases occur within the first year of treatment. Patients treated with clozapine, olanzapine and risperidone should undergo regular monitoring of blood glucose and body weight. Table 9.6 lists other medicines that have been associated with hyperglycaemia.

Table 9.6 Some other drugs associated with hyperglycaemia

Beta-adrenoceptor agonists, e.g. salbutamol
Calcium channel blockers
Ciclosporin
Diazoxide
Enoximone
Interferon alfa
Isoniazid
Phenytoin
Theophylline

Hypoglycaemia

Insulin

Hypoglycaemia is the most common adverse effect of insulin therapy. In the UK Diabetes Prospective Study (UKDPS) of patients with type 2 diabetes, 1.8% of patients per year had one or more major hypoglycaemic episodes while taking insulin.[51] This study also showed that hypoglycaemia is more common in patients receiving intensive treatment with insulin (i.e. treatment with the aim of maintaining fasting plasma glucose less than 6 mmol/L). The frequency of severe hypoglycaemia due to insulin seems to be similar in type 1 and type 2 patients. Hypoglycaemia may be due to inaccurate or excessive insulin dosing, heavy physical exercise, omission of meals or excess alcohol intake. Errors in injection technique may also cause variability in the subcutaneous absorption of insulin, causing an increase in the average dose and inadvertent hypoglycaemic episodes.[43]

Symptoms of hypoglycaemia vary from patient to patient. However, the main symptoms are hunger, restlessness, sweating, tachycardia, palpitations and pallor. These may progress to headache, confusion, drowsiness, fatigue, difficulty in finding words, yawning, blurred vision, diplopia, and numbness of fingers, toes or nose. If untreated, reduction in consciousness, deep respiration, cramps, hemiplegia and paralysis may rapidly proceed to coma.

Repeated hypoglycaemic episodes are known to reduce the patient's awareness of future hypoglycaemic symptoms. This is manifest in a reduction in the blood glucose concentrations at which activation of autonomic responses to hypoglycaemia occurs.[47] Awareness of hypoglycaemia may also be lower in patients on intensive insulin regimens.

Sulphonylureas

Hypoglycaemia is the most common adverse effect of therapy with sulphonylureas. It occurs as a direct effect of their mechanism of action – stimulation of insulin secretion, decreased hepatic glucose production and improved insulin sensitivity at the target receptors. The incidence of hypoglycaemia in patients taking sulphonylureas varies widely: an incidence of between 1.8 and 59% has been reported in the literature. In the UKDPS the incidence of hypoglycaemia in patients taking sulphonylureas was 17% and the cumulative incidence of severe hypoglycaemia (requiring medical assistance or admission to hospital) was 3.3% over 6 years. Severe sulphonylurea-induced hypoglycaemia may persist for several hours and must always be treated in hospital.[52]

The severity of hypoglycaemia associated with sulphonylureas is closely related to the drug's duration of action. Chlorpropamide and glibenclamide have a much longer duration of action and are associated with more severe and prolonged hypoglycaemia than the short-acting agents glipizide, gliclazide and tolbutamide. For this reason, long-acting agents should be avoided in the elderly.

Other antidiabetic drugs

Repaglinide and nateglinide stimulate release of insulin from the pancreas. Both may cause hypoglycaemia. In clinical trials hypoglycaemia was reported in up to 10% of patients taking nateglinide as monotherapy.

Rosiglitazone and pioglitazone are new agents which are members of the thiazolidinedione class of antidiabetic drugs. They act by reducing insulin resistance in adipose tissue, skeletal muscle and the liver. Both have been associated with hypoglycaemia.

Alcohol

Alcohol inhibits gluconeogenesis, and in individuals with insufficient glycogen reserve, such as during fasting or in those who are malnourished, symptoms may occur.[47] Alcohol may also enhance the effect of insulin on glucose in normal and mildly diabetic patients. Insulin-induced hypoglycaemia may also be prolonged by alcohol owing to suppression of lipolysis and plasma fatty acid levels by alcohol. Insulin overdosage in combination with alcohol may result in refractory hypoglycaemia due to the inhibitory effects of alcohol on counterregulation.

Disorders of fat metabolism

Cholesterol and triglycerides are lipophilic compounds. Cholesterol is transported in plasma as complexes with apoproteins called lipoproteins. Triglycerides are transported in plasma bound to albumin. There are five classes of lipoprotein, which vary in their properties and functions. Two of these, low-density lipoprotein (LDL) and very low-density lipoprotein (VLDL), are strongly associated with ischaemic heart disease. In contrast, high-density lipoprotein (HDL) appears to confer a protective effect. Triglycerides are also adversely associated with ischaemic heart disease. A variety of drug therapies can both increase and decrease serum lipid levels. Table 9.7 shows the effects of some drugs on serum lipid levels.[53] The mechanism of action for this adverse effect is poorly understood and is probably multifactorial.

Although some cardiovascular drugs, such as diuretics and beta-adrenoceptor blockers, may have a detrimental effect of the plasma lipid profile, overall they generally have a beneficial effect on cardiovascular morbidity and mortality. For other classes of drug it would be sensible to avoid those that increase total or LDL cholesterol and triglycerides in patients with cardiovascular disease where possible.

Table 9.7 Drugs causing raised LDL cholesterol and total serum cholesterol

Drugs causing raised LDL cholesterol and total serum cholesterol
Thiazide diuretics
Combined oral contraceptives
Danazol
Isotretinoin
Immunosuppressive agents, e.g. ciclosporin, azathioprine, corticosteroids
Protease inhibitors, e.g. ritonavir, saquinavir

Drugs causing decreased HDL cholesterol
Beta-adrenoceptor antagonists
Danazol

Drugs causing raised triglycerides
Thiazide diuretics
Beta-adrenoceptor antagonists
Combined oral contraceptives
Isotretinoin
Acitretin
Immunosuppressive agents (e.g. ciclosporin, azathioprine, corticosteroids)
Protease inhibitors (especially ritonavir, saquinavir)
Clozapine

Drugs causing increased HDL cholesterol
Angiotensin converting enzyme inhibitors
Unopposed oestrogens
Progestogens (high-dose only)
Immunosuppressive agents, e.g. ciclosporin, azathioprine, corticosteroids

Drugs causing decreased LDL and total cholesterol
Alpha-receptor blocking drugs
Unopposed oestrogens

CASE STUDY 9.1

AB, a 40-year-old woman, visits the pharmacy for her regular prescription for a salbutamol metered-dose inhaler and a beclometasone 250 μg metered-dose inhaler, which are prescribed for the treatment of asthma. She tells the pharmacist that she was discharged from hospital 2 days ago following an acute exacerbation and was given a 7-day course of prednisolone tablets. She is feeling much better now and is thinking of stopping taking the tablets.

What other information would the pharmacist need before advising her?

The British Thoracic Society asthma management guidelines advise that steroids may be stopped abruptly if the course was for less than 3 weeks and

→

CASE STUDY 9.1 (continued)

the patient is taking inhaled steroids. Patients at greatest risk of HPA suppression are those who have been treated for more than 3 weeks, have had repeated courses of systemic corticosteroids, received more than 40 mg prednisolone or the equivalent, or have received a short course of steroids within 1 year of stopping long-term steroids. A reducing course of corticosteroids should be considered in all of these patients. It is therefore important to find out what dose of prednisolone AB was prescribed, and how long she was taking the tablets in hospital before she was discharged. The pharmacist should also check the patient medication record, or ask the patient if she has had any other courses of prednisolone in the last year.

AB was in hospital for 4 days and was prescribed 40 mg prednisolone on the day of admission. This was the first time she had received prednisolone tablets.

What advice should the pharmacist now give her?

The pharmacist should advise that AB finish her course of prednisolone to ensure that her symptoms have completely resolved. As she has taken the tablets for less than 3 weeks and has had no other courses of steroids in the past, a reducing dose is unnecessary and she may stop the tablets straight away. The pharmacist should ensure that she is taking her steroid inhaler regularly and that her inhaler technique is adequate. If she has a peak flow meter and knows how to use it she should be advised to carry out regular recordings and report any deterioration to her GP.

CASE STUDY 9.2

CD is a 38-year-old man who attends his GP for his 6-monthly check-up. He has a long history of schizophrenia, for which he has undergone trials of a variety of different antipsychotics. He is now taking clozapine 300 mg daily and his symptoms are relatively well controlled. He has no other medical history but has a chaotic lifestyle. He drinks and smokes heavily, is obese, and has found dieting unsuccessful.

Routine blood tests during his visit to his GP show that his random blood glucose is 14 mmol/L. This measurement is confirmed on a subsequent visit and his GP diagnoses type 2 diabetes.

→

> **CASE STUDY 9.2** (continued)
>
> **Is CD's diabetes likely to be drug-induced, and what are the risk factors?**
>
> There is now good evidence that the atypical antipsychotics, in particular clozapine and olanzapine are associated with the development of glucose intolerance and diabetes. The mechanism for this adverse effect is not clearly defined, but as well as causing weight gain, clozapine, olanzapine and possibly quetiapine exert direct effects on glucose–insulin homoeostasis and induce metabolic abnormalities such as hyperinsulinaemia, which may lead to insulin resistance in the longer term. Recent studies have suggested that potential risk factors for glucose intolerance are an underlying diabetic condition, an increase in body weight and male gender.[49] Cigarette smoking and physical inactivity have also been independently associated with diabetes.[50]
>
> **What are the options for treatment?**
>
> Current evidence suggests that drug-induced diabetes is more likely with clozapine and olanzapine than with risperidone. There are few data on aripiprazole and amisulpride. It is generally recommended that if patients develop diabetes during treatment with atypical antipsychotics, they should be changed to an antipsychotic less likely to affect blood glucose. However, patients on clozapine are likely to be resistant to treatment with other antipsychotics. In this case the lowest effective dose of clozapine should be given and concomitant therapy with oral hypoglycaemics or insulin initiated. It should be noted that because of the nature of CD's mental illness, intensive follow-up is likely to be needed if he is started on insulin therapy.
>
> All patients commenced on clozapine, olanzapine and quetiapine should undergo monitoring of body weight and fasting glucose prior to the start of treatment, and at regular intervals during antipsychotic treatment.

References

1. Drury PL. Endocrinology. In: Kumar P, Clark M, eds. *Clinical Medicine*, 4th edn. Edinburgh: Churchill Livingstone, 1998: 895–958.
2. Gittoes NJ, Franklyn JA. Drug-induced thyroid disorders. *Drug Safety* 1995; 13: 46–55.
3. Quin JD, Thomson JA. Adverse effects of drugs on the thyroid gland. *Adv Drug React Toxicol Rev* 1994; 13: 43–50.
4. Martino E, Bartalena L, Bogazzi F, Braverman LE. The effects of amiodarone on the thyroid. *Endocr Rev* 2001; 22: 240–254.

5. Newman CM, Price A, Davies DW, Gray TA, Weetman AP. Amiodarone and the thyroid: A practical guide to the management of thyroid dysfunction induced by amiodarone therapy. *Heart* (British Cardiac Society) 1998; 79: 121–127.

6. Harjai KJ, Licata AA. Effects of amiodarone on thyroid function. *Ann Intern Med* 1997; 126: 63–73.

7. Yeung VTF, Cockram CS. Endocrine disorders. In: Davies DM, ed. *Davies's Textbook of Adverse Drug Reactions*, 5th edn. Oxford: Oxford University Press, 1998: 381–409.

8. Chow CC, Cockram CS. Thyroid disorders induced by lithium and amiodarone: an overview. *Adv Drug React Acute Pois Rev* 1990; 9: 207–222.

9. Becerra-Fernandez A. Autoimmune thyrotoxicosis during lithium therapy in a patient with manic–depressive illness. *Am J Med* 1995; 99: 575.

10. Roti E, Minelli R, Giuberti T, *et al.* Multiple changes in thyroid function in patients with chronic active HCV hepatitis treated with recombinant interferon-alpha. *Am J Med* 1996; 101: 482–487.

11. Davies PH, Franklyn JA. The effects of drugs on tests of thyroid function. *Eur J Clin Pharmacol* 1991; 40: 439–451.

12. Surks MI, Sievert R. Drugs and thyroid function. *N Engl J Med* 1995; 333: 1688–1694.

13. Martin FI, Tress BW, Colman PG, Deam DR. Iodine-induced hyperthyroidism due to nonionic contrast radiography in the elderly. *Am J Med* 1993; 95: 78–82.

14. Costa J. Corticotrophins and corticosteroids. In: Dukes MNG, ed. *Meyler's Side Effects of Drugs*, 14th edn. Edinburgh: Elsevier, 2000: 1364–1395.

15. Page RC. How to wean a patient off corticosteroids. *Prescribers' J* 1997; 37: 11–16.

16. Robinson DS, Geddes DM. Inhaled corticosteroids: Benefits and risks. *J Asthma* 1996; 33: 5–16.

17. Levin C, Maibach HI. Topical corticosteroid-induced adrenocortical insufficiency: Clinical implications. *Am J Clin Dermatol* 2002; 3: 141–147.

18. Anon. Drugs in the peri-operative period: 2: Corticosteroids and therapy for diabetes mellitus. *Drug Ther Bull* 1999; 37: 68–70.

19. British Thoracic Society. Scottish Intercollegiate Guidelines Network. British guideline on the management of asthma. *Thorax* 2003; 58(Suppl 1): 1–94.

20. Committee on Safety of Medicines. Medicines Control Agency. Focus on corticosteroids. Withdrawal of systemic corticosteroids. *Curr Probl Pharmacovigilance* 1998; 24: 5–9.

21. Kountz DS, Clark CL. Safely withdrawing patients from chronic glucocorticoid therapy. *Am Fam Phys* 1997; 55: 521–525.

22. Khosla S, Wolfson JS, Demerjian Z, Godine JE. Adrenal crisis in the setting of high-dose ketoconazole therapy. *Arch Intern Med* 1989; 149: 802–804.

23. Best TR, Jenkins JK, Murphy FY, *et al.* Persistent adrenal insufficiency secondary to low-dose ketoconazole therapy. *Am J Med* 1987; 82: 676–680.

24. Leuenberger P, Zellweger JP. Drugs used in tuberculosis and leprosy. In: Dukes MNG, Aronson JK, eds. *Meyler's Side Effects of Drugs*, 14th edn. London: Elsevier, 2000: 1005–1029.

25. Tan SY, Shapiro R, Franco R, Stockard H, Mulrow PJ. Indomethacin-induced prostaglandin inhibition with hyperkalemia. A reversible cause of hyporeninemic hypoaldosteronism. *Ann Intern Med* 1979; 90: 783–785.

26. Clive DM, Stoff JS. Renal syndromes associated with nonsteroidal anti-inflammatory drugs. *N Engl J Med* 1984; 310: 563–572.

27. Edes TE, Sunderrajan EV. Heparin-induced hyperkalemia. *Arch Intern Med* 1985; 145: 1070–1072.
28. Oster JR, Singer I, Fishman LM. Heparin-induced aldosterone suppression and hyperkalemia. *Am J Med* 1995; 98: 575–586.
29. Committee on Safety of Medicines. Medicines Control Agency. Suppression of aldosterone secretion by heparin. *Curr Probl Pharmacovigilance* 1999; 25: 6.
30. Schaffner A, Walter R. Antifungal drugs. In: Dukes MNG, ed. *Meyler's Side Effects of Drugs*, 14th edn. London: Elsevier, 2000: 922–946.
31. Thompson DF, Carter JR. Drug-induced gynecomastia. *Pharmacotherapy* 1993; 13: 37–45.
32. Turner HE. Gynaecomastia. *Medicine* 1997 2; 25: 41–43.
33. Lucas LM, Kumar KL, Smith DL. Gynecomastia. A worrisome problem for the patient. *Postgraduate Medicine* 1987; 82: 73–76.
34. Yeung VTF. Drug-induced gynaecomastia and galactorrhoea. *Adv Drug React Bull* 1993; 162: 611–614.
35. Dickson RA, Glazer WM. Neuroleptic-induced hyperprolactinemia. *Schizophrenia Res* 1999; 35(Suppl): S75–S86.
36. Hamner M. The effects of atypical antipsychotics on serum prolactin levels. *Ann Clin Psychiatry* 2002; 14: 163–173.
37. Wieck A, Haddad P. Hyperprolactinaemia caused by antipsychotic drugs. *Br Med J* 2002; 324: 250–252.
38. Yamreudeewong W, Henann NE, Rangaraj U. Drug-induced syndrome of inappropriate secretion of antidiuretic hormone. *J Pharm Tech* 1991; 7: 50–54.
39. Spigset O, Hedenmalm K. Hyponatraemia and the syndrome of inappropriate antidiuretic hormone secretion (SIADH) induced by psychotropic drugs. *Drug Safety* 1995; 12: 209–225.
40. Masood GR, Karki SD, Patterson WR. Hyponatremia with venlafaxine. *Ann Pharmacother* 1998; 32: 49–51.
41. Abdelrahman N, Kleinman Y, Rund D, Da'as N. Hyponatremia associated with the initiation of reboxetine therapy. *Eur J Clin Pharmacol* 2003; 59: 177.
42. Garrett CA, Simpson TA Jr. Syndrome of inappropriate antidiuretic hormone associated with vinorelbine therapy. *Ann Pharmacother* 1998; 32: 1306–1309.
43. Krans HMJ. Insulin, glucagon and hypoglycaemic agents. In: Dukes MNG, ed. *Side Effects of Drugs Annual* 4. Amsterdam: Excerpta Medica, 1980: 298–310.
44. Izzedine H, Fardet L, Launay-Vacher V, *et al.* Angiotensin-converting enzyme inhibitor-induced syndrome of inappropriate secretion of antidiuretic hormone: case report and review of the literature. *Clin Pharmacol Ther* 2002; 71: 503–507.
45. Joy MS, Hladik GA. Disorders of sodium, water, calcium and phosphorus homeostasis. In: Dipiro JT, ed. *Pharmacotherapy: A Pathophysiologic Approach*, 5th edn. New York: McGraw-Hill, 2002: 953–980.
46. Kinzie BJ. Management of the syndrome of inappropriate secretion of antidiuretic hormone. *Clin Pharm* 1987; 6: 625–633.
47. So WY, Chan JCN, Cockram CS. Disorders of metabolism 1. In: Davies DM, ed. *Davies's Textbook of Adverse Drug Reactions*, 5th edn. London: Chapman & Hall, 1998: 410–441.
48. McInnes GT. Diuretics. In: Dukes MNG, ed. *Meyler's Side Effects of Drugs*, 14th edn. London: Elsevier, 2000: 656–682.

49. Hedenmalm K, Hagg S, Stahl M, Mortimer O, Spigset O. Glucose intolerance with atypical antipsychotics. *Drug Safety* 2002; 25: 1107–1116.

50. Melkersson K, Dahl ML. Adverse metabolic effects associated with atypical antipsychotics: literature review and clinical implications. *Drugs* 2004; 64: 701–723.

51. Turner RC, Holman RR, Cull CA, *et al.* Intensive blood-glucose control with sulphonylureas or insulin compared with conventional treatment and risk of complications in patients with type 2 diabetes (UKPDS 33). *Lancet* 1998; 352: 837–853.

52. BMA/RPSGB. *British National Formulary,* 47th edn. London: Pharmaceutical Press, 2004.

53. Mantel-Teeuwisse AK, Kloosterman JM, Maitland-van der Zee AH, *et al.* Drug-induced lipid changes: a review of the unintended effects of some commonly used drugs on serum lipid levels. *Drug Safety* 2001; 24: 443–456.

Further reading

Committee on Safety of Medicines. Medicines Control Agency. Focus on cortico-steroids. Withdrawal of systemic corticosteroids. *Curr Probl Pharmacovigilance* 1998; 24: 5–9.

Gittoes NJ, Franklyn JA. Drug-induced thyroid disorders. *Drug Safety* 1995; 13: 46–55.

Hamner M. The effects of atypical antipsychotics on serum prolactin levels. *Ann Clin Psychiatry* 2002; 14: 163–173.

Mantel-Teeuwisse AK, Kloosterman JM, Maitland-van der Zee AH, *et al.* Drug-induced lipid changes: a review of the unintended effects of some commonly used drugs on serum lipid levels. *Drug Safety* 2001; 24: 443–456.

Newman CM, Price A, Davies DW, Gray TA, Weetman AP. Amiodarone and the thyroid: A practical guide to the management of thyroid dysfunction induced by amiodarone therapy. *Heart* (British Cardiac Society) 1998; 79: 121–127.

So WY, Chan JCN, Cockram CS. Disorders of metabolism 1. In: Davies DM, ed. *Davies's Textbook of Adverse Drug Reactions,* 5th edn. London: Chapman & Hall, 1998: 410–441.

Spigset O, Hedenmalm K. Hyponatraemia and the syndrome of inappropriate anti-diuretic hormone secretion (SIADH) induced by psychotropic drugs. *Drug Safety* 1995; 12: 209–225.

Yeung VTF. Drug-induced gynaecomastia and galactorrhoea. *Adv Drug React Bull* 1993; 162: 611–614.

10

Respiratory disorders

Karen Belton

Introduction

Adverse drug reactions (ADRs) affecting the respiratory system are uncommon but are often serious and sometimes fatal. This chapter reviews the types of respiratory adverse reaction that can occur and the drugs most commonly implicated.

Studies of ADRs leading to hospitalisation showed that 3–7% of all reactions and 12% of those considered life-threatening involved the respiratory tract.[1,2] Because these reactions are potentially serious it is important that they are recognised early, although this is not easy as many mimic naturally occurring respiratory disease. Often the symptoms are non-specific, such as cough, wheeze or dyspnoea. Changes in pulmonary function, as measured by spirometry or lung function tests, and the radiological abnormalities seen on chest X-ray are usually non-specific. A high degree of vigilance is needed to detect adverse reactions involving the respiratory tract. A wide variety of medicines can be responsible, and the underlying mechanisms are varied and often complex.

Nasal congestion

A number of drugs have been associated with nasal congestion (Table 10.1).[3] These can, by various mechanisms, cause dilation of the nasal vasculature leading to tissue oedema and nasal congestion. Aspirin and non-steroidal anti-inflammatory drugs (NSAIDs) can cause nasal congestion and rhinorrhoea in sensitive individuals, and sildenafil is reported to cause nasal congestion in between 4% and 19% of users.[4–6] However, the commonest drug cause is the prolonged use of topical nasal decongestants containing vasoconstrictors such as ephedrine, xylometazoline and

Table 10.1 Some drugs associated with nasal congestion

Some antihypertensive agents, e.g. methyldopa, prazosin, hydralazine, propranolol, enalapril
Antidepressant/antipsychotic/hypnotic agents, e.g. amitriptyline, thioridazine, clormethiazole
Hormonal preparations, e.g. oral contraceptives
Other, e.g. sildenafil

oxymetazoline.[7,8] These topical preparations cause vasoconstriction and decrease mucosal swelling by stimulating alpha-adrenergic receptors. With prolonged or repeated use of these decongestants, patients become tolerant; that is, more frequent applications and a greater dose are needed, and this often results in rebound swelling and congestion (rhinitis medicamentosa). This leads the patient to further use of the vasoconstrictor to obtain relief, and so a cycle of use and rebound congestion is set up. Several studies have shown that oxymetazoline and xylometazoline can cause rhinitis medicamentosa after just a few weeks' continued use.

The mechanisms responsible for rebound congestion are unclear. Theories proposed include desensitisation (down-regulation) of alpha-adrenoceptors and damage to the nasal mucosa. It was previously thought that benzalkonium chloride, a preservative commonly added to decongestant solutions, could increase the severity of rhinitis medicamentosa.[8] However, there is conflicting evidence for this,[9] and a recent review of the data concluded that nasal preparations containing benzalkonium chloride are safe and well tolerated.[10] The use of topical vasoconstrictors to treat nasal congestion should be limited to a short course of no more than 7 days' duration to minimise the risk of this problem. Patients with rhinitis medicamentosa should be advised to discontinue use of the topical decongestant, and short-term treatment with topical corticosteroids has been shown to accelerate recovery.[11,12]

Neonates are particularly at risk from the excessive use of decongestant nose drops because they are obligate nasal breathers and do not develop oral breathing until aged between 2 and 6 months. Nasal obstruction can therefore cause severe respiratory distress. Topical nasal decongestants should preferably be avoided in babies less than 3 months old.[3]

Airway obstruction

Bronchoconstriction, presenting as coughing, wheezing or worsening asthma, is the most common drug-induced respiratory problem. It can

Table 10.2 Proposed mechanisms of drug-induced airway obstruction and drugs commonly associated with them

Mechanism	Drug
Drug acts as antigen	Pencillins, cephalosporins
Direct release of mediators	Iodine-containing contrast media, IV anaesthetics, muscle relaxants
Drug alters synthesis of mediators	Aspirin, non-steroidal anti-inflammatory drugs
Drug inhibits breakdown of mediators	Anticholinesterases, ACE inhibitors
Antagonism of beta-adrenoceptor	Beta-blockers
Non-specific irritation	Some pharmaceutical excipients

ACE, angiotensin-converting enzyme.

be caused by many drugs and may be part of a more generalised reaction, e.g. anaphylaxis. Patients affected nearly always have pre-existing bronchial hyperreactivity (i.e. asthma or chronic obstructive airways disease).[13] These reactions can be caused by several mechanisms that ultimately result in the contraction of bronchial smooth muscle. Table 10.2 shows some of the proposed mechanisms and drugs commonly associated with each.[14]

Antibiotics

Penicillins are the most common cause of allergic drug reactions and anaphylaxis.[15] The reactions are frequently accompanied by bronchospasm, pruritus, urticaria and angio-oedema.[16,17] Although the true incidence of these reactions is difficult to determine, it has been estimated that allergic reactions overall have a prevalence of 2% per course of therapy,[18] and that bronchospasm and acute severe dyspnoea will occur once in every 1000–10 000 treatment courses.[19] There is almost always a history of a previous course of penicillin treatment with no sign of a reaction,[20] and patients sensitive to one penicillin should be considered sensitive to all penicillins. This reaction is most common in individuals with pre-existing asthma or other allergic conditions.

A proportion of penicillin-sensitive patients will also be allergic to other beta-lactam antibiotics, such as cephalosporins, carbapenems and monobactams. Studies suggest that anaphylactic reactions to cephalosporins are rare (frequency 0.0001–0.1%).[18,21] Patients with a history of penicillin allergy are recognised to have an increased risk of anaphylaxis with cephalosporins, but a precise incidence of cross-reactivity has not been established. It seems likely that early studies of allergy to cephalosporins and penicillins may have overestimated the degree of cross-reactivity. However, the issue is complicated by the fact that the specific haptens involved in cephalosporin hypersensitivity have not been identified. Overall, the available evidence suggests that the risk of an allergic reaction to cephalosporins in patients with a history of penicillin allergy may be up to eight times as high as the risk in those with no history of allergy to penicillin.[22] Skin testing for an allergy to penicillin may be helpful in patients with a history of penicillin allergy who have a clinical indication for a cephalosporin.

Aspirin and NSAIDs

Aspirin and NSAIDs are another common cause of bronchoconstriction. Aspirin-induced asthma was first recognised in 1902, shortly after the drug's introduction. Hypersensitivity is characterised by acute broncho-spasm in asthmatic individuals, which is often accompanied by conjunctival irritation, rhinorrhoea, nasal congestion, urticaria, and sometimes flushing of the face and neck.[23] A sensitive individual will exhibit any one or a combination of these symptoms, typically within 30 minutes to 3 hours after ingestion of aspirin or NSAIDs. Bronchoconstriction may be severe and often life-threatening, requiring hospital admission and sometimes mechanical ventilation.

There has been controversy about the prevalence of aspirin-induced asthma, with reported rates ranging from 4 to 44%.[24–27] A systematic review carried out to examine this issue concluded that the pooled incidence of aspirin sensitivity among asthmatic patients was 21% (95% confidence interval (CI) 14–29%), regardless of whether the patients had a history of aspirin-induced asthma or markers for an increased risk of the syndrome.[28] Cross-sensitivity to doses of over-the-counter NSAIDs was present in most patients with aspirin-induced asthma: ibuprofen 98%, naproxen 100% and diclofenac 93%. The incidence of cross-sensitivity to paracetamol among such patients was only 7%.

Cross-sensitivity between aspirin and NSAIDs of diverse structure argues against an immunological basis for the reaction.[16] It has not been possible to identify IgE (immunoglobulin E) antibodies against either aspirin or NSAIDs, hence these reactions may be termed anaphylactoid. The pathogenesis of aspirin-induced asthma has implicated both the lipoxygenase and the cyclooxygenase (COX) pathways.[16,23] By inhibiting the COX pathway, aspirin diverts arachidonic acid metabolites to the lipoxygenase pathway. This also leads to a decrease in the levels of prostaglandin E_2, the anti-inflammatory prostaglandin, along with an increase in the synthesis of leukotrienes.[23] Patients with sinusitis, allergic rhinitis, nasal polyps or chronic urticaria have a greater frequency of hypersensitivity, and women appear to be more susceptible than men.[26,29] It has been suggested that up to 25% of hospital admissions requiring ventilation for acute asthma are due to NSAID ingestion.[23]

Asthmatic patients affected by this problem should be advised to avoid preparations containing aspirin and NSAIDs that cross-react with aspirin. Studies have suggested that the inhibition of COX-1 is a key component of the reaction, and that highly selective COX-2 inhibitors may be well tolerated in patients with aspirin sensitivity.[30] However, pre-scribing information for COX-2 selective NSAIDs contraindicates their use in patients with a history of aspirin/ NSAID sensitivity. It is import-ant that patients with a previous history of bronchospasm, rhinorrhoea, rash or angio-oedema following aspirin or NSAID use be advised to avoid self-medication with all NSAIDs in the future.[31,32] Paracetamol is usually a suitable analgesic in these patients. Cross-reactivity has been demonstrated in some aspirin-sensitive patients, although this is unusual at therapeutic doses.[30] In patients who experience symptoms with para-cetamol, an opioid analgesic such as codeine may be recommended instead.

Desensitisation regimens have been carried out with some success in aspirin-sensitive patients with coexistent thromboembolic disease or arthritis, but patients need to continue aspirin therapy indefinitely to maintain a refractory state. If aspirin is discontinued for some days the patient can revert to a sensitive state, with the risk of an acute asthma attack on re-exposure to aspirin/NSAIDs. Pretreatment with leukotriene inhibitors such as zafirlukast and montelukast has been shown to attenu-ate aspirin-induced nasal and bronchial reactions.[23,26] Clopidogrel may be an alternative antiplatelet agent for asthmatic patients with aspirin-induced bronchoconstriction.

ACE inhibitors

Angiotensin-converting enzyme (ACE) inhibitors are associated with cough in 3–20% of all treated patients.[33,34] The mechanism is not proven, but is thought to involve the accumulation of prostaglandins, kinins (e.g. bradykinin) or substance P (the neurotransmitter present in respiratory C-fibres) as a direct result of ACE inhibition.[35]

The cough is typically dry, persistent and non-productive. Pulmonary function does not seem to be affected. It can begin within a week of starting therapy, but in many patients the onset is delayed for up to a year.

The cough usually disappears within several days of withdrawal of the ACE inhibitor, but can take as long as 4 weeks to subside. It usually recurs on rechallenge with the same or another ACE inhibitor.

The cough can be debilitating, leading to sleep disturbances, vomiting, sore throat and voice changes. It does not respond to treatment with antitussives. Sodium cromoglicate and nifedipine have been shown to ameliorate the cough in some studies.[35] Women may be affected more commonly than men, and asthma and chronic obstructive pulmonary disease (COPD) do not appear to be predisposing factors.[36] ACE inhibitors should generally be stopped in patients who experience a troublesome cough. The angiotensin-II receptor antagonists do not inhibit the breakdown of bradykinin, and cause significantly less cough.[37] These may be a suitable alternative for patients with ACE inhibitor-induced cough.

Beta-adrenoceptor blockers

Beta-adrenoceptor blockers can precipitate bronchoconstriction in patients with asthma or COPD and can interfere with the efficacy of adrenergic bronchodilators in such patients. The beta-adrenergic system has both beta$_1$ and beta$_2$ receptors: beta$_1$ stimulation results in an increase in rate and force of cardiac contraction, and beta$_2$ stimulation leads to bronchodilation.

Bronchoconstriction is due to antagonism of the beta$_2$-adrenoceptors in the bronchi. There are case reports of asthma exacerbation and bronchoconstriction with beta-blockers, including cases in association with their topical use.[37] Consequently, all beta-blockers have traditionally been considered contraindicated in patients with asthma and COPD because of fear of bronchoconstriction. Cardioselective beta-blockers, such as bisoprolol, atenolol and metoprolol, selectively block beta$_1$ receptors and have little or no effect on beta$_2$ receptors, except at high doses. As beta-blockers are now known to have important mortality benefits in cardiovascular disease, the extent of risk associated with their use in patients with COPD has recently been evaluated.[38] It was concluded that cardioselective beta-blockers do not produce a significant reduction in airway function or increase the risk of COPD exacerbations, and should not be withheld from patients with COPD.

General anaesthesia

Allergic reactions occurring during anaesthesia are an important problem; the incidence of life-threatening anaphylactic or anaphylactoid reactions occurring during anaesthesia has been estimated to be between 1 in 1000 and 1 in 25 000 anaesthetic procedures.[39] In the UK it has been estimated that about 100 deaths during anaesthesia each year may be due to hypersensitivity reactions.[40] These reactions are more common in women, with a female to male ratio of 2.5:1 reported.[41]

Bronchospasm occurs in up to 50% of affected patients. It may be either transient or severe, and in 3% of cases may be the only presenting feature. Neuromuscular blockers are thought to account for about 80% of these reactions.[39] Both depolarising agents, such as suxamethonium, and non-depolarising agents such as atracurium, have been implicated, although suxamethonium is the most frequent cause.[40] The mechanism may involve the release of mediators such as histamine or the development of specific antibodies.

Patients who may have experienced an allergic reaction during anaesthesia should be fully investigated to elucidate the cause. Skin-prick testing may be useful. Where the reaction was caused by a neuro-muscular blocker, cross-reactivity between drugs occurs in about 70% of patients.[41] The Association of Anaesthetists of Great Britain and Ireland produces a useful booklet giving guidance on these reactions.[41]

Other drugs

Radiocontrast media are a well-recognised cause of acute bronchospasm, usually as part of a generalised anaphylactic reaction. The rate of adverse reactions following administration of ionic contrast media is between 5 and 8%, and between 0.2 and 1% following administration of non-ionic contrast media.[42,43] Mild reactions are more common with ionic contrast media than with non-ionic, although reactions to both types can be life-threatening. The incidence is thought to be greater in asthmatic patients and those with known allergies to food or medicines.[44,45] In the UK the Royal College of Radiologists has issued advice on the management of reactions to intravenous contrast media.[42]

Some pharmaceutical excipients can cause hypersensitivity reactions featuring bronchospasm in susceptible individuals. Tartrazine was first identified as a cause of asthma in 1967. However, in double-blind placebo-controlled trials using pulmonary function testing, sensitivity to tartrazine was rare.[46]

A small number (approximately 3%) of patients who develop hypersensitivity reactions with aspirin may also show cross-reactivity to tartrazine.[47] Other excipients that have been implicated in these reactions include benzoates, phenylmercuric salts, parabens, benzalkonium chloride and metabisulphite. These reactions seem to occur almost exclusively in patients with pre-existing asthma.[46,48]

Parasympathomimetic drugs such as pilocarpine and carbachol, although now seldom used, have a direct effect on the vagal tone of the smooth muscles of the respiratory tract and can provoke bronchoconstriction. They should be used with caution in asthmatic patients.[49]

Hypersensitivity reactions to the nucleoside reverse transcriptase inhibitor abacavir occur in about 4% of patients treated, and respiratory disorders occur in 20% of those who experience hypersensitivity reactions.[50] Such reactions usually become apparent in the first 6 weeks of treatment, but may occur at any time. Possible respiratory symptoms include dyspnoea, cough and pharyngitis. Signs of pneumonia or bronchitis have been observed in a high proportion of fatalities. Patients who experience a hypersensitivity reaction with abacavir must not be re-exposed to the drug because of the risk of a more severe, life-threatening reaction.

Reflex bronchoconstriction

Paradoxical bronchoconstriction has been reported with a number of inhaled medicines, including beta-agonists, corticosteroids, ipratropium and cromoglicate. It is thought to result from non-specific irritation of the bronchial mucosa. The problem has occurred with both nebuliser solutions and metered-dose inhalers.[51] In the UK the Committee on Safety of Medicines (CSM) warned about the risk of worsening airways disease in association with nebulised bronchodilator solutions in 1988.[52] Formulation factors such as the hypotonicity of the solution or the presence of preservatives, such as benzalkonium chloride, were implicated. As most nebuliser solutions are now isotonic and preservative free, this problem is unusual.

Hydrofluorocarbon propellants in metered-dose inhalers are frequently implicated in bronchoconstriction, although in some cases the drug itself may be responsible.[53] Bronchoconstriction has been described with delivery of the long-acting bronchodilator salmeterol by metered-dose inhaler, but not after dry powder Diskhaler.[54] It has been suggested that salmeterol's relatively slow onset of action may expose such bronchoconstriction, whereas agents with a faster onset of action may attenuate any bronchoconstriction that occurs. Bronchospasm has been reported rarely after inhalation of zanamivir, the antiviral drug effective against influenza A or B infection, and this should be used with caution in patients with asthma or chronic bronchitis.[55] If such patients are prescribed zanamivir they should be advised to keep a fast-acting bronchodilator to hand.

Parenchymal lung disorders

Adverse drug reactions affecting the lung parenchyma form a heterogeneous group of inflammatory, infiltrative and fibrotic disorders. The two main mechanisms of these reactions are hypersensitivity and fibrosis (resulting from more direct toxicity). However, because these reactions share common clinical, radiographic and physiological features they are often grouped together. Hypersensitivity-type pneumonitis (sometimes termed alveolitis) and fibrotic pulmonary disease can therefore be regarded as part of a spectrum of closely related disease states.[49,56] The aetiology and pathogenesis of these conditions, however, are poorly understood, and not all drugs that cause pneumonitis are necessarily associated with fibrosis. Tables 10.3 and 10.4 show some of the drugs most frequently associated with hypersensitivity pneumonitis and pulmonary fibrosis.[33,57,58]

Hypersensitivity pneumonitis

In general, these reactions are of an allergic nature and may have a dramatic clinical presentation. They typically occur acutely, between a few hours and 7–10 days of starting therapy with the suspect drug.[59] The main symptoms are cough, breathlessness and wheeze, sometimes accompanied by bronchospasm. They require a prompt diagnosis and withdrawal of the suspect drug. With early detection and treatment there is a high chance of complete recovery.

Table 10.3 Drugs typically associated with interstitial pneumonitis

Amiodarone	Nitrofurantoin
Gold	Penicillamine
Methotrexate	Sulfasalazine

Table 10.4 Some drugs associated with pulmonary fibrosis

Amiodarone	Methysergide
Bleomycin	Mitomycin
Busulfan	Nitrofurantoin
Carmustine	Pergolide
Cyclophosphamide	Sulfasalazine
Gold	

An ADR may not be suspected with symptoms such as non-productive cough, breathlessness and wheeze. However, the presence of pulmonary infiltrates on X-ray and eosinophilia on a blood count (indicative of allergy) points towards this clinical diagnosis and the patient's recent drug therapy should be reviewed. The findings of other diagnostic techniques, such as bronchoscopic bronchoalveolar lavage, may help to confirm an iatrogenic cause. This technique involves the aspiration of buffered saline instilled into the bronchi via a bronchoscope. With this procedure it has proved possible to identify an increase in the total cell count (pleocytosis) in hypersensitivity pneumonitis and eosinophilia and/or lymphocytosis in the fluid obtained.[14] Pleural biopsy, demonstrating eosinophilia, may be a useful investigation in some situations. Withdrawal of the suspect drug will normally result in a good recovery, and treatment with a course of systemic corticosteroids will assist rapid symptom resolution.[14,33,60]

Nitrofurantoin

Nitrofurantoin is an important cause of respiratory reactions, causing both acute pneumonitis and, less commonly, chronic pulmonary fibrosis.[61] The frequency of acute severe pulmonary disease has been estimated at 1 in every 5000 first administrations,[62] and pulmonary reactions are among those most frequently reported for nitrofurantoin.[63] These reactions are more common in women between 40 and 50 years of age. The acute reaction tends to occur between 1 and 4 weeks of starting treatment,[14,63] and is usually accompanied by eosinophilia.[33] Symptoms include severe dyspnoea, tachypnoea, non-productive cough and fever. Recovery is usually rapid and complete after the drug is stopped.

The mechanism of this reaction is unclear, although it is thought to be a hypersensitivity-type reaction and an immune mechanism has been postulated.[64] However, it is also thought to involve a more direct toxic response, as nitrofurantoin produces free oxygen radicals that may damage the lung.[14]

Chronic respiratory reactions with nitrofurantoin are much less common: it is estimated that they occur 10–20 times less often than the acute type.[62] They have a much slower onset and usually occur during long-term prophylactic therapy of 6 months or more. Symptoms include cough, dyspnoea and fatigue; however, fever is uncommon in the chronic reaction. X-ray may show interstitial infiltrates, but fibrotic changes are rare. Recovery on drug withdrawal is usually good but not always complete; mortality is estimated at 1–10%.[64,65]

Methotrexate

Methotrexate may cause hypersensitivity pneumonitis in up to 7% of treated patients.[66] The onset is usually subacute, developing over several weeks, but may be delayed and can develop up to 4 weeks after therapy has been discontinued.[67] The most frequent symptoms are non-productive cough, dyspnoea and fever. Eosinophilia is common, and diffuse bilateral interstitial infiltrates can be seen on chest X-ray. The use of bronchoalveolar lavage (BAL) may be required to exclude infection. Corticosteroid therapy and methotrexate withdrawal will usually result in a good recovery; however, the mortality associated with the reaction has been estimated at between 10 and 25%.[33,68]

The UK CSM has issued recommendations on monitoring for pulmonary symptoms in patients receiving methotrexate.[69] These include advising patients to seek medical attention if they experience symptoms such as dyspnoea, dry cough and fever; monitoring patients for these symptoms at follow-up visits; and withdrawal of methotrexate and treatment with corticosteroids if pneumonitis is suspected.[69]

Gold

The incidence of pulmonary reactions to gold therapy is estimated at around 1%.[65] The time to onset is normally between 5 and 16 weeks after starting therapy,[65] but it can occur as late as a month after the last dose has been given.[37] Most patients will present with dyspnoea and non-productive cough progressing over several weeks. Rarely the reaction can present acutely with fever, wheeze and cough developing over several hours. Bilateral pulmonary infiltrates may be seen on X-ray,[70] and BAL would be expected to show a high total cell count with an increased percentage of lymphocytes.[37,70] The mechanism for the reaction is not well established, but it is thought (and the results of BAL suggest) to have an immunological basis.[71,72] However, histological examination using electron microscopy has shown a cellular presence of gold-containing lysosomes, suggesting a direct toxic effect. The rate of complete recovery on withdrawal of treatment is about 50%, mortality is estimated at about 7%, and the remaining patients will have some residual radiological and/or physiological effects.[71]

Pulmonary fibrosis

Direct toxicity of the causative drug causes cell damage, eliciting an inflammatory fibrotic response and resulting in the distortion and subsequent destruction of the alveoli. This type of fibrotic reaction is frequently correlated to the duration of therapy and/or the total cumulative dose received. In the case of cytotoxic agents the toxicity may be increased by a number of factors, including increasing patient age, decreased renal function, radiotherapy, oxygen therapy and other associated cytotoxic drug therapy.

The symptoms include malaise, a dry cough and increasing dyspnoea, which progress gradually over a period of weeks or months. Pulmonary function tests show reduced gas transfer and X-ray examination usually shows diffuse infiltrates. The withdrawal of the suspect drug, with or without corticosteroid treatment, does not always result in a complete resolution of the symptoms or cessation of the disease process. These reactions are associated with significant morbidity and mortality.[65]

Bleomycin

Pulmonary fibrosis is a well-recognised complication of bleomycin therapy. Bleomycin is deposited in both the skin and the lungs, and consequently its most serious side effects affect these two organs.[33] The reported incidence of pulmonary reactions with this drug ranges from 11 to 23%,[73] with the incidence of pulmonary fibrosis estimated at 10%.[33,60] Predisposing factors include impaired renal function, age over 70 years, concurrent radiotherapy, and administration of high concentrations of oxygen.[74] The relatively high oxygen tension in the lung facilitates the generation of superoxide radicals by bleomycin. Use of supplemental oxygen in patients receiving bleomycin should be avoided as far as possible and, if absolutely necessary, should be carefully monitored.[60]

The risk of pulmonary toxicity also rises with the total dose of bleomycin administered. At cumulative doses below 300 mg about 3–5% of patients are affected. At doses above 500 mg the rate of toxicity is estimated to be 20%.[75] However, rapidly fatal pulmonary toxicity has occurred with doses as low as 100 mg, whereas patients receiving doses over 500 mg have demonstrated no pulmonary toxicity.[75,76] It is recommended that the dose of bleomycin should be kept below 400 mg whenever possible, in order to minimise the risk.[75]

Symptoms such as cough, dyspnoea and malaise may progress over several weeks or months; however, some affected patients may remain asymptomatic.[60] Where symptoms occur, bleomycin should be withdrawn and oxygen therapy minimised. Corticosteroid therapy may be initiated, but there is little evidence to support this. Recovery may be incomplete and mortality is estimated to be around 1%.[14,37] Bleomycin is also associated with a hypersensitivity pneumonitis that is more amenable to treatment.[37]

Busulfan

Busulfan is another cytotoxic drug commonly associated with pneumonitis and fibrosis; the incidence is estimated at 4%.[37,60] Features are similar to those seen with bleomycin, but a critical dose level or specific predisposing factors have not been demonstrated. In contrast to bleomycin, drug withdrawal rarely causes resolution of symptoms and further progression of the fibrosis is common. Mortality has been reported to be as high as 80%.[60,77]

Amiodarone

Amiodarone can cause different patterns of pulmonary toxicity. It is associated with both pneumonitis and pulmonary fibrosis as well as with bronchiolitis obliterans organising pneumonia (BOOP). The incidence of pulmonary toxicity is reported to be about 5–10%.[78–80] Affected patients usually present with insidious evolving, non-specific symptoms such as cough, dyspnoea, weight loss and chest pain. The non-specific clinical symptoms due to amiodarone-induced pulmonary toxicity may be masked by symptoms of cardiac failure and delay recognition of the reaction. Several factors increase susceptibility to amiodarone lung damage, including dose, duration of therapy, advanced age and pre-existing pulmonary dysfunction.[58,79] The mechanism of toxicity is probably multifactorial, involving direct damage, immune-mediated hypersensitivity and phospholipid accumulation in lung tissue. In most cases the reaction is reversible if diagnosed at an early stage.

Clinical evidence suggests that the risk of a patient experiencing adverse effects with amiodarone increases as the dose and duration of therapy increase. Most amiodarone-induced pulmonary manifestations are found to occur when the dose exceeds 400 mg daily, administered for more than 2 months, or when a lower dose is given for more than 2 years.[58,79] However, several case studies and clinical trials of amiodarone have shown the possible occurrence of pulmonary toxicity during low-dose[80] and short-duration therapy, suggesting that dose and duration of treatment are not the only determinants of risk.[79] For example, lung toxicity has been described after short-term amiodarone therapy in patients treated on the intensive care unit for acute respiratory distress syndrome,[81] and after a short course of treatment following surgery for lung cancer.[82] Overall, the mortality associated with pulmonary adverse reactions is estimated at around 9–10%.[83,84] Management may consist of dose reduction and pulmonary monitoring in mild cases of toxicity, or complete withdrawal of amiodarone in more severe cases. However, the potential for recurrence of life-threatening arrhythmias on treatment discontinuation must be considered.

Up to 25% of patients with amiodarone-induced pulmonary damage may have bronchiolitis obliterans or BOOP.[14] BOOP is characterised by destruction of the small airways by a non-specific inflammation. This type of reaction needs to be differentiated from other pulmonary conditions, as it is associated with a more benign course and responds better to corticosteroids than the other infiltrative pulmonary diseases. Because of this, corticosteroid treatment is recommended for all patients with amiodarone-induced lung damage in case some areas of pneumonitis are of this nature. This treatment should probably be continued for at least 6 months after amiodarone is withdrawn, because of the drug's long half-life (55 days).[85]

Healthcare professionals should be aware of the risk of pulmonary toxicity with amiodarone. Patients should be counselled to report the development of symptoms such as cough, dyspnoea and chest pain promptly. A chest X-ray may be advisable before amiodarone therapy is started. During treatment, if pulmonary toxicity is suspected the chest X-ray should be repeated and lung function tests carried out.

Ergot derivatives

Pleuropulmonary fibrosis is a rare but well-recognised adverse effect of ergot-derived dopamine receptor agonists.[86,87] The reaction has an insidious onset and symptoms consist of cough, progressive dyspnoea and/or pleuritic pain. The mechanism for this reaction is not clear, and there is no evidence of a relationship to dose or treatment duration.[88] In April 2002 the UK CSM published data, collected via their yellow card scheme, of reported cases of fibrotic reactions involving the lungs, pericardium and retroperitoneum.[86] Pergolide appeared to be associated with a higher rate of such reactions than the other ergot derivatives; however, this could be due either to a true increase in incidence or to reporting biases. The CSM recommended that baseline investigations, such as chest X-ray and lung function tests, are undertaken prior to starting treatment, and that patients are regularly and carefully monitored for signs of fibrotic disorders during treatment.

Pulmonary oedema

Non-cardiogenic pulmonary oedema or adult respiratory distress syndrome (ARDS) is thought to be due to increased pulmonary vascular

Table 10.5 Some drugs associated with pulmonary oedema at therapeutic doses

Diamorphine	Naloxone
Epoprostenol	Protamine
Haloperidol	Ritodrine
Hydrochlorothiazide	Salbutamol (IV)
Indometacin	Terbutaline (IV)
Methadone	Vinorelbine

Table 10.6 Some drugs associated with pulmonary oedema in overdose

Aspirin	Dextropropoxyphene
Codeine	Dihydrocodeine
Colchicine	Tricyclic antidepressants

permeability, resulting in extravasation of fluid and proteinacious material into the alveoli.[57,89] The symptoms include acute breathlessness, cough and frothy sputum. Diffuse bilateral alveolar shadowing can be seen on chest X-ray.[58] The reaction seems to occur with therapeutic doses of some drugs and as a consequence of overdose with others[33,49,90–93] (Tables 10.5 and 10.6).

Hydrochlorothiazide

The thiazide diuretic hydrochlorothiazide can cause non-cardiogenic pulmonary oedema and interstitial pneumonitis.[37,94,95] Although it is estimated to be a rare adverse reaction, more than 30 cases have been described in the literature.[94] Most affected patients were women, and most had been prescribed the drug for hypertension or fluid retention. Onset is acute, occurring within a few hours of ingestion of hydrochlorothiazide, and symptoms include cough, dyspnoea, wheeze, chest pain, sweating, nausea and vomiting. In some cases the patient experienced recurrent episodes of pulmonary oedema before the link with drug therapy was made. The mechanism of the reaction is unknown, although an immunological basis has been suggested.[95] Supportive therapy with opioids, venous vasodilators and aminophylline (if bronchospasm is present) is the preferred management.[37] Patients who have experienced this problem should be advised to avoid hydrochlorothiazide in the future. Furosemide may be given if subsequent diuretic therapy is needed.

Intravenous beta-agonists

The use of intravenous beta-agonists to suppress uterine contractions (tocolytics) in premature labour is associated with pulmonary oedema. A recent study of over 62 000 pregnancies showed that, of those diagnosed with pulmonary oedema, 25.5% were attributable to the use of tocolytics.[96] A review of 58 cases of pulmonary oedema associated with ritodrine, salbutamol and terbutaline suggested that most cases occurred during or within 24 hours of drug use.[97] Symptoms improved rapidly when intravenous furosemide and oxygen were given. However, there were two maternal and three fetal deaths. Fluid overload is the single most important predisposing factor; others include multiple pregnancy, pre-existing cardiac disease, maternal infection and the use of multiple simultaneous tocolytics. Close monitoring of hydration is recommended in women receiving tocolytics.[98]

Pulmonary thromboembolism

Pulmonary thromboembolism occurs when a thrombus from the systemic veins embolises into the pulmonary arterial system. The clinical features of a large pulmonary embolism include sudden collapse, pleuritic pain, breathlessness, cyanosis and haemoptysis. Smaller emboli may present with increasing breathlessness and pleuritic pain. Conditions leading to the formation of thrombi in the systemic veins can thus predispose to pulmonary embolism. Hormonal contraceptives are a well-recognised cause. Recently there has been debate about the role of antipsychotic agents as a cause of venous thromboembolism and pulmonary embolism.[99–101]

CASE STUDY 10.1

MC is a 45-year-old man who comes into the pharmacy to ask for a more powerful decongestant. He developed a severe cold 2 months ago that was followed by a blocked nose. He began using an oxymetazoline nasal spray at night to help him breathe. He tells you that it worked really well for 2 weeks, but then his blocked nose worsened and he needed to use it more often. He now seems to be using it all the time, but is not getting much relief and would now like to purchase something more powerful to unblock his nose.

→

◗ **CASE STUDY 10.1** (continued)

What could be MC's problem?

Prolonged or repeated use of topical nasal congestants can lead to a tolerance of the nasal mucosa to their effects, causing a cycle of more frequent use and further nasal congestion. This condition is termed rhinitis medicamentosa and is among the most common causes of drug-induced nasal congestion. This condition can occur after just a couple of weeks' continued use of topical decongestants, and could be the cause of MC's problem.

What questions might you ask MC to clarify this suspicion?

As other medications may cause nasal congestion (Table 10.1) you may want to ask if he is taking any other medications, either bought over the counter or prescribed by his doctor.

His only other medication is aspirin, he has previously used this only occasionally. However, following a muscle sprain around 6 weeks ago, he has been using it regularly for pain relief.

Aspirin hypersensitivity is characterised by acute bronchospasm, often accompanied by urticaria, flushing, conjunctival irritation, rhinorrhoea and nasal congestion. Sensitive individuals may exhibit a combination, or any one, of these symptoms between 30 minutes and 3 hours after ingestion of aspirin. It most commonly presents for the first time in asthmatic individuals between the ages of 20 and 40, and is more common in women than in men.[102] It is unlikely that the aspirin is causing MC's problem, but it would be prudent to check that he does not have a history of asthma, nasal polyps, or any other accompanying symptoms, for example difficulty in breathing, flushing or a runny nose.

MC tells you that he is normally very fit and healthy and has no history of asthma or other accompanying symptoms. He has previously only suffered nasal congestion following a cold. From MC's history and the absence of accompanying symptoms, it seems that the most likely cause of his continued nasal congestion is rhinitis medicamentosa.

How can you help MC?

You should explain to MC the nature of this adverse effect and tell him that with continued use of the same, or an alternative, topical decongestant the congestion is likely to remain. This condition is managed by the withdrawal of topical decongestant. If he finds this difficult, owing to the extent of the congestion, it may be helpful to withdraw use of the decongestant gradually by decreasing the frequency of use.[3] MC should also be instructed that if he uses topical decongestants in the future he should limit this to a short course, i.e. not longer than 7 days, to prevent the problem recurring. He should be advised to contact his GP if the congestion does not resolve.

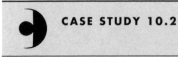

CASE STUDY 10.2

Mr L is a 65-year-old man with rheumatoid arthritis who is otherwise healthy. He has been taking methotrexate, 7.5 mg per week, for the last 3 months. Prior to starting methotrexate he was treated with oral gold for about 1 year, but this was stopped due to lack of response. At a routine outpatient rheumatology appointment Mr L complains of breathlessness, a dry cough, and feeling feverish for the past 3 weeks. He was previously warned that his gold therapy could cause lung problems and wonders if this could be the cause of his cough.

Could the symptoms be drug-induced?

Mr L's symptoms are non-specific and could be due to a number of causes: his medical notes should be reviewed for any history of respiratory problems. Respiratory infection, in particular should be excluded in a patient with these symptoms before an ADR is diagnosed.

Both gold and methotrexate can cause pneumonitis, characterised by dyspnoea, cough and fever. The incidence is thought to be lower with gold therapy than with methotrexate (1% compared to up to 7%).[65,66] Although Mr L is no longer taking gold, pneumonitis would be most likely to occur between 5 and 16 weeks after starting therapy, but has been reported to present up to a month after the last dose.[37] In Mr L's case it is unlikely that gold therapy is the cause of his symptoms due to the gap of 3 months since his last dose.

Methotrexate pneumonitis could be a possible cause for Mr L's symptoms. Most cases occur in patients with rheumatoid arthritis during the first year of treatment,[66,100] and previous therapy with gold is a known risk factor.[103] The most frequent symptoms are a non-productive cough, dyspnoea and fever.[66]

How can this be confirmed?

The diagnosis of methotrexate pneumonitis is generally one of exclusion. In particular, both sputum and blood cultures should be negative to exclude infection. Once other aetiologies have been excluded, in a patient with an appropriate history of methotrexate use, chest X-ray and pulmonary function tests may be helpful in diagnosing this condition. Diffuse bilateral infiltrates are normally seen on chest X-ray and a reduced vital capacity is often demonstrated by spirometry.[66,67] In addition, a reduced transfer factor for carbon monoxide is also a common feature.[67] A definite diagnosis will always be difficult because of the non-specific nature of the clinical features.

→

> **● CASE STUDY 10.2** (continued)
>
> **How should Mr L be managed?**
>
> If pneumonitis is suspected then methotrexate should be withdrawn and treatment with steroids initiated.[69] The long-term prognosis is usually good, but mortality has been reported to be between 10 and 25%. It is important to advise patients taking methotrexate to seek medical attention if they experience symptoms suggestive of pneumonitis.

References

1. Levy M, Kewitz H, Altwein W, *et al*. Hospital admissions due to adverse drug reactions: a comparative study from Jerusalem and Berlin. *Eur J Clin Pharmacol* 1980; 17: 25–31.
2. Ibanez L, Laporte JR, Carne X. Adverse drug reactions leading to hospital admission. *Drug Safety* 1991; 6: 450–459.
3. Simon PA. Acute and chronic rhinitis. In: Koda Kimble MA, Young LY, eds. *Applied Therapeutics: The Clinical Use of Drugs*, 7th edn. Philadelphia: Lippincott Williams & Wilkins, 2001: 23.1–23.31.
4. Moreira SG Jr, Brannigan RE, Spitz A, *et al*. Side-effect profile of sildenafil citrate (Viagra) in clinical practice. *Urology* 2000; 56: 474–476.
5. McMahon CG, Samali R, Johnson H. Efficacy, safety and patient acceptance of sildenafil citrate as treatment for erectile dysfunction. *J Urol* 2000; 164: 1192–1196.
6. Coelho OR. Tolerability and safety profile of sildenafil citrate (Viagra) in Latin American patient populations. *Int J Impot Res* 2002; 14(Suppl 2): S54–S59.
7. Diamond C. Ear, nose and throat disorders. In: Davies DM, Ferner RE, de Glanville H, eds. *Textbook of Adverse Drug Reactions*, 5th edn. London: Chapman & Hall, 1998: 643–668.
8. Graf P. Adverse effects of benzalkonium chloride on the nasal mucosa: allergic rhinitis and rhinitis medicamentosa. *Clin Ther* 1999; 21: 1749–1755.
9. Graf P. Benzalkonium chloride as a preservative in nasal solutions: re-examining the data. *Respir Med* 2001; 95: 728–733.
10. Marple B, Roland P, Benninger M. Safety review of benzalkonium chloride used as a preservative in intranasal solutions: an overview of conflicting data and opinions. *Otolaryngol Head Neck Surg* 2004; 130: 131–141.
11. Dykewicz MS, Fineman S, Skoner DP, *et al*. Diagnosis and management of rhinitis: complete guidelines of the Joint Task Force on Practice Parameters in Allergy, Asthma and Immunology. *Ann Allergy Asthma Immunol* 1998; 81: 478–518.
12. Ferguson BJ, Paramaesvaran S, Rubinstein E. A study of the effect of nasal steroid sprays in perennial allergic rhinitis patients with rhinitis medicamentosa. *Otolaryngol Head Neck Surg* 2001; 125: 253–260.

13. Hoigne RV, Braunschweig S, Zehnder D, *et al.* Drug-induced attack of bronchial asthma in inpatients: a 20-year survey of the Comprehensive Hospital Drug Monitoring Programme on adverse drug reactions, Berne/St. Gallen. *Eur J Clin Pharmacol* 1997; 53: 81–82.
14. Keaney NP. Drug induced lung disease. In: Walker R, Edwards C, eds. *Clinical Pharmacy and Therapeutics*, 3rd edn. London: Churchill Livingstone, 2002: 413–421.
15. Drain KL, Volcheck GW. Preventing and managing drug-induced anaphylaxis. *Drug Safety* 2001; 24: 843–853.
16. deShazo RD, Kemp SF. Allergic reactions to drugs and biologic agents. *JAMA* 1997; 278: 1895–1906.
17. Anon. Penicillin allergy. *Drug Ther Bull* 1996; 34: 87–88.
18. Yates AB, deShazo RD. Allergic and nonallergic drug reactions. *South Med J* 2003; 96: 1080–1087.
19. Neftel KA, Zoppi M, Cerny A, *et al.* Reactions typically shared by more than one class of bet-lactam antibiotic. In: Dukes MNG, Aronson JK, eds. *Meyler's Side Effects of Drugs*, 14th edn. Amsterdam: Elsevier, 2000: 791–809.
20. Szczeklik A, Nizankowska E. Drug induced asthma and bronchospasm. In: Akoun GM, White JP, eds. *Treatment Induced Respiratory Disorders*. Amsterdam: Elsevier, 1989: 189–209.
21. Kelkar PS, Li JTC. Current concepts: cephalosporin allergy. *N Engl J Med* 2001; 345: 804–809.
22. Kishiyama JL, Adelman DC. The cross-reactivity and immunology of beta-lactam antibiotics. *Drug Safety* 1994; 10: 318–327.
23. Babu KS, Salvi SS. Aspirin and asthma. *Chest* 2000; 118: 1470–1476.
24. Settipane GA. Aspirin and allergic diseases: a review. *Am J Med* 1983; 74(Suppl 6a): 102–109.
25. Power I. Aspirin-induced asthma (editorial). *Br J Anaesth* 1993; 71: 619–621.
26. Szczeklik A, Stevenson DD. Aspirin-induced asthma: advances in pathogenesis and management. *J Allergy Clin Immunol* 1999; 104: 5–13.
27. Bochenek G, Banska K, Szabo Z, *et al.* Diagnosis, prevention and treatment of aspirin-induced asthma and rhinitis. *Curr Drug Targets Inflamm Allergy* 2002; 1: 1–11.
28. Jenkins C, Costello J, Hodge L. Systematic review of prevalence of aspirin induced asthma and its implications for clinical practice. *Br Med J* 2004; 328: 434–437.
29. Oates JA, Fitzgerald GA, Branch RA, *et al.* Clinical implications of prostaglandin and thromboxane formation. *N Engl J Med* 1988; 319: 689.
30. Szczeklik A, Stevenson DD. Aspirin-induced asthma: advances in pathogenesis, diagnosis, and management. *J Allergy Clin Immunol* 2003; 111: 913–921.
31. Ayres JG, Fleming DM, Whittington RM. Asthma death due to ibuprofen. *Lancet* 1987; i: 1082.
32. Chan TYK. Severe asthma attacks precipitated by NSAIDs. *Ann Pharmacol* 1995; 29: 199.
33. Ozkan M, Dweik RA, Ahmad M. Drug-induced lung disease. *Cleveland Clin J Med* 2001; 68: 782–785, 789–795.
34. Israili ZH, Dallashall W. Cough and angioneurotic edema associated with angiotensin-converting enzyme inhibitor therapy. *Ann Intern Med* 1992; 117: 234–242.

35. Overlack A. ACE inhibitor-induced cough and bronchospasm: incidence, mechanisms, and management. *Drug Safety* 1996; 15: 72–78.
36. Packard KA, Wurdeman RL, Arouni AJ. ACE inhibitor-induced bronchial reactivity in patients with respiratory dysfunction. *Ann Pharmacother* 2002; 36: 1058–1067.
37. Ben-Noun L. Drug-induced respiratory disorders: incidence, prevention and management. *Drug Safety* 2000; 23: 143–164.
38. Andrus MR, Holloway KP, Clark DB. Use of beta-blockers in patients with COPD. *Ann Pharmacother* 2004; 38: 142–145.
39. Naguib M, Magboul MM. Adverse effects of neuromuscular blockers and their antagonists. *Drug Safety* 1998; 18: 99–116.
40. McKinnon RP, Wildsmith JAW. Histaminoid reactions in anaesthesia. *Br J Anaesth* 1995; 74: 217–228.
41. Association of Anaesthetists of Great Britain and Ireland and British Society for Allergy and Clinical Immunology. *Suspected Anaphylactic Reactions Associated with Anaesthesia*, 3rd edn. London: Association of Anaesthetists of Great Britain and Ireland and British Society for Allergy and Clinical Immunology, 2003.
42. Board of the Faculty of Clinical Radiology/The Royal College of Radiologists. *Advice on the Management of Reactions to Intravenous Contrast Media.* London: Royal College of Radiologists, 1996.
43. Cochran ST, Bomyea K, Sayre JW. Trends in adverse events after IV administration of contrast media. *AJR Am J Roentgenol* 2001; 176: 1385–1388.
44. Maddox TG. Adverse reactions to contrast material: recognition, prevention, and treatment. *Am Fam Phys* 2002; 66: 1229–1234.
45. Esplugas E, Cequier A, Gomez-Hospital JA, *et al.* Comparative tolerability of contrast media used for coronary interventions. *Drug Safety* 2002; 25: 1079–1098.
46. Golightly LK, Smolinske SS, Bennett ML, *et al.* Pharmaceutical excipients: adverse effects associated with inactive ingredients in drug products (Part I). *Med Toxicol Adv Drug Exp* 1988; 3: 128–165.
47. Virchow C, Szczeklik A, Bianco S, *et al.* Intolerance to tartrazine in aspirin-induced asthma: results of a multicenter study. *Respiration* 1988; 53: 20–23.
48. Uchegbu IF, Florence AT. Adverse drug events related to dosage forms and delivery systems. *Drug Safety* 1996; 14: 39–67.
49. Keaney NP. Respiratory Disorders. In: Davies DM, Ferner RE, de Glanville H, eds. *Textbook of Adverse Drug Reactions*, 5th edn. London: Chapman & Hall, 1998: 202–233.
50. Hetherington S, McGuirk S, Powell G, *et al.* Hypersensitivity reactions during therapy with the nucleoside reverse transcriptase inhibitor abacavir. *Clin Ther* 2001; 23: 1603–1614.
51. Nicklas RA. Paradoxical bronchospasm associated with the use of inhaled beta-agonists. *J Allergy Clin Immunol* 1990; 85: 959–964.
52. Committee on Safety of Medicines. Nebuliser solutions and paradoxical bronchoconstriction. *Curr Probl* 1988; 22: 2.
53. Finnerty JP, Howarth PH. Paradoxical bronchoconstriction with nebulized albuterol but not with terbutaline. *Am Rev Respir Dis* 1993; 148: 512–513.

54. Wilkinson JR, Roberts JA, Bradding P, *et al*. Paradoxical bronchoconstriction in asthmatic patients after salmeterol by metered dose inhaler. *Br Med J* 1992; 305: 931–932.
55. Williamson JC, Pegram PS. Neuraminidase inhibitors in patients with underlying airways disease. *Am J Respir Med* 2002; 1: 85–90.
56. Camus P. Pathophysiology of drug induced lung disease. In: Akoun GM, White JP, eds. *Treatment Induced Respiratory Disorders*. Amsterdam: Elsevier, 1989: 24–46.
57. Hill LE. Iatrogenic lung disease. In: D'Arcy PF, Griffin JP, eds. *Iatrogenic Diseases*, 3rd edn. Oxford: Oxford University Press, 1986.
58. Banerjee DJ, Honeybourne D. Drug induced pulmonary alveolar disease. *Adv Drug React Bull* 1996; 181: 687–690.
59. Dang-Vu B, Wilkinson W. Drug induced pulmonary disorders. In: Koda Kimble MA, Young LY, eds. *Applied Therapeutics: The Clinical Use of Drugs*, 7th edn. Philadelphia: Lippincott Williams & Wilkins, 2001: 24.1–24.15.
60. Abid SH, Malhotra V, Perry MC. Radiation-induced and chemotherapy-induced pulmonary injury. *Curr Opin Oncol* 2001; 13: 242–248.
61. D'Arcy PF. Nitrofurantoin. *Drug Intell Clin Pharm* 1985; 19: 540–547.
62. Krause M, Ruef C. Miscellaneous antibacterial drugs: lincomycins, macrolides, nitrofurantoin and polymyxins. In: Dukes MNG, Aronson JK, eds. *Meyler's Side Effects of Drugs*, 14th edn. Amsterdam: Elsevier, 2000: 871–895.
63. Tatley M. Pulmonary reactions with nitrofurantoin. (New Zealand Medicines and Medical Devices Safety Authority) *Prescriber Update* 2002; 23: 24–25.
64. Schattner A, Von der Walde J, Kozak N, *et al*. Nitrofurantoin-induced immune-mediated lung and liver disease. *Am J Med Sci* 1999; 317: 336–340.
65. White JP, Ward MJ. Drug-induced adverse pulmonary reactions. *Adv Drug React Acute Poisoning Rev* 1985; 4: 183–211.
66. Saravanan V, Kelly CA. Reducing the risk of methotrexate pneumonitis in rheumatoid arthritis. *Rheumatology* 2004; 43: 143–147.
67. Imokawa S, Colby TV, Leslie KO, *et al*. Methotrexate pneumonitis: review of the literature and histopathological findings in nine patients. *Eur Respir J* 2000; 15: 373–381.
68. Vial T, Chevrel G, Descotes J. Drugs acting on the immune system. In: Dukes MNG, Aronson JK, eds. *Meyler's Side Effects of Drugs*, 14th edn. Amsterdam: Elsevier, 2000: 1246–1337.
69. Committee on Safety of Medicines. Methotrexate and pneumonitis. *Curr Probl Pharmacovigilance* 2003; 29: 5.
70. Choulis NH, Dukes MNG. Metals. In: Dukes MNG, Aronson JK, eds. *Meyler's Side Effects of Drugs*, 14th edn. Amsterdam: Elsevier, 2000: 683–713.
71. Tomioka R, King TE Jr. Gold-induced pulmonary disease: clinical features, outcome, and differentiation from rheumatoid lung disease. *Am J Respir Crit Care Med* 1997; 155: 1011–1020.
72. Brion N, Legros V, Adnenifer C, *et al*. Pneumonitis induced by rheumatological drugs. In: Akoun GM, White JP, eds. *Treatment Induced Respiratory Disorders*. Amsterdam: Elsevier, 1989: 132–149.
73. Folb PI. Cytostatics and immunosuppressive drugs. In: Dukes MNG, Aronson JK, eds. *Meyler's Side Effects of Drugs*, 14th edn. Amsterdam: Elsevier, 2000: 1538–1595.

74. Cooper JAD, Matthay RA. Pneumonitis induced by cytotoxic drugs. In: Akoun GM, White JP, eds. *Treatment Induced Respiratory Disorders*. Amsterdam: Elsevier, 1989: 51–73.
75. Sleijfer S. Bleomycin-induced pneumonitis. *Chest* 2001; 120: 617–624.
76. Cooper JA Jr, White DA, Matthay RA. Drug-induced pulmonary disease. Part 1: cytotoxic drugs. *Am Rev Respir Dis* 1986; 133: 321–340.
77. Rosenow EC 3rd, Myers JL, Swensen SJ, *et al.* Drug-induced pulmonary disease. An update. *Chest* 1992; 102: 239–250.
78. Dusman RE, Stanton MS, Miles WM, *et al.* Clinical features of amiodarone-induced pulmonary toxicity. *Circulation* 1990; 82: 51–59.
79. Jessurun GA, Boersma WG, Crijns HJ. Amiodarone-induced pulmonary toxicity. Predisposing factors, clinical symptoms and treatment. *Drug Safety* 1998; 18: 339–344.
80. Ott MC, Khoor A, Leventhal JP, Paterick TE, Burger CD. Pulmonary toxicity in patients receiving low-dose amiodarone. *Chest* 2003; 123: 646–651.
81. Donaldson L, Grant IS, Naysmith MR, *et al.* Acute amiodarone-induced lung toxicity. *Intens Care Med* 1998; 24: 626–630.
82. Handschin AE, Lardinois D, Schneiter D, *et al.* Acute amiodarone-induced pulmonary toxicity following lung resection. *Respiration* 2003; 70: 310–312.
83. Wilson JS, Podrid PJ. Side effects from amiodarone. *Am Heart J* 1991; 121: 158–171.
84. Johnston GD. Positive inotropic drugs and drugs used in dysrhythmias. In: Dukes MNG, Aronson JK, eds. *Meyler's Side Effects of Drugs*, 14th edn. Amsterdam: Elsevier, 2000: 523–574.
85. Pollak PT, Bouillon T, Shafer SL. Population pharmacokinetics of long-term oral amiodarone therapy. *Clin Pharmacol Ther* 2000; 67: 642–652.
86. Committee on Safety of Medicines. Fibrotic reactions with pergolide and other ergot-derived dopamine receptor agonists. *Curr Probl* 2002; 28: 3.
87. Bleumink GS, van der Molen-Eijgenraam M, Strijbos JH, *et al.* Pergolide-induced pleuropulmonary fibrosis. *Clin Neuropharmacol* 2002; 25: 290–293.
88. Danoff SK, Grasso ME, Terry PB, *et al.* Pleuropulmonary disease due to pergolide use for restless legs syndrome. *Chest* 2001; 120: 313–316.
89. Reed CR, Glauser FL. Drug-induced noncardiogenic pulmonary edema. *Chest* 1991; 100: 1120–1124.
90. Cattan CE, Oberg KC. Vinorelbine tartrate-induced pulmonary edema confirmed on rechallenge. *Pharmacotherapy* 1999; 19: 992–994.
91. Brooks JC. Noncardiogenic pulmonary edema immediately following rapid protamine administration. *Ann Pharmacother* 1999; 33: 927–930.
92. Humbert M, Maitre S, Capron F, *et al.* Pulmonary edema complicating continuous intravenous prostacyclin in pulmonary capillary hemangiomatosis. *Am J Respir Crit Care Med* 1998; 157: 1681–1685.
93. Farber HW, Graven KK, Kokolski G, *et al.* Pulmonary edema during acute infusion of epoprostenol in a patient with pulmonary hypertension and limited scleroderma. *J Rheumatol* 1999; 26: 1195–1196.
94. Almoosa KF. Hydrochlorothiazide-induced pulmonary edema. *South Med J* 1999; 92: 1100–1102.
95. Bernal C, Patarca R. Hydrochlorothiazide-induced pulmonary edema and associated immunologic changes. *Ann Pharmacother* 1999; 33: 172–174.

96. Sciscione AC, Ivester T, Largoza M, *et al*. Acute pulmonary edema in pregnancy. *Obstet Gynecol* 2003; 101: 511–515.
97. Pisani RJ, Rosenow EC 3rd. Pulmonary edema associated with tocolytic therapy. *Ann Intern Med* 1989; 110: 714–718.
98. Committee on Safety of Medicines. Reminder: ritodrine and pulmonary oedema. *Curr Probl* 1995; 21: 7.
99. Waage IM, Gedde–Dahl A. Pulmonary embolism possibly associated with olanzapine treatment. *Br Med J* 2003; 327: 1384.
100. Curtin F. Schulz P. Psychotropic drugs and fatal pulmonary embolism: a comment. *Pharmacoepidemiol Drug Safety* 2004; 13: 659–660.
101. Selten JP, Buller H. Clozapine and venous thromboembolism: further evidence. *J Clin Psychiatry* 2003; 64: 609.
102. Simon RA. Adverse respiratory reactions to aspirin and nonsteroidal anti-inflammatory drugs. *Curr Allergy Asthma Rep* 2004; 4: 17–24.
103. Alarcon GS, Kremer JM, Macaluso M, *et al*. Risk factors for methotrexate-induced lung injury in patients with rheumatoid arthritis. A multicenter, case–control study. Methotrexate-Lung Study Group. *Ann Intern Med* 1997; 127: 356–364.

Further reading

Ben-Noun L. Drug-induced respiratory disorders: incidence, prevention and management. *Drug Safety* 2000; 23: 143–164.
Dang-Vu B, Wilkinson W. Drug induced pulmonary disorders. In: Koda Kimble MA, Young LY, eds. *Applied Therapeutics: The Clinical Use of Drugs*, 7th edn. Philadelphia: Lippincott Williams & Wilkins, 2001: 24.1–24.15.
Keaney NP. Drug induced lung disease. In: Walker R, Edwards C, eds. *Clinical Pharmacy and Therapeutics*, 3rd edn. London: Churchill Livingstone, 2002: 413 421.
Keaney NP. Respiratory disorders. In: Davies DM, Ferner RE, de Glanville H, eds *Textbook of Adverse Drug Reactions*, 5th edn. London: Chapman & Hall, 1998: 202–233.

11

Musculoskeletal disorders

Christine Randall

Introduction

Musculoskeletal diseases are the most common causes of physical disability, producing significant disability in 5% of the UK population. Musculoskeletal symptoms are very common and account for 20% of general practitioner (GP) consultations.[1] Since a wide range of medicines can cause musculoskeletal symptoms, they should always be considered in the differential diagnosis of patients presenting with such symptoms.[2]

Drug-induced musculoskeletal disorders can present as symptoms such as cramps, aches and pains in the limbs; these can be disabling, and can also be an early indication of potentially serious disorders.[3] For example, myalgia (muscle pain) is often a precursor of rhabdomyolysis. Other serious musculoskeletal disorders that can be associated with drug therapy include osteoporosis, fractures and tendon rupture. This chapter reviews the most common drug-induced musculoskeletal disorders.

Muscle disorders

Skeletal muscle accounts for around 45% of total body weight and has a high metabolic rate and blood flow. As a consequence it has a high exposure to drugs within the circulation.[4] Drugs can produce muscle damage in several ways, either directly on muscle cells possibly owing to high blood concentrations, or indirectly via electrolyte disturbances, excess energy requirements, inadequate delivery of energy or oxygen, or via an immunological reaction.[5] There is considerable variation among individuals in their susceptibility to adverse muscular effects. Muscle toxicity ranges from mild non-specific myalgia to myositis and rhabdomyolysis, and can be classified according to the presence or absence of muscle pain or by pathological features. As drug-induced muscle disorders are potentially reversible, their prompt recognition may reduce their damaging effects or even prevent a fatal outcome.

Myalgia and myositis

Myalgia (muscle pain) is clinically characterised by diffuse muscle pain, tenderness, cramps and/or muscle weakness and is a very common complaint. Proximal muscle groups of the legs are usually affected and symptoms often occur at night. Myalgia caused by drugs can affect the patient's quality of life and decrease compliance with therapy.[6] It may be accompanied by an increase in the enzyme creatine phosphokinase (CPK) in serum, which may be an indicator of muscle damage. The main source of CPK is skeletal muscle and the myocardium. Muscle pain with elevated CPK levels may also be the result of exercise or minor muscle damage from trauma.[4,7]

Myalgia may be an early symptom of drug-induced polyneuropathy, myopathy or extrapyramidal disorders (see Chapter 15).[3]

Mild muscle aches and pain can occasionally be caused by fluid retention; this has been described with oral contraceptives. Diuretics, calcium channel blockers and beta$_2$-agonists can cause muscle cramps. With diuretics, the problem may be related to electrolyte disturbances.

Suxamethonium causes myalgia in up to 50% of patients following surgery. The pain occurs mainly in the neck, shoulders, back and chest, and seems to be more common in women. The frequency and severity of muscle pain may be reduced by giving a small dose of a non-depolarising muscle relaxant just before suxamethonium.

Myositis (inflammatory myopathy), with or without serum CPK elevations, is usually self-limiting and is characterised by muscle weakness. Biopsy usually indicates cell damage with muscle fibre necrosis and inflammatory cell infiltration.[4,7]

Myopathy

Myopathy (serious muscle toxicity) can be clinically defined as muscle pain, tenderness and/or muscle weakness, accompanied by abnormal elevations in CPK. Myopathy should be considered when serum CPK levels are more than 10 times the upper limit of normal (ULN) or in patients with diffuse myalgia, muscle tenderness, and a marked increase in CPK. There is no associated organ damage. Drug-induced myopathy is characterised by a syndrome of muscle pain, tenderness and weakness, mainly of the proximal muscles of the upper limb, but at times it may be more generalised.[4,7] Muscle biopsy may reveal muscle fibre necrosis and regeneration. Factors that may contribute to myopathy include electrolyte disturbance (e.g. hypercalcaemia, hypokalaemia) or endocrine abnormalities. Clues to a drug-induced myopathy include the absence of pre-existing muscle dysfunction, gradual onset of muscular symptoms after start of the medication, lack of any other aetiology, and complete or partial resolution of the muscular symptoms after the causative agent is withdrawn.[8]

A focal myopathy consisting of local muscle inflammation may follow the intramuscular injection of any drug as a result of traumatic necrosis, haematoma formation or low-grade infection (needle myopathy). Muscle lesions of this type have been estimated to occur in up to 0.4% of hospitalised medical patients who receive at least one intramuscular injection.[5] Chronic focal myopathy can occur after repeated intramuscular injections, caused by needle trauma, the acidity/alkalinity of the injection, the inherent myotoxicity of the drug, or as a result of infection. It has been described after chronic intramuscular injection of opioids and antibiotics.[5]

Chronic use of oral corticosteroids, especially fluorinated corticosteroids, can cause proximal muscle weakness and atrophy.[5] Symptoms have been reported with daily doses of more than 10 mg (or equivalent) of prednisolone taken for at least 30 days.[3] Onset is usually insidious, but may develop rapidly. There is a relationship between the development of myopathy and the cumulative steroid dose, but not between the average daily dose and the duration of treatment.[5] In some cases a syndrome resembling lupus erythematosus has developed after stopping corticosteroids, but it has been suggested that stopping the corticosteroid therapy may have unmasked a pre-existing condition.[3]

Dose-related myopathy occurs in up to 20% of HIV-positive patients treated with zidovudine. Patients present with myalgia, fatigue and limb-girdle weakness which are sometimes associated with raised CPK levels. Zidovudine causes mitochondrial dysfunction by inhibiting mitochondrial DNA polymerase.[5]

Disruption of water and electrolyte homoeostasis can cause severe muscle damage. Hypokalaemia-related myopathy can be caused by laxative abuse, thiazide diuretics, carbenoxolone, mineralocorticoids and lithium.[5] Table 11.1 lists drugs that have been associated with myalgia or myopathy.

Rhabdomyolysis

Rhabdomyolysis is an acute, fulminating, potentially fatal skeletal muscle condition resulting from a toxic insult that leads to destruction of the muscle cell walls and the release of intracellular contents (enzymes and myoglobin) into the systemic circulation. Myoglobinaemia is the presence of myoglobin, an oxygen transport protein, in the blood; myoglobinuria is

Table 11.1 Some drugs that may cause myalgia or myopathy

Amiodarone	Minocycline
Beta-blockers	Mycophenolate mofetil
Carbimazole	Nicotinic acid
Ciclosporin	Opioids
Cimetidine	Penicillamine
Colchicine	Penicillins
Corticosteroids	Pentamidine
(oral, parenteral, inhaled)	Phenytoin
Danazol	Quinine, chloroquine
Diuretics	Quinolones
Ethanol	Statins
Fibrates	Suxamethonium
Interferon alfa	Tacrolimus
Isotretinoin	Taxanes (docetaxel, paclitaxel)
Itraconazole	Vincristine
Leflunomide	Zidovudine
Methotrexate	

the presence of myoglobin in the urine. Myoglobin and intracellular components are toxic, particularly to the kidney. Rhabdomyolysis has a number of different aetiologies, including excessive exertion, alcoholism, trauma, ischaemia, genetic susceptibility and drugs/toxins.[4]

The clinical presentation of rhabdomyolysis includes muscle swelling, tenderness and severe weakness, with dark brown (tea or cola coloured) urine due to myoglobin excretion. There is almost always associated organ damage, usually renal failure. CPK can rise to between 10 and more than 100 times the ULN. Up to 50% of patients with rhabdomyolysis may not admit to muscle pain.[9] Potentially life-threatening complications include hyperkalaemia, hypocalcaemia, myoglobinuric renal failure due to tubular necrosis, disseminated intravascular coagulation, cardiomyopathy, respiratory failure and severe metabolic acidosis.[4] If left untreated rhabdomyolysis can be fatal; mortality has been reported to be approximately 10%.[10] Alcohol and opioids are the drugs most often implicated in rhabdomyolysis.[11] Risk factors include increasing age, multisystem disease, hypothyroidism, acute illness, major surgery, low body weight and female gender.[12]

The management of rhabdomyolysis requires discontinuation of the causative agent followed by treatment to prevent renal failure, including intravenous fluids and alkalinisation of the urine using sodium bicarbonate infusion. This is followed by treatment to correct electrolyte abnormalities.[4]

Statin myopathy

Hydroxymethyl glutaryl coenzyme A (HMG-CoA) reductase inhibitors, or statins, are known to cause a wide range of muscular symptoms, varying from mild aching to severe pain. In most cases the level of CPK in the blood is increased.[12] Myotoxicity with statins is a class effect, although the incidence varies for individual agents within the class.

Mild symptoms (myalgia) occur in 2–7% of patients treated with statins, and these are usually associated with a minimal elevation of CPK (3–10 times the ULN).[12,13] Myopathy is less common, occurring in 0.1–0.2% of patients in clinical trials, and can present with or without symptoms; the CPK is usually more than 10 times the ULN.[12,13] There appears to be no relationship between the magnitude of the CPK elevation and the intensity of symptoms. Statin-associated rhabdomyolysis is very rare, occurring in 0.05% of patients in one study, with fatal rhabdomyolysis estimated to occur in less than 1 case per million prescriptions.[6,11,14] It usually presents with severe muscle pain, stiffness, weakness, fever, malaise and dark urine. CPK is often greater than 40 times the ULN.

Statin-related myotoxicity is dose related and factors that increase statin blood levels may enhance their myotoxic effect. Approximately half of all cases of statin-induced rhabdomyolysis are associated with a drug interaction that leads to increased blood levels of the drug.[15] Most clinically important drug interactions are attributable to the concurrent use of a statin that is metabolised by CYP3A4 (e.g. simvastatin) and agents that are potent inhibitors or substrates of this enzyme (e.g. azole antifungal agents, macrolide antibiotics, ciclosporin, protease inhibitors, diltiazem).[15] However, myotoxicity is a well-recognised complication of statins used in combination with fibrates, which do not inhibit CYP3A4. One explanation is that fibrates inhibit a hepatic glucuronidation pathway involved in the metabolism of most statins, in particular cerivastatin.[6,12] Cerivastatin, a potent lipophilic second-generation statin, was voluntarily withdrawn from the world market in August 2001 because of its adverse effects on muscle.[16,17] It was associated with a 10 times higher rate of rhabdomyolysis than first-generation statins, such as simvastatin. Of all deaths related to cerivastatin-induced rhabdomyolysis, 25% were associated with a cerivastatin–gemfibrozil interaction. Despite Europe-wide regulatory action in June 2001 to contraindicate this combination and reduce the maximum cerivastatin dose to 0.4 mg, the company suspended marketing and distribution at short notice.

The mechanism of statin-induced myopathy is not clear. Proposed mechanisms include the indirect inhibition of adenosine triphosphate (ATP) by inhibition of the production of coenzyme Q, leading to cell death and the disruption of cell membrane fluidity, followed by the risk of wall rupture and cell death.[13,18]

The UK Committee on Safety of Medicines (CSM) issued a statement in 2002 reminding prescribers that myopathy, including rhabdomyolysis, is a rare but clinically important adverse effect of statin therapy.[19] The CSM recommends that:

- Dosage instructions are closely adhered to;
- Care is taken with patients who may be at increased risk of developing myopathy, e.g. those with underlying muscle disorders, renal impairment, hypothyroidism, alcoholism, use of other lipid-lowering therapy, concomitant CYP450 3A4 inhibitors (baseline CPK should be considered) (Table 11.2);
- Patients are made aware of the risk of myopathy and asked to report any muscle symptoms and/or dark urine;
- CPK levels should be monitored in any patient experiencing muscle symptoms, and treatment stopped if CPK >5 times ULN.

Patient counselling on the risks and warning signs of myopathy is extremely important.[4] A first line of defence to improve safety and reduce the incidence of adverse reactions is to thoroughly educate patients on what symptoms to report immediately to their doctor, i.e. muscle aches, pain, tenderness or weakness, especially if accompanied by malaise, fever or dark

Table 11.2 Factors that can increase the risk of statin-induced myopathy

Patient characteristics
Increasing age
Female sex
Renal insufficiency
Hypothyroidism
Diet (grapefruit juice)
Concomitant medications
Diabetes
Hepatobiliary dysfunction

Statin properties
High dose
Lipophilicity
High bioavailability
Limited protein binding
Potential for drug interactions metabolised by CYP450 pathways
  (particularly CYP3A4)

urine.[20] Patients developing symptoms of muscle toxicity should have their statin therapy withdrawn and be monitored carefully. If myopathy is not recognised and treatment is continued, it can proceed to rhabdomyolysis and acute renal failure, so it is important that healthcare professionals are aware of this rare adverse effect.

Table 11.3 lists substances that may interact with statins to increase the risk of myopathy and rhabdomyolysis.

Eosinophilia–myalgia syndrome

Eosinophilia–myalgia syndrome (EMS) is characterised by severe, incapacitating myalgia and a raised blood eosinophil count (more than 1.0×10^9 cells/L).[21] Other features include arthralgia, rash, cough, dyspnoea, oedema, abnormal liver function tests and fever. Following the first documented case in 1989, over 1500 cases, some fatal, were reported in 1 year in the US. Almost all the affected patients had taken dietary supplements containing tryptophan. The median dose ingested was 1.5 g daily for periods ranging between a few weeks and several years. Women were more frequently affected than men: more than 80% of initial reports involved women. The course of the disease was variable: in some patients it resolved quickly after discontinuation of tryptophan preparations, but in most cases it was chronic, severe and disabling. In some cases, symptoms progressed after drug withdrawal. A contaminant in the tryptophan manufacturing process is believed to have been responsible, but this has not been confirmed.[22] In 1990, the CSM recommended the withdrawal of products containing tryptophan in the UK, despite only a few reports of EMS in Europe.[23] Tryptophan was later reintroduced for the adjunctive treatment of severe and disabling resistant depression. It should only be prescribed by hospital specialists and treatment must be closely monitored.

Table 11.3 Some substances that may interact with statins to increase the risk of myopathy and rhabdomyolysis

Azole antifungals (itraconazole, miconazole)	HIV protease inhibitors (ritonavir, saquinavir, indinavir, nelfinavir)
Ciclosporin	Macrolide antibiotics
Colchicine	Nefazodone
Digoxin	Nicotinic acid
Diltiazem	Risperidone
Fibrates	Verapamil
Grapefruit juice	Warfarin

Bone

Bone is a metabolically active tissue, with 10–15% of bone surfaces remodelling at any one time in adults.[24] Bone metabolism is regulated by parathyroid hormone (PTH), activated vitamin D and sex hormones. PTH has an important role in extracellular calcium homoeostasis and acts on the skeleton to stimulate bone turnover. PTH levels rise with age, leading to age-related bone loss. Activated vitamin D regulates extracellular calcium homoeostasis, intestinal calcium absorption and calcium resorption in the kidney. Sex hormones are important regulators of bone remodelling; estrogens act indirectly via local cytokines, whereas androgens act directly on the osteoblasts, leading to osteoblast proliferation and increased bone formation.[25] Medicines can interfere with bone regulation by three main mechanisms: increased bone turnover, suppression of new bone formation and inhibition of normal mineralisation.[26] These mechanisms are influenced by effects on the metabolism of calcium, phosphate and vitamin D, leading to metabolic bone diseases such as osteoporosis and osteomalacia.[27]

Osteoporosis

Osteoporosis, commonly referred to as 'thinning of the bones', is characterised by microarchitectural deterioration of bone tissue and low bone mass, resulting in increased bone fragility and susceptibility to fracture. In 1994 the World Health Organization (WHO) defined osteoporosis in terms of bone mass; bone is considered to be osteoporotic when bone mineral density (BMD) is 2.5 standard deviations (SD) or more below the young adult mean value.[25] A BMD between 1 and 2.5 SD below the young adult mean is classed as osteopenia (low bone mass). Clinical risk factors for osteoporosis are shown in Table 11.4.[25]

Osteoporosis is estimated to affect one in three women and one in 12 men at some time in their lives. Osteoporosis is asymptomatic at onset, but gradual bone loss leads to fractures that are acutely painful. Fractures are often at clinically relevant sites such as the femoral head and vertebrae. Vertebral compression and collapse lead to back pain or spinal deformity, spontaneous fractures of the ribs, pelvis and other bones. All lead to debility and a reduced quality of life.

Corticosteroids have been known for over 50 years to have adverse effects on bone. They are by far the most common cause of iatrogenic osteoporosis, accounting for the condition in 13% of male and 10% of female sufferers, and causing fractures in up to 50% of patients who take

Table 11.4 Clinical risk factors for osteoporosis

Female sex, increased further in postmenopausal women, women with a premature
   menopause, and women who had a hysterectomy before age 45, with at least
   one conserved ovary
Smokers
High alcohol intake
Low body mass index
Physical inactivity
A family history of the disease
Long-term steroid use (i.e. those taking 7.5 mg prednisolone (or equivalent) daily
   or more for 6 months or longer)

---

them long term.[25,26] Three major mechanisms contribute to corticosteroid-
induced osteoporosis:

- Effects on calcium homoeostasis lead to reduced intestinal absorption and increased urinary elimination of calcium.
- Bone formation is inhibited owing to decreased osteoblast activity
   and a reduction in osteoblast lifespan.
- Reduction in sex hormone production, resulting in decreased intestinal calcium absorption and increased urinary excretion.[25,26,28]

Trabecular bone, found mostly in the lumbar spine, hip and distal
radius, is affected earlier and more severely than cortical bone, contained in the midshaft of long bones.[26] Bone loss associated with corticosteroid use is most rapid in the first 6–12 months of treatment, with
an average 5% bone loss in the first year.[26,28,29] Significant loss is
measurable after 3 months.[30] A study in patients with rheumatoid
arthritis showed that after a 20-week course of prednisolone 10 mg daily
there was an 8% loss of BMD compared to 1% with placebo.[30,31] After
a year of corticosteroid treatment the rate of loss decelerates and
plateaus at a loss of 1–2% per year.[28,29,31] Young patients lose bone
faster than older patients, but it is postmenopausal women who are
most at risk of fracture.[29] The risk of fractures associated with corticosteroid treatment varies with dose, duration of treatment, underlying
disease state and gender. Non-vertebral fractures increased by 54%
in the first year of treatment in patients taking ≥7.5 mg prednisolone
daily in one study, and in an epidemiological study the relative risk of
hip fracture in women increased by 59% and in men by 67%.[31]
Vertebral fractures have been shown to occur in 17% of patients within
1 year of starting corticosteroid therapy when no preventative treatment is

given.[29] Although it is clear that bone loss is a dose-related adverse effect, it is not clear whether the cumulative dose or the daily dose of corticosteroid is most important. Prednisolone doses of 1–5 mg daily may cause bone loss, but at doses $\geqslant$5 mg daily bone loss is significant and rapid.[26,30]

Patients with a cumulative dose of more than 30 g prednisolone appear to have a high incidence of fracture (53%) and osteopenia (78%).[26] One epidemiological study showed that the excess risk of fracture disappeared within 1 year of stopping therapy.[31]

The use of inhaled as opposed to oral corticosteroids reduces adverse effects, including bone loss. However, inhaled corticosteroids do have systemic effects: a meta-analysis observed a dose-related reduction in BMD in patients using high-dose inhaled corticosteroids (>1.5 mg daily of oral prednisolone equivalent, 0.75 mg daily of inhaled fluticasone propionate). A study comparing users of inhaled corticosteroids with users of inhaled bronchodilators (controls) found the relative risk of vertebral, hip and non-vertebral fracture was 51%, 22% and 15% higher, respectively, in corticosteroid users than in bronchodilator users. The effect was dose dependent, doses of beclometasone of $\geqslant$0.7 mg daily resulting in a relative risk of hip fracture 80% higher than that for the controls.[30]

Prevention and management of corticosteroid-induced osteoporosis has been addressed in a document produced by the Bone and Tooth Society, the National Osteoporosis Society and the Royal College of Physicians.[32] The advice applies to individuals who will be exposed to corticosteroids for 3 months or more. Individuals at high risk, for example those aged 65 years or over and those with a prior fragility fracture (a fracture occurring with minimal trauma after the age of 40 years), should be advised to commence bone-protective therapy when starting glucocorticoids. In these individuals measurement of BMD is not necessary before starting therapy, but in others measurement of BMD is recommended for assessment of fracture risk. Other secondary causes of osteoporosis should be excluded if there is prior history of fracture. General measures to reduce bone loss should be taken, such as reduction of the glucocorticoid dose to a minimum, consideration of alternative formulations or routes of administration, and prescription of alternative glucocorticoid-sparing immunosuppressive agents (for example azathioprine). Good nutrition, an adequate dietary calcium and vitamin D intake and appropriate weight-bearing physical activity should be encouraged, and tobacco use and excessive alcohol use avoided.[32] The therapeutic options for the prophylaxis and treatment of corticosteroid-induced osteoporosis are the same: a bisphosphonate (e.g. alendronate, cyclical etidronate, risedronate) is the first choice; alternatives include raloxifene, calcitriol or testosterone in men.[30] Hormone replacement therapy (HRT) is no longer considered a first-line treatment but may be considered if other therapies are not tolerated, are contraindicated or are ineffective.[33] Most patients benefit from supplementation with calcium (1500 mg/day) and vitamin D (800 IU/day).

Osteoporosis and fractures have been reported in patients treated long term with heparin.[26] Symptomatic vertebral fractures have been demonstrated in 2.2% of women receiving long-term heparin prophylaxis.[26] Up to one-third of patients treated long term with heparin have a subclinical reduction in BMD. Studies show that the critical dose of heparin is more than 15 000 units daily for longer than 3 months.[26] Fractures occur in the vertebra and the ribs. Osteoporosis associated with heparin seems to be related to daily dose rather than duration of therapy, and is mainly associated with unfractionated heparin, although a case of vertebral fracture in a young woman treated with low molecular weight heparin has been reported.[34] The bone loss appears to be reversible in about 70% of patients, with improvement occurring within 6–12 months of stopping heparin. It has been suggested that, where possible, bone density should be monitored in patients being treated for longer than 3 months.[27] The mechanism of heparin-induced osteoporosis is not clear, but it is multifactorial. Increased bone resorption and decreased bone formation have been implicated, but the results of published studies are conflicting.

Hyperthyroidism leads to high bone turnover with an increase in trabecular bone and a decrease in cortical bone. A meta-analysis showed that postmenopausal women treated with an average daily dose of 171 μg of levothyroxine for 9.9 years showed a mean reduction in BMD of 9% compared to controls. Luteinising-hormone-releasing hormone agonists (LHRH-a), such as leuprorelin and goserelin, down-regulate pituitary LHRH receptors, causing a decrease in testosterone in men and in oestrogen in women, with the subsequent development of osteoporosis. Significant trabecular bone loss has been reported (5–10% within 6 months) with little or no change in cortical bone density. Men treated with LHRH-a develop a reduction in vertebral BMD within the first year of treatment and have a 5% incidence of osteoporotic fractures.[26] Chronic opioid use may also lead to hypogonadism, resulting in lowered BMD. Opioids may also increase fracture risk by interfering directly with bone formation.[35] Drugs associated with osteoporosis are shown in Table 11.5.

Table 11.5 Some drugs that may cause osteoporosis

Antiepileptics	Luteinising-hormone-releasing
Aromatase inhibitors	hormone agonists
Ciclosporin	Methotrexate
Corticosteroids	Opioids
Heparin	Thyroid hormones
Lithium	Warfarin

Osteomalacia

Osteomalacia is a condition that results from a lack of vitamin D or a disturbance of its metabolism; in children it is often referred to as rickets. Severe calcium deficiency or hypophosphataemia can also lead to osteomalacia. The main histological feature is an accumulation of increased amounts of demineralised bone matrix and a decrease in the rate of bone formation. The main symptoms are bone pain, often involving the spine, ribcage, shoulder girdle and pelvis, commonly with tenderness and muscle weakness.[36] Patients with osteomalacia may also experience fractures, either spontaneously or as a consequence of trauma.

Long-term administration of antiepileptics can cause bone disease, with features of osteomalacia. This adverse effect has been attributed to induction of the hepatic cytochrome P450 enzymes that metabolise vitamin D (colecalciferol and calcifediol), leading to its increased catabolism. This leads to hypocalcaemia, hypophosphataemia, increased serum parathyroid, calcitonin deficiency and impaired calcium absorption.[28,37] The more potent enzyme-inducing antiepileptics, such as phenytoin, phenobarbital and carbamazepine, are more commonly associated with bone loss than the non-enzyme-inducing sodium valproate.[26,37] The effect on bone of the newer antiepileptics gabapentin, lamotrigine and felbamate is not yet known.[26] This complication is most likely to affect patients with other factors contributing to vitamin D deficiency, such as poor diet or lack of exposure to sunlight, which may be found, for example, in patients with epilepsy living in institutions.[36,37]

Aluminium is thought to cause osteomalacia in a number of ways: inhibition of bone mineralisation, impairment of osteoblast proliferation and reduction of PTH production. The incidence of aluminium deposition in bone has been reported to be as high as 50% in chronic dialysis-dependent patients compared to 5% in chronic renal failure patients not being dialysed.[26] The problem was first documented in patients with chronic renal failure on haemodialysis.[38] The high aluminium content of water used in the dialysis fluid was subsequently

Table 11.6 Some drugs that may cause osteomalacia

Aluminium salts	Heavy metals
Barbiturates	Phenytoin
Bisphosphonates	Rifampicin
Carbamazepine	Saccharated iron oxide
Exchange resins (colestyramine, colestipol)	Total parenteral nutrition
Fluoride	

found to be responsible. Patients developed symptoms of osteomalacia not responsive to vitamin D. The use of aluminium salts as phosphate binders in patients with chronic renal failure can also lead to osteomalacia.[36] The prevalence of aluminium-induced bone disease in renal patients has reduced markedly since these two problems were recognised. Prolonged ingestion of large quantities of aluminium-containing antacids has resulted in osteomalacia in patients with normal renal function.[26]

Histological osteomalacia may occur in association with chronic fluoride, etidronate, pamidronate and aluminium ingestion and gallium nitrate toxicity.[36] Osteomalacia is also a potential complication of long-term parenteral nutrition, with metabolic bone disease reported to affect 42–100% of home-treated patients.[39] There are many possible contributing factors, including inadequate calcium and phosphate supplementation, aluminium overload and hypercalciuria.[40] Patients on long-term parenteral nutrition should be carefully monitored. Table 11.6 lists some drugs that may cause osteomalacia.

Avascular bone necrosis (osteonecrosis)

Avascular necrosis of bone, or osteonecrosis, is a common clinical problem accounting for 10% or more of joint replacements in the USA. It results in collapse of the bone structure, leading to joint pain, bone destruction and loss of function.[41] Osteonecrosis occurs when there is impairment of blood supply to a specific region of bone as a result of local trauma or non-traumatic systemic conditions.[41] The condition can occur at all ages, but 75% of patients with osteonecrosis are between 30 and 60 years old and it is seen predominantly in males (male:female ratio = 7:3).[41] There are several predisposing factors, including exposure to high barometric pressures (e.g. in divers), sickle cell disease, radiotherapy, alcohol misuse and drug therapy. Pain is almost always the presenting symptom and may initially be mild or vague; however, trauma will precipitate sudden and severe pain. The most common site of involvement is the femoral head, but the knee, small bones in the hands and feet, wrists, ankles, vertebrae and less commonly the facial bones are all affected. Clinical features and imaging studies are used to diagnose and stage osteonecrosis. Conventional X-rays are used, but early lesions are often missed. Radiographs become positive only after the development of a 'crescent sign' or a sclerotic rim of reactive bone at the interface between ischaemic and viable bone.[41] Newer techniques, including MRI (magnetic resonance imaging), selective angiography and skeletal scintigraphy, are used to evaluate early disease.[41] Criteria for diagnosing drug-induced osteonecrosis include:[42]

- A high index of suspicion;
- A definite history of drug intake before symptoms;
- Clinical evidence of avascular necrosis;
- Radiological evidence.

Management of confirmed osteonecrosis is difficult, primarily palliative, and does not halt or slow the progression of the disease. Attempts to promote healing by resting the joint are relatively unsuccessful. Surgical treatment options include bone grafting, core decompression, osteotomy, hemiarthroplasty and total hip replacement.[41]

The most common iatrogenic cause of osteonecrosis is systemic corticosteroid use, with osteonecrosis of the femoral head occurring in 5–40% of patients on long-term therapy.[43,44] Osteonecrosis has been observed in patients treated with steroids for a variety of clinical problems and can develop in as little as 2 weeks, although onset of symptoms rarely occurs before 6 months and may take up to 3 years.[28,41] Screening in the first year of long-term corticosteroid treatment to aid early diagnosis is therefore critically important to limit damage.[43,45] Patients with systemic lupus erythematosus and rheumatoid arthritis appear to be most at risk, but the problem can occur in patients taking corticosteroids for chronic diseases, including inflammatory bowel disease, organ transplant recipients, and patients receiving chemotherapy for Hodgkin's lymphoma. In corticosteroid-induced cases dose appears to be a major risk factor, with high doses in the first weeks of treatment being more important than the cumulative dose.[28,43] In patients with rheumatoid arthritis on low-dose corticosteroids the incidence of osteonecrosis is low, whereas in patients with lupus who have been treated with high doses for a much shorter period, the incidence is considerably higher.[28] Although the risk appears to increase with both the dose and duration of corticosteroid treatment, it is difficult to predict which patients will develop osteonecrosis, as there may be a degree of genetic susceptibility.[28,41] The risk decreases after corticosteroid therapy is stopped.

Avascular necrosis of the jaw can occur in association with use of the bisphosphonates pamidronate and zoledronate for the treatment of hypercalcaemia of malignancy, often after removal of a painful tooth.[46–50] A retrospective review from one oral surgery unit identified 63 cases of refractory osteomyelitis or osteonecrosis of the jaw in patients on chronic bisphosphonate therapy.[48] Fifty-six patients had been receiving intravenous bisphosphonate for over a year for malignant disease, seven had been receiving chronic oral bisphosphonates for the treatment of osteoporosis. Typical presenting features were pain and either a non-healing extraction socket or an exposed jawbone. However, nine patients (14%) had no history of a recent dentoalveolar procedure. Lesions presented in the maxilla in 38% of cases and the mandible in 63%. The pathogenesis of osteonecrosis associated with bisphosphonates is not clear, but may be related to osteoclast inhibition mediated by bisphosphonates.[48]

Risk factors for osteonecrosis of the jaw (ONJ) include chemotherapy, corticosteroid therapy and dental procedures, e.g. tooth extraction. The manufacturer of disodium pamidronate and zoledronate now includes a warning about ONJ in the Summary of Product Characteristics.[51,52]

> Osteonecrosis of the jaw has been reported in cancer patients treated with bisphosphonates. Many of these patients were also receiving chemotherapy and corticosteroids. The majority of reported cases have been associated with dental procedures such as tooth extraction. Many affected patients had signs of local infection, including osteomyelitis.
>
> A dental examination with appropriate preventive dentistry should be considered prior to treatment with bisphosphonates in patients with concomitant risk factors (e.g. cancer, chemotherapy, corticosteroids, poor oral hygiene).
>
> While on treatment, these patients should avoid invasive dental procedures if possible. For patients who develop osteonecrosis of the jaw while on bisphosphonate therapy, dental surgery may exacerbate the condition. For patients requiring dental procedures, there are no data available to suggest whether discontinuation of bisphosphonates reduces the risk of osteonecrosis of the jaw. The clinical judgement of the treating physician should guide the management plan of each patient based on individual benefit–risk assessment.

Dentists and oncologists should be aware of the early signs and symptoms of ONJ, which include ulceration, irritation and pain.[53] Effective management of the bony lesions of ONJ is still unclear. Some lesions respond to local irrigation, debridement and antibiotics, whereas others do not heal even after large bony resections and hyperbaric oxygen therapy.[54]

Adrenocorticotrophic hormone (ACTH), heparin, interferon alfa, antineoplastic drugs and non-steroidal anti-inflammatory drugs (NSAIDs) have also been implicated in osteonecrosis.[42]

Joints

Diseases of the joints (arthropathy or arthrosis) include arthralgia (joint pain) and arthritis (joint inflammation). Mild arthralgia may accompany almost any drug-induced skin eruption, and more severe joint pain with swelling is an essential component of 'serum sickness', which may be drug-induced (e.g. penicillin or barbiturates).

Arthropathy, including arthralgia, of small peripheral joints has been reported after some vaccinations. Whether rubella vaccination can cause chronic arthropathy or musculoskeletal symptoms has been the subject of much controversy. Rubella vaccination, like natural rubella infection, is associated with acute joint symptoms; adult women are more likely to be affected than men or children (female:male ratio 3.0, average age 45 years).[55–57] The most recent epidemiological studies suggest that any increased risk is small, with an incidence of 2.9 cases per million vaccinations. The mean time to onset is 10–11 days following vaccination.[57,58]

The use of intravesical BCG (bacillus Calmette–Guérin) for immunotherapy in cancer patients has been linked with arthralgias of the lower limb joints, occurring in 0.5–5% of patients, and aseptic arthritis in 0.4–0.8% of cases.[28] Following intradermal BCG the clinical presentation of arthritis is different from that seen with intravesical administration, with a symmetrical polyarthritis of the hands resembling rheumatoid arthritis occurring after a period of 32 weeks on average.[28,59]

There have been reports of inflammatory polyarthritis after vaccination with hepatitis B vaccine. Many of the affected individuals were rheumatoid factor positive and developed transient or persistent arthritis shortly after the second or third vaccination.[28] An epidemiological study found that the incidence of chronic arthritis following hepatitis B vaccination was 0.56 cases per million vaccinations, predominantly in females (female:male ratio = 3.5) with a mean age of 33 years. The reactions occurred a mean of 16 days after vaccination.[57] One theory suggests that these individuals may be genetically susceptible to rheumatoid arthritis, with hepatitis B vaccine triggering its development.[28] Influenza vaccine has also been reported to cause joint complications.[60,61] Table 11.7 lists some

Table 11.7 Some drugs associated with arthralgia and arthritis

Aromatase inhibitors	Procainamide
BCG vaccine (intravesical)	Quinidine
Calcium channel blockers	Quinolone antibiotics
Carbimazole	Quinopristin-dalfopristin
Hepatitis B vaccine	Rubella vaccine
Isoniazid	Terbinafine
Mirtazapine	

drugs associated with arthralgia or arthritis.[62–67] There is no evidence that rheumatoid arthritis is ever drug induced, but a number of drugs have been reported to trigger or exacerbate the condition, including sodium aurothiomalate, hepatitis B vaccine, interferon, interleukin, levamisole, granulocyte and granulocyte–macrophage colony–stimulating factors.[3,28]

Severe joint pain may also be caused by the arthritis of acute gout, which can be precipitated by certain medicines. The underlying mechanism of drug-induced hyperuricaemia and gout is decreased uric acid excretion. At low doses salicylate intake is accompanied by the accumulation of organic acids that compete with urate for tubular secretion. Gout, resulting from hyperuricaemia, may also be induced by diuretics (thiazide and loop), ethambutol, pyrazinamide, levodopa, thiamine, cyanocobalamin, retinoids, fibrates, cimetidine, rantidine, nicotinic acid and intravenous fructose. Ciclosporin causes increased uricaemia in about 50% of patients treated. Gouty arthritis affects 5–30% of patients receiving ciclosporin after renal or heart transplants.[28] Urate concentrations greater than 100 mg/L require antihyperuricaemic therapy such as allopurinol or colchicine.

Musculoskeletal adverse effects associated with quinolones are rare: myalgia (0.8%), arthralgia, arthritis (0.4%) and tendonitis have been reported. In studies in young dogs, prolonged administration of high doses of quinolone antibiotics caused erosions of articular cartilage and permanent damage to the weight-bearing joints.[68] All quinolone antibiotics have been associated with arthropathies in humans. The lesions are described as non-erosive bilateral symmetric arthropathies that frequently affect the lower extremities.[28] The mechanism of quinolone arthrotoxicity has not been confirmed. The problem is more common in adolescents and adults under 30 years of age. During long-term treatment (>3 months) the incidence may be as high as 45%.[28] Quinolones are therefore contraindicated in children, in growing adolescents, and during pregnancy. Stiffness, pain and synovial swelling within the first few days of therapy are the main symptoms. These usually resolve on stopping treatment. Limited outcome data after exposure during human pregnancy have so far been reassuring (see Chapter 4).

Vasculitis may present with polyarthralgia and polyarthritis. This uncommon disease may arise spontaneously or be induced by drugs (see Chapter 5).

Connective tissue

Tendinopathy may complicate corticosteroid treatment, if infiltration of the periarticular tissues occurs or intra-articular injections are used. The Achilles tendon is most often involved, but the patellar tendon can also rupture.

Quinolone tendinopathy

There have been case reports of tendonitis with quinolones since they were first introduced in the mid-1980s. The first case of Achilles tendon rupture in a quinolone-treated patient was reported in 1991.[69] Since then there have been many case reports of quinolone-associated tendonitis, with over 2000 cases reported worldwide to the WHO Collaborating Centre in Uppsala.[70] The incidence is difficult to evaluate, but is estimated to be 15–20 per 100 000 persons treated, or 0.14–0.4%.[71–73] The Achilles tendon is most often affected because of its weight-bearing role, but other tendons, including those of the quadriceps muscle and the rotator cuff, may be affected.[74] Tendon rupture is possible and is often bilateral, may be partial or complete, spontaneous, or occur after activity.[28] Rupture is estimated to occur in up to 30% of reported tendonitis cases.[74] A case–control study using the UK General Practice Research Database estimated the relative risk of Achilles tendon rupture to be 6.4 in patients aged 60–79 years and 20.4 in patients 80 years or over. The adverse effects of quinolones on the tendon can occur within hours of the initial dose but may be delayed for up to 6 months; the median time to onset is estimated to be 6 days.[73,75] Tendon effects have been reported with all quinolones but at varying frequencies, with levofloxacin being implicated most frequently.[28,70] Predisposing factors include:[28,70,72,75,76]

- Age over 60 years;
- Corticosteroid therapy – concomitant use of oral corticosteroids increased the relative risk of Achilles tendon ruptures (all ages) from 4.2 to 14.5;[77]
- Renal failure and/or haemodialysis;
- Renal transplant recipients;

- Diabetes mellitus;
- Rheumatoid arthritis;
- Gout;
- Chronic lung disease.

Tendon injury manifests most commonly with a sudden onset of severe pain. Other signs and symptoms include tenderness to palpation, oedema, and difficulty with movement in the affected areas. Diagnosis is made primarily by physical examination, but ultrasound and MRI scanning are also used.[72] Treatment consists of immediate discontinuation of the quinolone and immobilisation of the tendon.[28] Surgical repair may be required if rupture has occurred. Healing can take up to 3 months for tendonitis and 6 months for tendon rupture.[28,75]

In 2002 the CSM issued a reminder about tendinopathy associated with quinolones.[78] Prescribers were reminded that:

- Quinolones are contraindicated in patients with a history of tendon disorders related to quinolone use.
- Elderly patients and those on corticosteroids are at increased risk.
- If tendonitis is suspected quinolones should be stopped immediately and appropriate treatment initiated.

Retroperitoneal fibrosis

Retroperitoneal fibrosis is a disorder characterised by fibrous tissue proliferation behind the peritoneum, with minimal inflammation. Fibrosis may also occur around the lungs and pericardium. Patients commonly describe persistent pain in the loin and groin area, oliguria, pain on micturition, myalgia and oedema. Although early withdrawal of the precipitating drug results in symptom improvement, the non-specific nature of the symptoms means that diagnosis is often delayed, with subsequent irreversible damage. Fibrotic reactions are well recognised adverse effects of ergot alkaloids. Retroperitoneal fibrosis has been observed in patients being treated for migraine with ergotamine and methysergide. More recently it has been reported in patients with Parkinson's disease treated with the ergot-derived dopamine receptor agonists pergolide, cabergoline and lisuride.[79–81] The CSM has reported on reactions identified via the yellow card scheme and has issued advice on fibrotic reactions associated with the ergot-derived dopamine receptor agonists (Box 11.1).[82]

Several beta-blockers have also been associated with retroperitoneal fibrosis, including atenolol, propranolol, oxprenolol and sotalol.[83] Other medicines have been linked with retroperitoneal fibrosis (Table 11.8), but a causal relationship has not been established for them all.

> **Box 11.1** CSM advice on fibrotic reactions associated with ergot-derived dopamine receptor agonists
>
> The CSM has advised that ergot-derived dopamine receptor agonists bromocriptine, cabergoline, lisuride and pergolide have been associated with pulmonary, retroperitoneal and pericardial fibrotic reactions. Before starting treatment with these ergot derivatives it may be appropriate to measure the erythrocyte sedimentation rate and serum creatinine and to obtain a chest X-ray. Patients should be monitored for dyspnoea, persistent cough, chest pain, cardiac failure, and abdominal pain or tenderness. If long-term treatment is expected, then lung function tests may also be helpful.

Table 11.8 Some drugs that may cause retroperitoneal fibrosis

Aspirin	Ergotamine
Beta-blockers	Haloperidol
Bromocriptine	Lisuride
Cabergoline	Methysergide
Codeine	Pergolide

Drug-induced lupus

Systemic lupus erythematosus (SLE) is an autoimmune disease of the connective tissue, the cause of which remains unknown. Up to 10% of cases are estimated to be caused by drugs.[84] Since a syndrome resembling SLE was first reported with sulfadiazine in 1945, over 80 medications have been implicated.[84–88] The various terms used for this condition include lupus-like syndrome, drug-induced lupus erythematosus, drug-related lupus and lupus erythematosus medicamentosa.

Drug-induced lupus develops between 1 month and 5 years after starting the causative drug. Although symptom onset can be rapid, patients frequently present with mild lupus-like symptoms, which typically worsen the longer the implicated drug is taken. There have been occasional reports of fatalities. Features resemble those of naturally occurring SLE and include arthralgia and/or arthritis (80–90%), myalgia (up to 50%), fever, pleurisy and pericarditis. However, features characterising SLE are seldom seen in drug-induced lupus, such as malar (butterfly) or discoid rash, oral ulcers, alopecia, and renal or neurological disorders. Cutaneous manifestations feature in only about 25% of cases of drug-induced lupus, but erythema multiforme-like lesions, papular skin lesions and purpura do occur.[28] Laboratory tests show that some patients

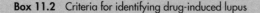

> **Box 11.2** Criteria for identifying drug-induced lupus
>
> - Continuous treatment with suspect drug for at least 1 month and usually much longer.
> - Common presenting symptoms are arthralgias, myalgias, malaise, fever, serositis (pleurisy and pericarditis).
> - Abnormal laboratory profile: presence of anti-histone antibodies (present in up to 80% of drug-induced SLE cases).
> - No previous history of lupus.
> - Symptom improvement within days or a few weeks of discontinuation of the suspect drug.

also have mild leukopenia, thrombocytopenia, anaemia and elevated erythrocyte sedimentation rate (ESR). Autoantibodies are raised in SLE: antinuclear antibodies are raised in over 95% of cases of both idiopathic and drug-induced SLE.[89] Antihistone antibodies are commonly associated with drug-induced SLE (in over 80% of patients), although they are also detected in 20–30% of idiopathic SLE.[28] Antibodies to double-stranded DNA are found in <1% of cases of drug-induced SLE but over 50% patients with idiopathic SLE. Gender does not appear to be an important factor in drug-induced lupus, with both sexes being affected equally, whereas more females than males are affected by idiopathic SLE. Again in contrast to idiopathic SLE, drug-induced lupus often occurs in older age groups.[90] Drug-induced lupus must be distinguished from drug-induced autoimmunity, in which drug therapy results in asymptomatic development of autoantibodies, elevated immunoglobulin levels and other laboratory abnormalities. Although a large number of patients develop laboratory features of autoimmunity, such as the production of antinuclear antibodies (ANA), a very small proportion develop drug-induced lupus. There are no specific diagnostic criteria for drug-induced lupus, but the criteria listed in Box 11.2 generally apply. Drug withdrawal is usually followed by resolution of symptoms and laboratory abnormalities within days or weeks, although they may persist for months or years in some patients.[91] Patients may require short-term treatment with low-dose corticosteroids.[86,87] The prompt resolution of symptoms is of particular value in supporting the diagnosis of drug-induced lupus.

The mechanism behind drug-induced lupus is not yet fully understood; it has been suggested that certain drugs act as immunogens in genetically predisposed individuals. There is a strong suggestion that the problem is mediated by drug metabolites. Several lupus-inducing drugs are known to undergo oxidative metabolism by activated neutrophils, including procainamide, hydralazine, phenytoin, quinidine, dapsone, propylthiouracil and carbamazepine. This hypothesis is in keeping with the finding that individuals with rapid acetylator status are less likely to develop drug-induced lupus with procainamide or hydralazine. N-acetylation of these drugs in the liver is known to compete with neutrophil-mediated N-oxidation, blocking the generation of oxidised drug metabolites.[87] Further research into the mechanisms underlying drug-induced lupus is in progress.

Although many medicines have been implicated as a cause of lupus-like illness, for some of these the risk may be very low or the causality uncertain (Table 11.9). By far the highest-risk drugs are procainamide and hydralazine. About 20% of patients treated with procainamide and about 5–8% of those treated with hydralazine during 1 year of therapy at standard doses develop symptoms.[87] The risk of drug-induced lupus is greater in slow acetylators and those who possess the HLA-DR4 genotype (see Chapter 3). Pleuritis and pericarditis are frequent characteristics of procainamide-induced lupus and glomerulonephritis, and rash may be seen in hydralazine-induced lupus. Patients taking long-term hydralazine or procainamide should be carefully monitored: every 3 months a full blood count should be carried out and ESR and ANA measured.

Table 11.9 Some drugs associated with systemic lupus erythematosus

Most frequent offenders	Unproven or isolated reports
Carbamazepine	Amiodarone
Chlorpromazine	Beta-blockers
Etanercept	Disopyramide
Hydralazine	Doxycycline
Infliximab	Ethosuximide
Isoniazid	Griseofulvin
Methyldopa	Nitrofurantoin
Minocycline (and other tetracyclines)	Oral contraceptives
Penicillamine	Phenytoin
Procainamide	Primidone
Quinidine	Rifampicin
Sulfasalazine	Statins
	Thiazide diuretics
	Ticlopidine

For other drugs associated with lupus-like disease the incidence is probably considerably less than 1% of patients treated. Quinidine can be considered moderate risk, whereas chlorpromazine, penicillamine, methyldopa, carbamazepine, isoniazid, captopril, propylthiouracil and minocycline incur a relatively low risk. Other drugs have been noted to exacerbate pre-existing SLE; the onset of problems usually occurs within hours of drug exposure.[87]

Minocycline-induced lupus

Minocycline, the most widely prescribed systemic antibiotic for acne, has been linked with drug-induced lupus.[84,91,92] There are over 100 cases reported in the literature.[84,91,92] Over three-quarters of the affected patients have been young women, although this may reflect usage, as acne is more frequently treated in young women. A review of 57 published cases reports a median duration of treatment, at doses between 50 mg and 200 mg, of 19 months before symptoms emerged.[84] In a Welsh case series of 23 patients (20 female, 3 male; 22 acne, 1 rheumatoid arthritis) the median period of treatment before symptoms began was 22.5 months. Although minocycline is increasingly being used as a second-line drug in rheumatoid arthritis, this is the only published report of minocycline-induced lupus among these patients.[92] In a further case series from Scotland the 20 patients involved (15 female, 5 male) took minocycline for a mean of 25 months prior to developing symptoms.[91] Arthralgia/arthritis was a feature in all reported cases and fever, myalgia and malaise were all common, with rash, pleuritic pain and hepatitis seen in some cases. Although laboratory tests showed an increased ESR in most patients, antihistone antibodies were present in only four of 40 patients in whom they were measured. In most patients the syndrome resolved rapidly after minocycline was discontinued. In some cases there was a long period before the link with minocycline therapy was made. Supervised rechallenge was carried out in 10 patients once the symptoms had resolved.[92] In seven of these patients malaise and polyarthralgia developed within 12 hours of consuming a single 100-mg dose of minocycline; in the remaining three, symptoms developed after 26, 36 and 72 hours. The rapid response to rechallenge was seen even in patients who had discontinued minocycline years earlier, suggesting that minocycline-induced lupus is associated with the development of long-term immunological memory. Healthcare professionals should be aware of this adverse effect and have a high index of suspicion in young patients taking minocycline who develop features of autoimmune syndromes.

TNF-alpha inhibitor-induced lupus

Tumour necrosis factor (TNF)-alpha is a proinflammatory cytokine with a role in the pathogenesis of a number of conditions, including rheumatoid arthritis and Crohn's disease. The anti-TNF-alpha therapies infliximab (chimeric anti-TNF-alpha antibody) and etanercept (soluble TNF-alpha receptor) were first marketed in the UK in 2000. Since then there have been a number of reports linking them to SLE.[93–99] In an animal model TNF-alpha has been shown to delay the onset and progression of SLE, implying a potentially protective role in suppressing autoimmunity.[98,100] The blockade of TNF-alpha may predispose an individual to the appearance of autoantibodies and clinical autoimmune syndromes.[98] In published reports of etanercept-induced SLE all patients presented with a skin reaction (erythema, scaling, malar rash, photosensitivity). Other symptoms included malaise, pericarditis, fever, muscle pain, polyarthralgia and synovitis. The timing of onset and resolution of skin abnormalities relative to the period of etanercept therapy strongly support a drug-induced aetiology. Most patients developed abnormalities 3–14 months after commencing treatment and improved rapidly on stopping.[93] Symptoms reported with infliximab-induced SLE include inflammatory arthritis, arthralgia, symmetrical synovitis involving hands, wrists, ankles, knees and elbow, malar rash and photosensitivity. Symptoms first appeared between 2 and 8 months after the initial dose, and resolution usually occurred 2–6 months after withdrawal. Cases of infliximab-induced SLE occurring in clinical trials suggest that the incidence is between 0.2% and 0.3%.[97,98] No renal or neurological symptoms of SLE have so far been reported with either etanercept or infliximab.[100] The anti-TNF-alpha agents appear to share the potential to induce SLE and lupus-like syndromes as a result of common biologic action rather than as a consequence of immunogenicity.[98]

CASE STUDY 11.1

Mrs D is a 72-year-old woman who has hypertension, asthma and chronic obstructive pulmonary disease (COPD). She takes bendroflumethiazide 2.5 mg daily, prednisolone 5 mg daily and salbutamol two puffs four times daily. She is allergic to penicillin. Last week she started a 10-day course of levofloxacin

→

◗ CASE STUDY 11.1 (continued)

500 mg daily for a lower respiratory chest infection. After 5 days of treatment she started to experience muscle pains in her lower legs, which were tender to touch and slightly swollen. The pain became so bad that Mrs D was unable to walk without help. Getting up the following day she heard a 'snap' and experienced severe pain in the calf area of her left leg.

Could Mrs D's symptoms be related to her medication?

Tendinopathies are a well-recognised but rare adverse effect associated with quinolone antibiotics. The incidence of quinolone-induced tendonitis is between 0.1% and 0.4%. Tendon rupture occurs in around 30% of theses cases. Tendon effects have been reported with all quinolones, but levofloxacin appears to be implicated in a higher proportion of cases. The Achilles tendon is most often affected because of its weight-bearing role, but other tendons, including those of the quadriceps muscle and the rotator cuff, may be affected. The symptoms described by Mrs D suggest that her Achilles tendon has ruptured.

What are the risk factors?

There are a number of risk factors that increase the risk of tendinopathy with quinolone antibiotics, including:

- Age over 60 years;
- Corticosteroid therapy;
- Renal failure and/or haemodialysis;
- Renal transplant recipients;
- Diabetes mellitus;
- Rheumatoid arthritis;
- Gout;
- Chronic lung disease.

In one epidemiological study concomitant use of oral corticosteroids increased the relative risk of Achilles tendon rupture (all ages) from 4.2 to 14.5 compared to no exposure to quinolones.[76] The risk of tendinopathy also increases gradually with age, the relative risk being estimated as 6.4 in patients aged 60–79 years and 20.4 in patients aged 80 or older.[76] Mrs D's risk factors include her age, concomitant prednisolone therapy and chronic lung disease.

How would the diagnosis of Achilles tendon rupture be made?

Diagnosis of tendon rupture is primarily by physical examination. It usually occurs 3–6 cm above the bony insertion and there may be a palpable gap at this position. Rupture can also be confirmed using X-ray, ultrasound and MRI.

→

CASE STUDY 11.1 (continued)

How should tendon disorders associated with quinolone antibiotics be managed?

Quinolone antibiotics should be discontinued immediately any tendinopathy is suspected. Immobilisation of ruptured tendons is advised; this can be achieved using a plaster cast. Weight-bearing activity should be avoided. In cases of complete rupture surgical repair of the tendon may be required. Analgesics should be used for pain control. Recovery from tendon injury is slow: it can take up to 3 months for tendonitis to resolve and up to 6 months for healing of a ruptured tendon.

Should any measures be taken to prevent further episodes of quinolone-associated tendinopathy?

The CSM have issued advice about tendon damage associated with quinolone antibiotics:

- Quinolones are contraindicated in patients with a history of tendon disorders related to quinolone use.
- Elderly patients and those on corticosteroids are at increased risk.
- If tendonitis is suspected quinolones should be stopped immediately and appropriate treatment initiated.

Mrs D should be told that she must avoid quinolone antibiotics in the future. This information should be recorded in her medical notes. If the reaction has been identified in hospital it is important that primary healthcare providers are informed that Mrs D's tendon rupture is suspected to have been caused by levofloxacin.

Tendon rupture is a serious adverse reaction and cases suspected to have been associated with quinolone antibiotics should be reported to the CSM on a yellow card.

 CASE STUDY 11.2

Mr C is a 48-year-old man who has recently been diagnosed with hypertension (blood pressure (BP) 145/95) and is to be monitored monthly. He is a smoker and is overweight, with a body mass index of 28. His total serum cholesterol

→

> **CASE STUDY 11.2** (continued)

concentration is 6.2 mmol/L. It is decided that Mr C should start simvastatin 10 mg at night. Advice on how to reduce cholesterol in his diet is provided and he is advised to stop smoking.

What should be done before initiating simvastatin therapy?

Before starting statin therapy patients should have hypothyroidism controlled if present, and liver function should be assessed. If patients have any of the following risk factors associated with myopathy they should have creatine phosphokinase (CPK) measured:[19]

- Underlying muscle disorders, renal impairment, hypothyroidism or alcohol misuse;
- Concomitant use of other lipid-lowering agents, e.g. fibrates or nicotinic acid;
- Concomitant use of cytochrome P450 3A4 inhibitors, including ciclosporin, macrolide antibiotics, azole antifungals, protease inhibitors.

Mr C should be advised to return to the surgery if he experiences any muscle pain, tenderness or weakness, especially if accompanied by malaise, fever or dark urine.

Mr C comes to the surgery 14 weeks later complaining of slight muscle pains and weakness, although the muscle pain does not particularly trouble him. At his last routine visit his BP (still high) and liver function (normal) were measured. His cholesterol level was falling slowly and his simvastatin dose had been increased incrementally from an initial 10 mg to 40 mg at month 3.

Could Mr C's muscle pains have been caused by the simvastatin?

Mild muscle pain occurs in 2–7% of patients taking statins and is usually associated with a minimal elevation of CPK (3–10 times the upper limit of normal – ULN). Statin-related myotoxicity is dose related and therefore factors that increase blood levels may enhance their myotoxic effect. The timing of the onset of myalgia suggests that it may be related to the recent increase in simvastatin dose.

What investigations should be carried out?

Mr C should have his CPK levels measured. If the level is >5 times the ULN or myopathy is suspected then statin treatment should be stopped. If the CPK levels are <5 times the ULN then simvastatin may be continued.

CPK levels were 4.8 times ULN and it was decided to continue simvastatin and to monitor the CPK. Mr C was advised to return if the muscle pains became any worse.

→

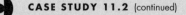

CASE STUDY 11.2 (continued)

Five weeks later Mr C returned, describing terrible muscle pain and cramps. He also felt generally unwell and described his urine as tea coloured. Initially Mr C associated the increased muscle pains with using the gym. During the week prior to presenting with muscle pain Mr C had toothache and his dentist had given him a 7-day course of erythromycin.

What is the cause of Mr C's new symptoms?

Mr C may have developed rhabdomyolysis. Rhabdomyolysis presents as muscle swelling, tenderness and severe weakness with dark brown (tea or cola coloured) urine due to myoglobin excretion. The CPK levels rise to at least 10 times the ULN and can rise to more than 100 times the ULN. Rhabdomyolysis is potentially life-threatening owing to the complications of hyperkalaemia, hypocalcaemia, myoglobinuric renal failure due to tubular necrosis, disseminated intravascular coagulation, cardiomyopathy, respiratory failure and severe metabolic acidosis. Approximately half of the cases of statin-induced rhabdomyolysis are associated with a statin–drug interaction that leads to increased statin blood levels. Macrolide antibiotics, including erythromycin, are potent inhibitors of CYP 3A4. They interact with statins metabolised by CYP 3A4 (simvastatin, atorvastatin) to produce a significant rise in statin blood levels. Mr C has recently had a dose increase of simvastatin and has also been taking erythromycin, suggesting that statin-related myopathy is possible.

How should Mr C be managed now?

The simvastatin should be stopped immediately and treatment to prevent renal failure started, including intravenous fluids, alkalinisation of the urine using sodium bicarbonate infusion followed by treatment to correct electrolyte abnormalities.

In future Mr C may need to be treated with an alternative lipid-lowering therapy, e.g. fibrates, nicotinic acid, ezetimibe.

References

1. Griffiths ID. Musculoskeletal disorders: Introduction. Rheumatology. Part 1. *Medicine* 2002; 30: 1–2.
2. Anon. Drug induced aches and pains. *Adv Drug React Bull* 1971; 30: 88–90.
3. Shetty HMG, Routledge PA, Davies DM. Disorders of muscle, bone and connective tissue. In: Davies DM, Ferner RE, de Glanville H, eds. *Davies's Textbook of Adverse Drug Reactions*, 5th edn. London: Chapman & Hall, 1998: Chapter 18.
4. Evans M, Rees A. Effects of HMG-CoA reductase inhibitors on skeletal muscle. *Drug Safety* 2002; 25: 649–663.

5. Sieb JP, Gillessen T. Iatrogenic and toxic myopathies. *Muscle Nerve* 2003; 27: 142–156.
6. Thompson PD, Clarkson P, Karas RH. Statin-induced myopathy. *JAMA* 2003; 289: 1681–1690.
7. Ucar M, Mjorndal T, Dahlquist R. HMG-CoA reductase inhibitors and myotoxicity. *Drug Safety* 2000; 22: 441–457.
8. Van Gerpen JA, McKinley KL. Leuprolide-induced myopathy. *J Am Geriatr Soc* 2002; 50: 1746.
9. Lewin JJ, Nappi JM, Taylor MH. Rhabdomyolysis with concurrent atorvastatin and diltiazem. *Ann Pharmacother* 2002; 36: 1546–1549.
10. Black C, Jick H. Etiology and frequency of rhabdomyolysis. *Pharmacotherapy* 2002; 22: 1524–1526.
11. Lane R, Phillips M. Rhabdomyolysis. *Br Med J* 2003; 327: 115–116.
12. Hamilton-Craig I. Statins and muscle damage. *Aust Prescriber* 2003; 26: 74–75.
13. Langford NJ, Kendall MJ. Rhabdomyolysis with HMG CoA reductase inhibitors: a class effect? *J Clin Pharm Ther* 2001; 26: 391–395.
14. Rosenson RS. Current overview of statin-induced myopathy. *Am J Med* 2004; 116: 408–416.
15. Ballantyne CM, Corsini A, Davidson MH, *et al.* Risk for myopathy with statin therapy in high-risk patients. *Arch Intern Med* 2003; 163: 553–564.
16. Farmer JA. Learning from the cerivastatin experience. *Lancet* 2001; 358: 1383–1385.
17. Committee on Safety of Medicines. Cerivastatin (Lipobay) withdrawn. *Curr Probl Pharmacovigilance* 2001; 27: 9.
18. Lee AJ, Maddix DS. Rhabdomyolysis secondary to a drug interaction between simvastatin and clarithromycin. *Ann Pharmacother* 2001; 35: 26–31.
19. Committee on Safety of Medicines. HMG CoA reductase inhibitors and myopathy. *Curr Probl Pharmacovigilance* 2002; 28: 8–9.
20. Maxa JL, Melton LB, Ogu CC, *et al.* Rhabdomyolysis after concomitant use of cyclosporine, simvastatin, gemfibrozil, and itraconazole. *Ann Pharmacother* 2002; 36: 820–823.
21. Swygert LA, Maes EF, Sewel LE, *et al.* Eosinophilia–myalgia syndrome. Results of national surveillance. *JAMA* 1990; 264: 1698–1703.
22. Belongia EA, Hedberg CW, Gleich GJ, *et al.* An investigation of the eosinophilia-myalgia syndrome associated with tryptophan use. *N Engl J Med* 1990; 323: 357–365.
23. Committee on Safety of Medicines. Update on L-tryptophan and eosinophilia–myalgia syndrome. *Curr Probl* 1990; Number 29.
24. Robinson D, Geddes DM. Inhaled corticosteroids: benefits and risks. *J Asthma* 1996; 33: 5–16.
25. Ligget NW, Reid DM. The incidence, epidemiology and aetiology of osteoporosis. *Hosp Pharmacist* 2000; 7: 62–68.
26. Tannirandorn P, Epstein S. Drug-induced bone loss. *Osteoporosis Int* 2000; 11: 637–659.
27. Jones G, Sambrook PN. Drug-induced disorders of bone metabolism. Incidence, management and avoidance. *Drug Safety* 1994; 10: 480–489.
28. Vergne P, Bertin P, Bonnet C, *et al.* Drug-induced rheumatic disorders. Incidence, prevention and management. *Drug Safety* 2000; 23: 279–293.

29. Boling EP. Secondary osteoporosis: Underlying disease and the risk for glucocorticoid-induced osteoporosis. *Clin Ther* 2004; 26: 1–14.

30. McIlwain HH. Glucocorticoid-induced osteoporosis: pathogenesis, diagnosis, and management. *Prev Med* 2003; 36: 243–249.

31. van Staa TP, Leufkens HGM, Cooper C. The epidemiology of corticosteroid-induced osteoporosis: a meta-analysis. *Osteoporosis Int* 2002; 13: 777–787.

32. Royal College of Physicians. *Glucocorticoid-Induced Osteoporosis: Guidelines for Prevention and Treatment.* London: Royal College of Physicians, 2002.

33. Duff G, Chairman of CSM. *Further Advice on Safety of HRT: Risk:Benefit Unfavourable for First-Line use in Prevention of Osteoporosis CEM/CMO/ 2003/19, Gateway ref: 2421.*

34. Sivakumaran M, Ghosh K, Zaidi Y, *et al.* Osteoporosis and vertebral collapse following low-dose, low molecular weight heparin therapy in a young patient. *Clin Lab Haematol* 1996; 18: 55–57.

35. Daniell HW. Opioid osteoporosis. *Arch Intern Med* 2004; 164: 338.

36. Reginato AJ, Coquia JA. Musculoskeletal manifestations of osteomalacia and rickets. *Best Pract Res Clin Rheumatol* 2003; 17: 1063–1080.

37. Fitzpatrick LA. Pathophysiology of bone loss in patients receiving anticonvulsant therapy. *Epilepsy Behav* 2004; 5: S3–S15.

38. Goodman WG, Duarte MEL. Aluminium: effects on bone and role in the pathogenesis of renal osteodystrophy. *Miner Electrolyte Metab* 1991; 17: 221–232.

39. Hurley DL, McMahon HM. Long term parenteral nutrition and metabolic bone disease. *Endocrinol Metab Clin North Am* 1990; 19: 113.

40. Klein GL, Coburn JW. Total parenteral nutrition and its effect on bone metabolism. *Crit Rev Clin Lab Sci* 1994; 31: 135.

41. Assouline-Dyan Y, Chang C, Greenspan A, *et al.* Pathogenesis and natural history of osteonecrosis. *Semin Arthritis Rheum* 2002; 32: 94–124.

42. Prathapkumar KR, Smith I, Attara GA. Indomethacin induced avascular necrosis of head of femur. *Postgrad Med J* 2000; 76: 574–575.

43. Koo K-H, Kim R, Kim Y-S, *et al.* Risk period for developing osteonecrosis of the femoral head in patients on steroid treatment. *Clin Rheumatol* 2002; 21: 299–303.

44. Nasser SMS, Ewan PW. Depot corticosteroid treatment for hayfever causing avascular necrosis of both hips. *Br Med J* 2001; 322: 1589–1591.

45. Clinkscales A, Cleary JD. Steroid–induced avascular necreosis. *Ann Pharmacother* 2002; 36: 1105.

46. Marx RE. Pamidronate (Aredia) and zoledronate (Zometa) induced avascular necrosis of the jaws: a growing epidemic. *J Oral Maxillofac Surg* 2003; 61: 1115–1118.

47. Migliorati CA. Bisphosphonates and oral cavity avascular bone necrosis. *J Clin Oncol* 2003; 21: 4253–4254.

48. Ruggiero SL, Mehrotra B, Rosenberg TJ, *et al.* Osteonecrosis of the jaws associated with the use of bisphosphonates: A review of 63 cases. *J Oral Maxillofac Surg* 2004; 62: 527–534.

49. Pogrel MA. Bisphosphonates and bone necrosis. *J Oral Maxillofac Surg* 2004; 62: 391–392.

50. Schwartz HC. Osteonecrosis and bisphosphonates: correlation versus causation. *J Oral Maxillofac Surg* 2004; 62: 763–764.

51. Aredia. Summary of Product Characteristics, January 2005. Novartis Pharmaceuticals UK Ltd.

52. Zometa. Summary of Product Characteristics, December 2004. Novartis Pharmaceuticals UK Ltd.

53. Hellsten JW, Marek CL. Bis-phossy jaw, phossy jaw, and the 21st century: Bisphosphonate-associated complications of the jaws. *J Oral Maxillofac Surg* 2004; 62: 1563–1565.

54. Greenberg MS. Intravenous bisphosphonates and osteonecrosis. *Oral Surg Oral Med Oral Pathol Oral Radiol Endod* 2004; 98: 259–260.

55. Slater PE. Chronic arthropathy after rubella vaccination in women. *JAMA* 1997; 278: 594–595.

56. Weibel RE, Benor DE. Chronic arthropathy and musculoskeletal symptoms associated with rubella vaccines. *Arthritis Rheum* 1996; 39: 1529–1534.

57. Geirer DA, Geier MR. A one year follow up of chronic arthritis following rubella and hepatitis B vaccination based upon analysis of the Vaccine Adverse Events Reporting System (VAERS) database. *Clin Exp Rheumatol* 2002; 20: 767–771.

58. Ray P, Black S, Shinefield H. Risk of chronic arthropathy among women after rubella vaccination. *JAMA* 1997; 278: 551–556.

59. Missiuox D, Hermabessiere J, Sauvezie B. Arthritis and iritis after bacillus Calmette–Guerin therapy. *J Rheumatol* 1995; 22: 2010.

60. Thurairajan G, Hope-Ross MW, Situnayake RD, *et al*. Polyarthropathy, orbital myositis and posterior scleritis: an unusual adverse reaction to influenza vaccine. *Br J Rheumatology* 1997; 36: 120–123.

61. Liozon E, Ittig R, Vogt N, *et al*. Polymyalgia rheumatica following influenza vaccination. *J Am Geriatr Soc* 2000; 48: 1533–1534.

62. Donnellan PP, Douglas SL, Cameron DA, *et al*. Aromatase inhibitors and arthralgia. *J Clin Oncol* 2001; 19: 2767.

63. Smith KM. Arthralgia associated with calcium-channel blockers. *Am J Health-Syst Pharm* 2000; 57: 55–57.

64. Jolliet P, Veyrac G, Bourin M. First report of mirtazapine-induced arthralgia. *Eur Psychiatry* 2001; 16: 503–505.

65. Olsen KM, Rebuck JA, Rupp ME. Arthralgias and myalgias related to Quinupristin-dalfopristin administration *Clin Infect Dis* 2001; 32: 83–86.

66. Carver PL, Whang E, VandenBussche HL, *et al*. Risk factors for arthralgias or myalgias associated with quinupristin-dalfopristin therapy. *Pharmacotherapy* 2003; 23: 159–164.

67. van Puijenbroek EP, Egberts ACG, Meyboom RHB, *et al*. Association between terbinafine and arthralgia, fever and urticaria: symptoms or syndrome? *Pharmacoepidemiol Drug Safety* 2001; 10: 135–142.

68. Stahlman F. Safety profile of the quinolones. *J Antimicrob Chemother* 1990; 26(Suppl D): 31–44.

69. van der Linden PD, Nab HW, Simonian S, *et al*. Fluoroquinolone use and the change in incidence of tendon ruptures in the Netherlands. *Pharm World Sci* 2001; 23: 89–92.

70. Leone R, Venegoni M, Motola D, *et al*. Adverse drug reactions related to the use of fluoroquinolone antimicrobials. *Drug Safety* 2003; 26: 109–120.

71. Harrell RM. Fluoroquinolone-induced tendinopathy: What do we know? *South Med J* 1999; 92: 622–625.

72. Khaliq Y, Zhane GG. Fluoroquinolone-associated tendinopathy: A critical review of the literature. *Clin Infect Dis* 2003; 36: 1404–1410.
73. van der Linden PD, van Puijenvroek EP, Feenstra J, *et al.* Tendon disorders attributed to fluoroquinolones: A study on 42 spontaneous reports in the period 1988 to 1998. *Arthritis Care Res* 2001; 45: 235–239.
74. de la Red G, Mejia JC, Cervera R, *et al.* Bilateral Achilles tendonitis with spontaneous rupture induced by levofloxacin in a patient with systemic sclerosis. *Clin Rheumatol* 2003; 22: 367–368.
75. Mathis AS, Chan V, Gryszkiewicz M, *et al.* Levofloxacin-associated Achilles tendon rupture. *Ann Pharmacother* 2003; 37: 1014–1017.
76. Haddow LJ, Sekhar MC, Hajela V, *et al.* Spontaneous Achilles tendon rupture in patients treated with levofloxacin. *J Antimicrob Chemother* 2003; 51: 747–748.
77. van der Linden PD, Sturkenboom MCJM Herings RMC, *et al.* Fluoroquinolones increase the risk of Achilles tendon rupture, especially in elderly patients on oral corticosteroids. *Br J Clin Pharmacol* 2001; 52: 626P–627P.
78. Committee on Safety of Medicines. Reminder: Fluoroquinolone antibiotics and tendon disorders. *Curr Probl Pharmacovigilance* 2002; 28: 3–4.
79. Mondal BK. Pergolide-induced retroperitoneal fibrosis. *Int J Clin Pract* 2000; 54: 403.
80. Shaunak S, Wilkins A, Pilling JB, *et al.* Pericardial, retroperitoneal, and pleural fibrosis induced by pergolide. *J Neurol Neurosurg Psychiatry* 1999; 66: 79–81.
81. Bleumink GS, van der Molen-Eijgenraam M, Strijbos JH, *et al.* Pergolide-induced pleuropulmonary fibrosis. *Clin Neuropharmacol* 2002; 25: 290–293.
82. Committee on Safety of Medicines. Fibrotic reactions with pergolide and other ergot-derived dopamine agonists. *Curr Probl Pharmacovigilance* 2002; 28: 3.
83. Lim PO, MacDonald TM. Antianginal drugs and beta-adrenoceptor antagonists. In: Dukes MNG, Aronson JK eds. *Meyler's Side Effects Of Drugs*, 14th edn. Amsterdam: Elsevier, 2000: Chapter 18.
84. Shepherd J. Severe complication of a commonly prescribed drug: Minocycline-induced lupus. *J Am Board Fam Pract* 2002; 15: 239–241.
85. Price EJ, Venables VJW. Drug-induced lupus. *Drug Safety* 1995; 12: 283–909.
86. Pramatarov KD. Drug-induced lupus erythematosus. *Clin Dermatol* 1998; 16: 368–377.
87. Rubin RL. Etiology and mechanisms of drug-induced lupus. *Curr Opin Rheumatol* 1999; 11: 357–363.
88. Brogan BL, Olsen J. Drug-induced rheumatic syndromes. *Curr Opin Rheumatol* 2003; 15: 76–80.
89. Wallach J ed. Laboratory tests for collagen/vascular/rheumatic diseases. In: *Interpretation of Diagnostic Tests,* 7th edn. Philadelphia: Lippincott Williams & Wilkins, 2000: Chapter 16.
90. Patel GK, Anstey AV. Rifampicin-induced lupus erythematosus. *Clin Exp Dermatol* 2001; 26: 260–262.
91. Gordon MM, Porter D. Minocycline induced lupus: Case series in the West of Scotland. *J Rheumatol* 2001; 28: 1004–1006.
92. Lawson TM, Amos N, Bulgen D, *et al.* Minocycline-induced lupus: clinical features and response to rechallenge. *Rheumatology* 2001; 40: 329–335.
93. Shakoor N, Michalska M, Harris CA, *et al.* Drug-induced systemic lupus erythematosus associated with etanercept therapy. *Lancet* 2002; 359: 579–580.

94. Cairns AP, Duncan MKJ, Hinder AE, *et al*. New onset systemic lupus erythematosus in a patient receiving etanercept for rheumatoid arthritis. *Ann Rheum Dis* 2002; 61: 1031–1032.
95. Debandt M, Vittecoq O, Descamps V, *et al*. Anti-TNF-alpha-induced systemic lupus syndrome. *Clin Rheumatol* 2003; 22: 56–61.
96. Swale VJ, Perrett CM, Denton CP, *et al*. Etanercept-induced systemic lupus erythematosus. *Clin Exper Dermatol* 2003; 28: 604–607.
97. Ali Y, Shah S. Infliximab-induced systemic lupus erythematosus. *Ann Intern Med* 2002; 137: 625–626.
98. Klapman JB, Ene-Stroescu D, Becker MA, *et al*. A lupus-like syndrome associated with infliximab therapy. *Inflamm Bowel Dis* 2003; 9: 176–178.
99. Sarzi-Puttini P, Ardizzone S, Manzionna G, *et al*. Infliximab-induced lupus in Crohn's disease: a case report. *Dig Liver Dis* 2003; 35: 814–817.
100. Khanna D, McMahon M, Furst DE. Safety of tumour necrosis factor-alpha antagonists. *Drug Safety* 2004; 27: 307–324.

Further reading

Assouline-Dyan Y, Chang C, Greenspan A, *et al*. Pathogenesis and natural history of osteonecrosis. *Semin Arthritis Rheum* 2002; 32: 94–124.
Evans M, Rees A. Effects of HMG-CoA reductase inhibitors on skeletal muscle. *Drug Safety* 2002; 25: 649–663.
Khaliq Y, Zhane GG. Fluoroquinolone-associated tendinopathy: A critical review of the literature. *Clin Infect Dis* 2003; 36: 1404–1410.
Sieb JP, Gillessen T. Iatrogenic and toxic myopathies. *Muscle Nerve* 2003; 27: 142–156.
Tannirandorn P, Epstein S. Drug-induced bone loss. *Osteoporosis Int* 2000; 11: 637–659.
Thompson PD, Clarkson P, Karas RH. Statin-induced myopathy. *JAMA* 2003; 289: 1681–1690.
Vergne P, Bertin P, Bonnet C, *et al*. Drug-induced rheumatic disorders. Incidence, prevention and management. *Drug Safety* 2000; 23: 279–293.

12

Blood disorders

Moira McMurray and Fiona Maclean

Introduction

This chapter reviews the main types of drug-induced blood disorder, the symptoms, and the medicines most commonly implicated. Although such blood disorders (dyscrasias) are comparatively rare, they are always serious and have a high incidence of morbidity and mortality. As with other adverse drug reactions (ADRs) their exact incidence is not easy to determine, mainly because of difficulties in assessing the risk with particular drugs and in proving a causal relationship. There are no definitive tests to prove an aetiological link and although rechallenge, whether deliberate or inadvertent, provides the strongest evidence, it is not recommended. Reliable evidence on causative links can be derived from statistically significant epidemiological data.[1] Any suspected ADR involving the blood should be reported to the appropriate regulatory authority.

Like other ADRs, those affecting the blood can be divided into type A and type B reactions. Type A reactions are predictable from the known pharmacology of the drug. Bone marrow suppression by cytotoxics and other immunosuppressants is a common type A effect. Although serious and potentially fatal, appropriate monitoring and advances in management with antimicrobials, growth factors and stem cell rescue limit the impact of this kind of reaction. This chapter focuses on type B (unpredictable) reactions. Healthcare professionals should be aware of the characteristic symptoms associated with haematological ADRs, the medicines most commonly implicated, and those that require routine blood-count monitoring. Patients receiving high-risk medicines should be made aware of the symptoms of blood dyscrasias and counselled to seek advice immediately should any of these develop. In practice, patients will often present with a sore throat, mouth ulcers, bruising or bleeding, fever, malaise, rash or non-specific illness. Early recognition of these indicators of a potentially fatal reaction is crucial.

The high incidence of blood dyscrasias with some medicines, for example the antipsychotic remoxipride, has led to their withdrawal from the market. For others the risk of a haematological reaction is high enough to warrant regular, routine monitoring of the blood count (Table 12.1). This list is not exhaustive and does not include cytotoxic and other myelosuppressant drugs. There are other medicines with a known risk of blood dyscrasias for which regular monitoring is not considered worthwhile, such as the antithyroid drugs carbimazole and propylthiouracil. In European populations the estimated incidence of agranulocytosis with antithyroid drugs is about 0.3 per 1000 patient-years. However, the onset of the reaction can be so rapid that regular monitoring is unlikely to be of value. Instead, it is recommended that patients report any symptoms

Table 12.1 Some drugs requiring regular blood count monitoring

Amphotericin
Apomorphine (when given with levodopa)
Azathioprine
Ceftriaxone
Chloramphenicol
Chlorpromazine
Clozapine
Co-trimoxazole (prolonged)
Gold
Heparin (for >5 days)
Indometacin (prolonged)
Interferon alfa
Interferon beta
Leflunomide
Linezolid (for >10–14 days, pre-existing myelosuppression, severe renal insufficiency or with concomitant drugs that may adversely affect blood counts)
Mefenamic acid (prolonged)
Mianserin
Nalidixic acid (for >2 weeks)
Penicillamine
Phenylbutazone (for >7 days)
Phenytoin
Pyrimethamine (prolonged)
Rifampicin (prolonged, or if patient has hepatic disorder)
Sulfasalazine
Tacrolimus
Ticlopidine (discontinued 2003)
Tryptophan
Zidovudine

suggestive of infection, especially sore throat. The full blood count should be checked if there is clinical evidence of infection.[2]

In man, normal haemopoiesis takes place only in the bone marrow. One type of undifferentiated stem cell (pluripotential) develops into a number of progenitor cells which are responsible for the three main marrow cell lines: erythroid (red cells); granulocytic and monocytic (white cells); and megakaryocytic (platelets).[3]

The normal ranges of blood components are shown in Table 12.2. A reduction below the normal range in the peripheral blood cell count of any particular cell type is known as a cytopenia. Reductions may be caused either by a decrease in the production rate of that cell type or by a reduced life span of the cells in the circulation.[4] Drugs can cause blood dyscrasias by acting at different stages of haemopoiesis, from the stem cell through to the mature cell. The number of cell types affected depends on where in the process the effect takes place. Damage to a stem cell will affect most cell lines, whereas damage to the mature cell may be specific to that cell line. There is therefore considerable overlap in the drugs implicated in the different types of blood dyscrasias. Damage to the earliest progenitor cells usually takes more than 2 weeks for recovery, whereas damage to one of the later precursors is associated with recovery within a few days.[5]

Some patients may be genetically susceptible to the effects of certain medicines, resulting in an increased risk of an adverse event affecting the blood. Examples include the increased risk of clozapine-induced agranulocytosis in patients with particular phenotypes of human leukocyte antigen (HLA) (see Chapter 3); azathioprine and mercaptopurine myelotoxicity in patients deficient in the enzyme thiopurine methyltransferase (TPMT); and methotrexate toxicity in patients with polymorphism in

Table 12.2 Normal ranges of blood components

Component	Males and Females	
Haemoglobin	13.5–17.5 g/dL (males)	11.5–15.5 g/dL (females)
Red cells	4.5–6.5×10^{12}/L (males)	3.9–5.6×10^{12}/L (females)
White cells total	4.0–11.0×10^9/L	
Neutrophils	2.5–7.5×10^9/L	
Lymphocytes	1.5–3.5×10^9/L	
Monocytes	0.2–0.8×10^9/L	
Eosinophils	0.04–0.44×10^9/L	
Basophils	0.01–0.1×10^9/L	
Platelets	150–400×10^9/L	

the methylene tetrahydrofolate gene. Chloramphenicol toxicity is also considered to have a genetic basis.[6]

Depending on the type of cell line affected and the severity of the reaction, haematological ADRs usually manifest as one or more of the following: signs of anaemia, bleeding and/or bruising, and infection (often fever, sore throat, mouth ulcers). For many of the type B reactions the underlying mechanisms are either toxic or immune in nature.[5]

Aplastic anaemia

Aplastic anaemia describes a peripheral blood picture with suppression of red cells (anaemia), white cells (leukopenia) and platelets (thrombocytopenia) due to hypoplasia of the bone marrow. Aplastic anaemia is defined by the peripheral blood featuring two of the following three criteria: haemoglobin $<10\,$g/dL; platelets $<50 \times 10^9$/L; and neutrophils $<1.5 \times 10^9$/L. There are also defined criteria for the severity of the condition. In severe aplastic anaemia the bone marrow cellularity is $<25\%$ of normal, or 25–50% of normal with $<30\%$ residual haemopoietic cells. Two of the following three criteria must also be fulfilled: neutrophils $<0.5 \times 10^9$/L; platelets $<20 \times 10^9$/L; and reticulocytes $<1\%$. Very severe aplastic anaemia is as above but with a neutrophil count $<0.2 \times 10^9$/L. The neutrophil count appears to be the most important prognostic factor.[7]

The incidence in Europe and America has been estimated at between 2 and 5 per million of the population per year.[8] The lower limit of 2 per million would equate to 100–150 new cases in the UK each year.[7] Aplastic anaemia can be congenital, but most idiopathic cases are acquired from drugs, chemicals, radiation or viral infection.[9] This reaction is rarer than agranulocytosis or thrombocytopenia, but in contrast to these it often persists and worsens despite drug withdrawal. It is characterised by symptoms and signs of anaemia, infection and bleeding. The onset of drug-induced aplastic anaemia can be acute or, more commonly, chronic. Acute cases usually present with severe bleeding and sometimes with infection. When the onset is insidious, weakness, fatigue and pallor are the predominant symptoms.

It was previously thought that there were many different mechanisms of aplastic anaemia, including direct stem cell toxicity. However, it is now believed that most cases have an immune origin and result from T-cell-mediated organ-specific destruction of bone marrow haemopoietic cells. These immune responses may be linked to a viral infection or to drug or chemical exposure.[10] A number of drugs are associated with an unpredictable (type B) aplastic anaemia (Table 12.3).

Table 12.3 Some drugs strongly associated with aplastic anaemia

Group	Example
Antidiabetics	Chlorpropamide, tolbutamide
Antiepileptics	Carbamazepine, phenytoin, felbamate, lamotrigine
Anti-inflammatory drugs	Diclofenac, gold, indometacin, penicillamine, phenylbutazone, piroxicam, sulindac, sulfasalazine
Antimalarials	Pyrimethamine
Antimicrobials	Chloramphenicol, co-trimoxazole, sulfonamides, linezolid
Antiplatelets	Ticlopidine (discontinued 2003)
Antipsychotics	Chlorpromazine
Antithyroid drugs	Carbimazole, propylthiouracil

However, it is often difficult to prove a causal association, particularly because there may be a significant delay between exposure to the medicine and development of the reaction. The reaction can occur months after the causative drug has been stopped.[8] It is also more likely to occur after two or more exposures to the drug than after the initial exposure. Chloramphenicol was one of the first agents to be associated with aplastic anaemia.[11] Large doses produce mild, reversible bone marrow depression in all patients; this mainly affects red cells and is thought to be due to mitochondrial injury.[12] This is a predictable, type A reaction.

The type B aplastic anaemia is rare, unpredictable, and frequently irreversible and fatal. It has been reported to occur days, months or even years after an initial exposure to chloramphenicol, and in some cases has terminated in leukaemia.[13] The incidence is thought to be between 1 in 25 000 and 1 in 60 000. There is some evidence that genetic predisposition is involved. It is thought that the nitrobenzene ring on the chloramphenicol molecule undergoes nitroreduction in susceptible individuals to a toxic intermediate that causes stem cell damage.[6] In the UK, systemic chloramphenicol is reserved for life-threatening infections. Regular blood count monitoring before and during treatment with systemic chloramphenicol is essential.

The link between ocular chloramphenicol and aplastic anaemia is controversial.[14] Several published studies do not support the view that the use of chloramphenicol eye drops because of the risk of aplastic anaemia is inadvisable.[15,16] A recent epidemiological estimate of the risk found that, although an association between ocular chloramphenicol and aplastic anaemia could not be excluded, the absolute risk was very low, of the order of less than 1 per million treatment courses.[17] The *British*

National Formulary states that chloramphenicol is the drug of choice for superficial eye infections.[18]

Since the use of systemic chloramphenicol has declined, non-steroidal anti-inflammatory drugs (NSAIDs), as a therapeutic group, are thought to be the most frequent cause of drug-induced aplastic anaemia.[8] Because of its association with aplastic anaemia and agranulocytosis, the use of phenylbutazone is restricted to hospital treatment of ankylosing spondylitis unresponsive to other therapy.[19]

Many of the second-line or disease-modifying antirheumatic drugs (DMARDs) have the potential to cause haematological toxicity, including aplastic anaemia. Patients receiving gold, penicillamine, sulfasalazine, leflunomide or immunosuppressants must undergo regular blood monitoring. Platelet and neutrophil counts usually fall first in these patients, so regular monitoring may help avoid the development of aplastic anaemia.[20]

The antiepileptic agent felbamate is available only for restricted use on the US market because of associated cases of aplastic anaemia and acute liver failure. By 1997, 34 cases of felbamate-associated aplastic anaemia had been reported, 13 of which had been fatal. It should only be used for patients with epilepsy refractory to other antiepileptics, especially those with the Lennox–Gastaut syndrome, and full blood counts should be carried out before treatment and regularly during treatment.[21] Aplastic anaemia can occur after felbamate has been discontinued, so patients should continue to be monitored. Felbamate does not have marketing authorisation in the UK.

The antiplatelet agent ticlopidine, which was discontinued in the UK in 2003, has also been associated with aplastic anaemia. By early 1998, 19 cases had been reported in the literature.[22] A more recent review of two new and 55 additional cases postulates that the real incidence is higher. Many cases presented initially as agranulocytosis and/or thrombocytopenia, which may have in fact have been aplastic anaemia but were not accompanied by examination of bone marrow for confirmation. In more than 95% of cases the onset occurred between 3 weeks and 3 months of initial exposure to ticlopidine. The review proposed a direct cytotoxic effect on the progenitor stem cell.[23]

The diagnosis of aplastic anaemia is assisted by examination of peripheral blood and bone marrow. It is important to exclude other conditions that may also present with a pancytopenia, including certain forms of leukaemia.[7] Management involves two main principles: supporting and protecting the patient to improve the chance of a spontaneous recovery, and accelerating the recovery process. Any drug therapy that may be implicated in the reaction must be stopped. Supportive care involves transfusion of blood and platelet concentrates, antibiotic and antifungal treatment or prophylaxis, and possibly the use of recombinant human haemopoietic growth factors such as granulocyte colony-stimulating factor (G-CSF). These help to stabilise the patient in terms of bleeding and infection in the short term to allow time for spontaneous recovery.

Longer-term treatment, in specialist haematology centres, involves immunosuppressive therapy or replacing the bone marrow by a bone marrow transplant or stem cell transplant. The decision on treatment depends on the severity of the disease, the age and health of the patient and the availability of a histocompatible sibling.[7] In suitable patients who have a matched sibling donor, transplantation offers the chance of cure. In one experienced centre survival rates of 90% have been reported, although survival rates generally are 75–80%.[24,25] However, as there is only a one in four chance of histocompatibility for each sibling, this is not an option for 70% of patients. Transplants from matched unrelated donors have lower success rates.[10]

Immunosuppressive therapy is used in patients who are not suitable for a transplant because of age or lack of a donor. Immunosuppression with a course of antilymphocyte globulin achieves a response in about half of acquired cases, but recovery is slow and may be incomplete.[18] Ciclosporin has produced an improvement in some patients with aplastic anaemia, and a 50% response rate in patients refractory to antilymphocyte globulin has been reported. Improved response in terms of haematological parameters, quality of response and early mortality were achieved when antithymocyte globulin was used in combination with ciclosporin. Response rates of 70–80% have been reported with the combination, with 5-year survival rates of 80–90% in responding patients.[10]

Administration of recombinant human growth factors (granulocyte colony-stimulating factor (G-CSF) or granulocyte–macrophage colony-stimulating factor (GM-CSF)) tends to increase the neutrophil count only and the effect is usually transient. When used alone, they have generally not produced a sustained response and they do not improve response or survival rates in patients receiving immunosuppressive therapy.[10] Their use after bone marrow transplantation can reduce the neutropenic period.[26] In patients with refractory aplastic anaemia growth factors may offer an alternative, and blood counts have improved in patients treated with G-CSF and erythropoietin.[27]

The anabolic steroid nandrolone is licensed for the treatment of aplastic anaemia but its use is controversial because of its uncertain efficacy. Another anabolic steroid, oxymetholone, (unlicensed in the UK) has also been used, with mixed results.[18] When some marrow function remains anabolic steroids may increase cell lines, but there is no evidence of improved patient survival.[8] High-dose corticosteroids can induce a response, but other treatments are preferred.[26]

Agranulocytosis

Some medicines can cause a reduction in the total white cell count (leukopenia), but selective reduction in granulocytes, which include neutrophils, eosinophils and basophils, is more common. Agranulocytosis is defined as a profound decrease in the number of circulating granulocytes, resulting in a neutrophil count of less than 0.5×10^9/L. Patients with neutropenia of this severity are susceptible to serious and sometimes fatal infection. More modest reductions in the neutrophil count are referred to as neutropenia or granulocytopenia.[28]

Agranulocytosis is usually drug-induced but a few clinical conditions may occasionally be responsible, including viral infection, nutritional deficiencies, lymphomas or leukaemia, immune disorders or congenital or chronic neutropenia. In Europe, the incidence of non-chemotherapy drug-induced agranulocytosis is approximately 3.4 to 5.3 cases per million per year.[29] The aetiology is believed to be either autoimmune or direct toxicity to the bone marrow cells.[30] It is difficult to determine whether a drug-induced agranulocytosis is immune or toxic in nature in the individual patient, and some drugs are thought to be able to cause agranulocytosis by more than one mechanism.[29]

Immune-mediated destruction of neutrophils or suppression of granulopoiesis is probably the most common mechanism, and this may result in severe neutropenia of rapid onset, often with a single dose, or in a patient who has taken the medicine before. This mechanism is believed to be involved in agranulocytosis caused by sulfonamides, antithyroid agents, quinidine and phenytoin.[30] Complete recovery may occur 2–3 weeks after the drug is withdrawn, but the patient is then sensitised so that further drug exposure initiates a prompt recurrence.

Agranulocytosis may also arise from direct marrow toxicity, which in some cases may result from a genetic alteration of drug handling. The atypical antipsychotic clozapine is associated with a 2–3% incidence of neutropenia. The aetiology of clozapine-induced agranulocytosis is thought to be toxic, and there is an element of genetic susceptibility with an increased risk in patients with certain HLA phenotypes (see Chapter 3).[29] Clozapine remains available in the UK for the treatment of schizophrenia only in patients unresponsive to or intolerant of conventional antipsychotic drugs. Its use is restricted to patients registered with mandatory blood monitoring programmes. This ensures that clozapine is not given if the total white cell count falls below $3 \times 10^9/L$, or if the neutrophil count is less than $1.5 \times 10^9/L$. Monitoring must continue throughout treatment and for at least four weeks after discontinuation. Databases are maintained of all patients who have developed abnormal leukocyte or neutrophil counts who should then not be re-exposed to clozapine.[31]

Chlorpromazine has been shown to produce a dose-dependent inhibition of granulopoiesis. Severe, symptomatic and potentially fatal agranulocytosis is believed to occur in about 0.1 per cent of patients taking chlorpromazine in standard doses. This effect is usually delayed in onset.[32]

Antithyroid drugs (i.e. carbimazole and propylthiouracil) appear to incur a relatively high risk of agranulocytosis; some studies have estimated this risk to be in the order of 1.9 to 3 per 10 000 users per year[33,34]. The UK Committee on Safety of Medicines estimated the incidence at 0.3 per 1000 patient years of treatment in European populations.[2]

Ticlopidine has been associated with agranulocytosis and the initial clinical trials with ticlopidine in the UK were suspended because of neutropenia. The incidence of neutropenia was 2.4 per cent, with 0.85 per cent of patients described as severely neutropenic (less than $0.45 \times 10^9/L$). Most cases tended to develop within the first 3 months of treatment.[22] There is clearly an overlap between agranulocytosis and aplastic anaemia with ticlopidine, and it is unclear whether cases of agranulocytosis may have developed into aplastic anemia.[23]

Dapsone is associated with a unique risk pattern for agranulocytosis. When dapsone is used to treat leprosy the risk of agranulocytosis is virtually zero, and when used for malaria, in combination with maloprim, the incidence is estimated at 1 in 10–20 000. However, the risk is increased 25–33-fold when dapsone is used in patients with dermatitis herpetiformis, possibly owing to immune responsiveness and the high doses used in these patients.[35]

Medicines most strongly associated with agranulocytosis are listed in Table 12.4; there is considerable overlap with those implicated in aplastic anaemia.

The potential severity of agranulocytosis is indicated by an analysis of reports to the UK Committee on Safety of Medicines during the period 1963–1993.[36] There were 912 cases of agranulocytosis, 30% of which had a fatal outcome. Of 1499 cases of neutropenia, 3.5% were fatal. Six drug classes accounted for half the reports of agranulocytosis and a third of the reports of neutropenia. These were antithyroid drugs, beta-lactam

Table 12.4 Some drugs strongly associated with agranulocytosis

Group	Examples
Antidepressants	Imipramine, clomipramine, desipramine, mianserin
Antiepileptics	Carbamazepine, phenytoin
Anti-inflammatory drugs	Gold, leflunomide, penicillamine, sulfasalazine, non-steroidal anti-inflammatory drugs
Antimalarials	Pyrimethamine
Antimicrobials	Penicillins, cephalosporins, co-trimoxazole, chloramphenicol, sulfonamides, linezolid, dapsone
Antipsychotics	Chlorpromazine, thioridazine, clozapine
Antithyroid drugs	Carbimazole, propylthiouracil
Cardiovascular drugs	Captopril, procainamide, ticlopidine (discontinued 2003)

antibiotics, NSAIDs, phenothiazines, sulfonamides and tricyclic antidepressants. The individual drugs most commonly implicated were carbimazole, co-trimoxazole, chlorpromazine, clozapine, mianserin, phenylbutazone, sulfasalazine and thioridazine.

A Dutch population-based case–cohort study found the highest relative risk of drug-associated agranulocytosis with thyroid inhibitors, co-trimoxazole, sulfasalazine, clomipramine and dipyrone in combination with analgesics.[34] Examination of 90 cases of drug-induced agranulocytosis in one French centre found that antibiotics, antithyroid drugs and antiaggregative platelet agents (mainly ticlopidine) were the most frequent causative agents.[37]

Patients with drug-induced agranulocytosis usually become suddenly unwell, with fever and sometimes rigors, sore throat, mouth ulcers, headache and malaise. Most patients develop septicaemia and some have evidence of pneumonia, oropharyngeal candidiasis or skin infection. Any patient with suspected drug-induced agranulocytosis should be admitted to hospital immediately for full blood-count monitoring. A full drug history, including exposure to over-the-counter medicines, should be taken. If agranulocytosis is confirmed, any medicine that might be implicated should be stopped immediately. Examination of the bone marrow is useful to exclude any other underlying cause and to predict the likely duration of neutropenia. In most cases there is spontaneous recovery within 2 weeks of drug withdrawal. Patients who are febrile or have other evidence of infection should be treated promptly with broad-spectrum antibiotics, including one with good activity against *Pseudomonas aeruginosa*.[28] When an antibiotic is suspected of causing the agranulocytosis, consideration should be given to cross-reactivity when selecting an agent for management.[29] Antifungal therapy should be added if fever continues after 3–4 days of antibiotic therapy and there is some evidence that prophylactic use may be of benefit.[28]

A decade ago, European mortality rates from agranulocytosis were 10–16%, but improved management has reduced this to less than 5%.[29] Death is more likely when agranulocytosis is severe or prolonged, and in such cases recombinant human growth factors have been used to accelerate neutrophil recovery. The efficacy of these agents (G-CSF or GM-CSF) in this situation has been described in numerous case reports in which therapy appears to have improved the recovery time.[38,39] One small randomised study in patients with antithyroid-induced agranulocytosis found that G-CSF did not significantly reduce the mean duration of haematological recovery.[40] Recombinant human growth factors are not licensed for this indication.

Patients prescribed medicines with a significant risk of causing agranulocytosis should be advised to see the doctor immediately if fever, sore throat, mouth ulcers or excessive tiredness develop. They should be aware that a blood test will be necessary and that the medicine will be stopped if the white blood cell count is low. If patients are unable to see their GP immediately, they should go to the local hospital accident and emergency department.[28]

Thrombocytopenia

Thrombocytopenia is defined as a reduction in the platelet count to less than 150×10^9/L. The main presenting feature is haemorrhage, which is most commonly seen in the skin, giving rise to purpura and petechiae, and in the gastrointestinal and genitourinary tracts. Cerebral haemorrhage is the most common cause of death. Haemorrhage is unlikely to develop unless the platelet count is below 20×10^9/L.[41] In thrombocytopenia the bleeding time is prolonged, although coagulation tests (e.g. international normalised ratio, prothrombin time) remain normal.

Thrombocytopenia can result from a reduction in platelet production due to suppression or failure of the bone marrow. The platelet count usually falls 7–10 days after initiation of the offending drug. An autoimmune mechanism may also be responsible: autoimmune antibodies reduce the lifespan of platelets in the circulation from 7–10 days to several hours.[42] Table 12.5 lists the drugs most commonly associated with thrombocytopenia.

A study in Denmark from 1969 to 1991 found the most commonly implicated drugs were sodium aurothiomalate, co-trimoxazole, quinidine,

Table 12.5 Some drugs associated with thrombocytopenia

Effect	Examples
Decreased platelet production	Chloramphenicol, co-trimoxazole, idoxuridine, phenylbutazone, penicillamine
Increased platelet consumption	Acetazolamide, chlorpropamide, diazepam, digoxin, furosemide, glycoprotein IIb/IIIa inhibitors, gold, heparin, methyldopa, oxprenolol, penicillins, quinine, quinidine, rifampicin, sodium valproate, sulfonamides, thiazide diuretics, tolbutamide, trimethoprim

valproate and penicillamine. NSAIDs were the class of drug most commonly involved.[43] Different drugs appear to produce different clinical pictures of thrombocytopenia. Severe thrombocytopenia was associated with gold salts, NSAIDs, sulfonamides, antibiotics, quinine and quinidine. Valproic-acid-induced thrombocytopenia tended to be dose dependent, gradual in onset and mild in severity.[44]

Removal of the responsible drug is often sufficient to restore the platelet count within several days. Platelet transfusions may be needed if the count is very low ($<10 \times 10^9$/L).[1] In pyrexial patients the risk of haemorrhage is higher and platelet transfusion should be given at a higher threshold. Corticosteroids may also be beneficial in immune-mediated cases. Future exposure to the likely causative agent should be avoided. Aspirin and NSAIDs should be avoided as they reduce the effectiveness of the remaining platelets.[45]

More recently, the glycoprotein (GP) IIb/IIIa inhibitors have been associated with thrombocytopenia, with the highest risk in patients treated with abciximab. The mechanism is unclear, but may be due to the formation of a neoepitope on the platelet surface after binding of the drug. When this neoepitope binds to preformed antibodies, the platelets are phagocytosed.[46] The thrombocytopenia typically develops within 24 hours of starting treatment with the GP IIb/IIIa inhibitor, with platelets decreasing to below 50×10^9/L. Affected patients are at increased risk of developing bleeding complications, and if these occur platelet transfusions are recommended. On drug withdrawal, the platelet count usually recovers within 2–3 days. As these agents are often used in combination with heparin, heparin-induced thrombocytopenia should be ruled out. It is also important to exclude a diagnosis of pseudothrombocytopenia before giving platelets or reducing the concomitant heparin dose, which may increase the risk of a new arterial occlusion.[46]

Heparin is probably the drug best recognised as a cause of thrombo-cytopenia, of which there are two distinct types. The first is heparin-associated thrombocytopenia, which is a non-thrombogenic, non-immune form that can affect 25% of treated patients. It usually occurs during the first few days of heparin administration and is mild, with the platelet count not usually below 100×10^9/L. It is caused by a direct interaction between heparin and platelets that does not involve antibodies. Affected patients usually have no complications and the thrombocytopenia resolves on stop-ping heparin.[47] The second type, heparin-induced thrombocytopenia (HIT), is less frequent, occurring in about 2% of patients receiving unfractionated heparin. It is much more serious and can present as thrombocytopenia alone (HIT) or as thrombocytopenia plus thrombotic syndrome (HITTS) in 25–50% of affected patients.[45] Thrombotic events can include myocardial infarction, stroke, arterial and venous throm-bosis and pulmonary embolus. The onset of the reaction is usually 5–10 days after starting heparin. Patients usually have mild to moderate thrombocytopenia (platelet count of $20–150 \times 10^9$/L). The mechanism involves immune destruction and activation of platelets by antibodies that bind to heparin-platelet factor 4 (PF4) complexes, leading to platelet aggregation and thrombocytopenia. This can trigger platelet activation, coagulation activation and thrombin generation.[48] The diag-nosis of HIT is based on the occurrence of one or more HIT-associated clinical events and the detection of HIT antibodies in plasma or serum.[48]

Early recognition and management is necessary to prevent throm-botic complications. If this reaction is suspected, all heparin, including line flushes, should be stopped. Because the risk of thrombosis remains high, a suitable alternative anticoagulant must be considered until the platelet count has recovered. Thrombosis has occurred in 20–50% of patients with isolated HIT only when heparin is stopped.[47] Warfarin should not be used because of the risk of warfarin-induced venous limb gangrene.[49] Platelet transfusions should be avoided in these patients, as they may pre-cipitate thrombotic events.[49] Low molecular weight heparins are less commonly associated with HIT than unfractionated heparin, but as there is a high risk of *in vivo* cross-reactivity, they should also be avoided in HIT patients.[48]

There have been a number of recent advances in the options available to treat these patients. The heparinoid danaparoid is available in the UK. It may have a role in HIT patients when there is no evidence of cross-reactivity; however, cross-reactivity occurs *in vitro* in about 20% of cases, and although *in vivo* cross-reactivity is rare, it can occur.[50] Two direct thrombin inhibitors are also suitable alternatives: lepirudin, which is licensed in the UK for anticoagulation in patients with HIT who require antithrombotic treatment, and argatroban, which is available in the US and may soon be available in Europe. Both agents are potent inhibitors of free and clot-bound thrombin and they do not cross-react with HIT antibodies. Lepirudin is cleared by the kidneys and accumulates in patients with renal impairment. In contrast, argatroban is metabolised in the liver and excreted in the bile. In patients with HIT who require antithrombotic treatment, those who have renal impairment would be best treated with argatroban, whereas lepirudin is suitable in those with hepatic impairment.[50]

Pure red cell aplasia

Pure red cell aplasia (PRCA) is characterised by anaemia with a marked reduction in reticulocytes (immature red cells). There is an absence of nucleated red cell precursors in an otherwise normal bone marrow.[1] In most cases the mechanism remains unclear, with possible immune or toxin-mediated cell destruction. Patients experience weakness, lethargy and pallor. About 5% of reported cases are thought to be drug-induced, and there is overlap with drugs associated with aplastic anaemia. Over 30 drugs have been implicated as a cause of PRCA by one or two case reports, but those implicated in several reports include phenytoin, aza-thioprine and isoniazid. Other associated drugs include penicillamine, chlorpropamide and chloramphenicol.[1] More recently, epoetin has been linked with PRCA. After an initial response to epoetin, 13 affected patients became severely anaemic and dependent on transfusions. In all patients, neutralising antibodies against the protein moiety of epoetin were detected.[51] In 2002, the UK Committee on Safety of Medicines reported 40 confirmed or suspected worldwide cases of PRCA in patients treated with epoetin alfa. This corresponds to a reporting rate of less than 1 in 10 000 treated patients.[52]

Management of PRCA involves supportive care with red cell trans-fusion.[1] Some patients will respond to corticosteroid therapy and others to immunosuppressants such as cyclophosphamide.[53]

Haemolytic anaemia

Haemolytic anaemia is anaemia resulting from an increased rate of red cell destruction. Anaemia may not develop until the rate of red cell destruction has increased severalfold, as initially erythropoiesis will increase to compensate. The red cell normally survives for about 120 days, but in haemolytic anaemia the lifespan may be reduced to only a few days.[54]

Immune or metabolic mechanisms may be responsible for drug-induced haemolytic anaemia. The immune type may be further divided according to four proposed mechanisms. The first involves antibody formation against a drug that can bind to the red blood cell membrane. When the antibodies combine with the erythrocyte-bound drug, the complement mechanism on the red cell membrane is activated, resulting in cell lysis. This form of haemolytic anaemia has been associated with penicillins and cephalosporins.[55]

The second mechanism involves the drug binding to a plasma protein, forming an immunogenic conjugate. When this conjugate binds to its resulting antidrug antibody an immune complex is formed. This adheres to red blood cells, activating complement in the membrane, causing intravascular haemolysis with haemoglobinaemia and haemoglobulinuria and even renal failure. Isoniazid, methotrexate, quinidine, quinine, rifampicin, sulphonylureas and diclofenac have been implicated.[54]

Thirdly, the formation of immunogenic drug–red blood cell complexes causes *in vivo* sensitisation to the drug. The specificity of the produced antibodies arises from the drug and defined red blood cell antigens.[55]

Autoimmune haemolysis is the basis of the fourth mechanism: the drug alters immune regulation so that autoantibodies are expressed against normal red blood cell antigens. This is more common than immune complex formation and has been associated with methyldopa, levodopa, mefenamic acid and azapropazone.[4]

More recently, ribavirin therapy in patients with chronic hepatitis C has been associated with haemolytic anaemia. A meta-analysis of 17 studies suggested a 9% excess risk of developing anaemia during ribavirin therapy.[56]

The Coombs' test, which detects the presence of antibodies on red cells, can distinguish these immune mechanisms from other disorders that reduce the lifespan of red blood cells.

Red blood cells can also be damaged by drugs that have an oxidant effect on the cell membrane. These metabolic effects can occur in normal individuals but are more common in those deficient in glucose-6-phosphate dehydrogenase (G6PD), an enzyme required for the stability of red blood cells. Many medicines have been associated with haemolysis in G6PD deficiency, but only a few of these have proven haemolytic potential. Drugs that should be avoided in susceptible patients include nitrofurantoin, nalidixic acid, sulfamethoxazole and sulfasalazine.[57] The *British*

National Formulary gives further details of medicines that incur a risk of haemolysis in most G6PD-deficient individuals.[18]

Patients with haemolytic anaemia usually present acutely with symptoms of anaemia. They often have jaundice, haemoglobinuria (which may be marked enough to make the urine black in colour), and some will have renal impairment. Any implicated drug therapy should be withdrawn. Red cells usually return to normal within 2–3 weeks. Corticosteroid therapy is sometimes beneficial, and some patients will require dialysis.[55]

Megaloblastic anaemia

Megaloblastic anaemia results from impaired DNA synthesis while protein and RNA synthesis remain normal. It is usually due to folate or vitamin B_{12} deficiency. The mechanisms through which drugs cause megaloblastic anaemia are either inhibition of DNA synthesis, for example cytotoxic agents and zidovudine, or reduction of vitamin B_{12} or folate levels, for example trimethoprim and antiepileptics. Table 12.6 lists implicated drugs.

The condition is characterised by a high mean cell volume (macrocytosis) and disordered maturation of haemopoietic cells. As a result, patients generally develop progressive symptoms of anaemia, but in severe cases may also have leukopenia and thrombocytopenia. Neurological symptoms, such as neuropathy, may also be present, with the legs more likely to be affected than the arms.[58]

When given at therapeutic doses, folate reductase inhibitors such as trimethoprim and pyrimethamine do not normally induce megaloblastic anaemia but may worsen folate deficiency. Methotrexate-induced cases are dose related, therefore treatment with high doses requires rescue therapy with calcium folinate. If megaloblastic anaemia develops in patients on antiepileptics, folic acid supplements are recommended.[59]

Table 12.6 Some drugs associated with megaloblastic anaemia

Aciclovir	Pentamidine
Alcohol	Proguanil
Antiepileptics	Pyrimethamine
Cycloserine	Sulfasalazine
Methotrexate	Triamterene
Nitrofurantoin	Trimethoprim
Oral contraceptives	

● **CASE STUDY 12.1**

Mrs D is a 65-year-old woman who was admitted to the Accident and Emergency Unit at her local hospital. She presented with fever, lethargy and shortness of breath, and had felt generally unwell for several weeks. On examination she had a dry cough but no spit, chest pain or urinary symptoms. Her temperature was 37.7°C, blood pressure 136/70 mmHg, oxygen saturation 95%, and there was good air entry to both lungs. Her past medical history included rheumatoid arthritis, for which she was prescribed azathioprine. Her other medication was folic acid, lansoprazole and ferrous sulphate. Mrs D's full blood count was:

White cell count 1.0 (4.0–11.0 × 10^9/L)
Neutrophils 0.5 (2.5–7.5 × 10^9/L)
Haemoglobin 8.5 (11.5–15.5 g/dL)
Platelets 18 (150–400 × 10^9/L).

What drug-induced disorder could the symptoms suggest?

Fever, lethargy and sore throat are possible features of a blood dyscrasia. This is confirmed by the full blood count, which shows pancytopenia. The most likely cause is azathioprine, an immunosuppressant drug prescribed for rheumatoid arthritis. The *British National Formulary* recommends that patients receiving azathioprine should undergo regular blood monitoring every week for the first 4 weeks of therapy, and thereafter at least every 3 months. Patients should also be counselled at the outset of therapy to report immediately any signs or symptoms of bone marrow suppression.

Mrs D was diagnosed with pancytopenia and sepsis secondary to azathioprine therapy. The drug was stopped immediately and she was referred to the haematologists. She was commenced on gentamicin, Tazocin and filgrastim.

Do you agree with this course of action, and what monitoring is required?

Mrs D is pyrexial and neutropenic. Disturbances in the production of neutrophils lead to an increased risk of life-threatening infection, and the depth, duration and rate of fall of the neutrophil count influence this.[2] Until a source of the temperature is identified, she should be commenced on empirical broad-spectrum antibiotic therapy. Her temperature and clinical signs of infection will be monitored during antibiotic therapy.

Platelet and blood transfusions will support Mrs D until her bone marrow recovers, but she needs neutrophils to mount a response to infection. Filgrastim (G-CSF, granulocyte colony-stimulating factor) is a haematopoietic growth

→

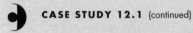

CASE STUDY 12.1 (continued)

factor that supports the growth and development of neutrophils.[60] Although unlicensed in drug-induced neutropenia, it may be given daily as a subcutaneous injection until a sustained increase in the neutrophil count is seen. A daily full blood count is necessary to monitor response.

A week after admission Mrs D's full blood count was:

White cell count $3.3 \times 10^9/L$
Neutrophils $2.1 \times 10^9/L$
Haemoglobin $9.2\,g/dL$
Platelets $39 \times 10^9/L.$

Filgrastim and IV antibiotics were stopped. The rheumatologist will be asked to review her requirement for a DMARD.

CASE STUDY 12.2

Dr B is a 50-year-old man who attended his GP surgery for a routine appointment. He presents with shortness of breath, fatigue, and looks mildly jaundiced. He claims his urine is dark in colour. He has Parkinson's disease and is prescribed co-beneldopa.

His blood count showed:

Haemoglobin 4.8 (13.5–17.5 g/dL)
Reticulocytes 453 (25–100 $\times$ 10^9/L).

Liver function tests showed a bilirubin of 59 µmol/L (3–16 µmol/L) and lactate dehydrogenase (LDH) was 1582 IU (70–250 IU/L).

What do Mr B's symptoms and blood count suggest, and what might be the cause?

Shortness of breath and fatigue are possible features of anaemia, which is confirmed by the full blood count. There are different types of drug-induced anaemia, and Mr B's jaundiced appearance, coupled with the bilirubin and LDH levels, suggests haemolytic anaemia. Drug-induced haemolytic anaemia is often the result of an alteration of immune regulation where autoantibodies are expressed against red blood cell antigens. The main sites of red cell

→

> **CASE STUDY 12.2** (continued)

destruction are the spleen and liver. When red cells are destroyed haem is converted to bilirubin. In normal states the liver converts this to a water-soluble glucuronide, which is excreted. However, if the supply of bilirubin exceeds the liver's upper limit for the rate of glucuronidation, unconjugated bilirubin plasma levels rise. LDH rises as a result of red cell lysis.

Mr B is prescribed co-beneldopa, which is a combination of benserazide and levodopa. Levodopa has been associated with haemolytic anaemia, and the *British National Formulary* recommends haematological surveillance in patients on prolonged therapy. Autoimmune haemolytic anaemia is considered a serious and potentially life-threatening disease, and Mr B was admitted to hospital for haematological support and neurological review of his Parkinson's disease.

How is this managed?

The suspected causative agent should be stopped, and if the haemoglobin continues to fall, red cell transfusion may be necessary. The bone marrow cannot respond to anaemia if there is a lack of iron, vitamin B or folic acid. Any deficiency in these must first be corrected. Folic acid 5 mg a day is usually required. Corticosteroids are generally used first-line, 1 mg/kg/day of prednisolone for 2–3 weeks, then reduced, according to response, over about 3 months.

Mr B's blood counts recovered gradually as below:

Day 12

Haemoglobin	10.7 g/dL
Reticulocytes	237 10^9/L
Total bilirubin	27 μmol/L
LDH	756 IU/L

Day 20

Haemoglobin	14.3 g/dL
Reticulocytes	44 10^9/L
Total bilirubin	10 μmol/L

References

1. Carey PJ. Drug-induced myelosuppression: diagnosis and management. *Drug Safety* 2003; 26: 691–706.
2. Committee on Safety of Medicines. Reminder: Agranulocytosis with antithyroid drugs. *Curr Probl Pharmacovigilance* 1999; 25: 1–4.

3. Hoffbrand AV, Pettit JE. Blood cell formation (haemopoiesis). In: Hoffbrand AV, Pettit JE, eds. *Essential Haematology*, 3rd edn. Oxford: Blackwell Scientific, 1993: 1–27.

4. Carey PJ. Drug-induced haemocytopenias. *Adv Drug React Bull* 1995; 175: 663–666.

5. Patton WN, Duffull SB. Idiosyncratic drug-induced haematological abnormalities. Incidence, pathogenesis, management and avoidance. *Drug Safety* 1994; 11: 445–462.

6. Yunis M. Chloramphenicol toxicity: 25 years of research. *Am J Med* 1989; 87: 44–48.

7. Killick SB, Marsh JCW. Aplastic anaemia: management. *Blood Rev* 2000; 14: 157–171.

8. Gordon-Smith EC. Aplastic anaemia and other causes of bone marrow failure. In: Weatherall DJ, Ledingham JGG, Warrell DA, eds. *Oxford Textbook of Medicine*, 3rd edn. Oxford: Oxford Medical Publications, 1996: 3441–3449.

9. Young NS. Aplastic anaemia. *Lancet* 1995; 346: 228–232.

10. Young NS. Acquired aplastic anemia. *Ann Intern Med* 2002; 136: 534–546.

11. Rich ML, Ritterhoff RJ, Hoffman RJ. A fatal case of aplastic anaemia following chloramphenicol therapy. *Ann Intern Med* 1950; 33: 1459–1467.

12. Yunis M. Chloramphenicol-induced bone marrow suppression. *Semin Hematol* 1973; 10: 225–234.

13. Holt D, Harvey D, Hurley R. Chloramphenicol toxicity. *Adv Drug React Toxicol Rev* 1993; 12: 83–95.

14. Rayner SA, Buckley RJ. Ocular chloramphenicol and aplastic anaemia. Is there a link? *Drug Safety* 1996; 14: 273–276.

15. Wiholm BE, Kelly JP, Kaufman D, *et al*. Relation of aplastic anaemia to use of chloramphenicol eye drops in two international case–control studies. *Br Med J* 1998; 316: 666.

16. Lancaster T, Swart AM, Jick H. Risk of serious haematological toxicity with use of chloramphenicol eye drops in a British general practice database. *Br Med J* 1998; 316: 667.

17. Laporte J-R, Vidal X, Ballarin E, *et al*. Possible association between ocular chloramphenicol and aplastic anaemia – the absolute risk is very low. *Br J Clin Pharmacol* 1998; 46: 181–184.

18. British Medical Association, Royal Pharmaceutical Society of Great Britain. *British National Formulary*. London: Pharmaceutical Press, 2005.

19. Inman WHW. Study of fatal bone marrow depression with special reference to phenylbutazone and oxyphenbutazone. *Br Med J* 1977; i: 1500.

20. Jackson GH, Proctor SJ. Disorders of blood cells. In: Davies DM, ed. *Textbook of Adverse Drug Reactions*, 4th edn. Oxford: Oxford University Press, 1991: Chapter 22.

21. Pellock JM, Brodie MJ. Felbamate: 1997 Update. *Epilepsia* 1997; 38: 1261–1264.

22. Yeh SP, Hsueh EJ, Wu H, *et al*. Ticlopidine-associated aplastic anemia. A case report and review of literature. *Ann Hematol* 1998; 76: 87–90.

23. Symeonidis A, Kouraklis-Symeonidis A, Seimeni U, *et al*. Ticlopidine-induced aplastic anemia: Two new case reports, review and meta-analysis of 55 additional cases. *Am J Hematol* 2002; 71: 24–32.

24. Storb R, Etzioni R, Anasetti C. Cyclophosphamide combined with antithymocyte globulin in preparation for allogeneic marrow transplants in patients with aplastic anaemia. *Blood* 1994; 84: 941–949.

25. Deeg HJ, Leisenring W, Storb R, *et al*. Long-term outcome after marrow transplantation for severe aplastic anemia. *Blood* 1998; 91: 3637–3645.
26. Young NS, Barrett AJ. The treatment of severe acquired aplastic anaemia. *Blood* 1995; 12: 3367–3377.
27. Bessho M, Hirashima K, Asano S, *et al*. Treatment of the anemia of aplastic anemia patients with recombinant human erythropoietin in combination with granulocyte colony-stimulating factor: a multicenter randomised controlled study. *Eur J Haematol* 1997; 58: 265–272.
28. Anon. Drug-induced agranulocytosis. *Drug Ther Bull* 1997; 35: 49–52.
29. Andres E, Kurtz J-E, Maloisel F. Nonchemotherapy drug-induced agranulocytosis: experience of the Strasbourg teaching hospital (1985–2000) and review of the literature. *Clin Lab Haematol* 2002; 24: 99–106.
30. Heimpel H. Drug-induced agranulocytosis. *Med Toxicol* 1988; 3: 449–462.
31. Novartis. *Clozaril Summary of Product Characteristics*. December 2002.
32. Vincent PC. Drug-induced aplastic anaemia and agranulocytosis. Incidence and mechanisms. *Drugs* 1986; 31: 52–63.
33. International Agranulocytosis and Aplastic Anaemia Study. Risk of agranulocytosis and aplastic anaemia in relation to use of antithyroid drugs. *Br Med J* 1988; 297: 262–265.
34. van der Klauw MM, Goudsmit R, Halie R, *et al*. A population-based case–cohort study of drug-associated agranulocytosis. *Arch Intern Med* 1999; 159: 369–374.
35. Coleman MD. Dapsone-mediated agranulocytosis: risks, possible mechanisms and prevention. *Toxicology* 2001; 162: 53–60.
36. Committee on Safety of Medicines. Drug-induced neutropenia and agranulocytosis. *Curr Probl Pharmacovigilance* 1993; 19: 10–11.
37. Andres E, Maloisel F, Kurtz J-E, *et al*. Modern management of non-chemotherapy drug-induced agranulocytosis: a monocentric study of 90 cases and review of the literature. *Eur J Intern Med* 2002; 13: 324–328.
38. Sprinkkelman A, de Wolf JTM, Vellenga E. The application of haemapoietic growth factors in drug-induced agranulocytosis: a review of 70 cases. *Leukemia* 1994; 8: 2031–2036.
39. Beauchesne MF, Shalansky SJ. Nonchemotherapy drug induced agranulocytosis: a review of 118 patients treated with colony-stimulating factors. *Pharmacotherapy* 1999; 19: 299–305.
40. Fukata S, Kuma K, Sugawara M. Granulocyte colony stimulating factor (G-CSF) does not improve recovery from antithyroid drug induced agranulocytosis: a prospective study. *Thyroid* 1999; 9: 29–31.
41. Machin SJ. Purpura. In: Weatherall DJ, Ledingham JGG and Warrell DA, eds. *Oxford Textbook of Medicine*, 3rd edn. Oxford: Oxford University Press, 1996: 3630–3637
42. Liesner RJ, Machin SJ. Platelet disorders. *Br Med J* 1997; 314: 809–812.
43. Pedersen-Bjergaard U, Andersen M, Hansen PB. Thrombocytopenia induced by noncytotoxic drugs in Denmark 1968–91. *J Intern Med* 1996; 239: 509–515.
44. Pedersen-Bjergaard U, Andersen M, Hansen PB. Drug-specific characteristics of thrombocytopenia caused by non-cytotoxic drugs. *Eur J Clin Pharmacol* 1998; 54: 701–706.
45. Magee P, Beeley L. Drug-induced blood disorders. In: Walker R, Edwards C, eds. *Clinical Pharmacy and Therapeutics*. London: Churchill Livingstone, 1994: Chapter 46.

46. Greinacher A, Eichler P, Lubenow N, *et al*. Drug-induced and drug dependent immune thrombocytopenia. *Rev Clin Exp Hematol* 2001; 5: 166–200.
47. Dager WE, White RH. Treatment of heparin-induced thrombocytopenia. *Ann Pharmacother* 2002; 36: 489–503.
48. Warkentin TE. Heparin-induced thrombocytopenia: pathogenesis and management. *Br J Haematol* 2003; 121: 535–555.
49. Warkentin TE, Barkin RL. Newer strategies for the treatment of heparin-induced thrombocytopenia. *Pharmacotherapy* 1999; 19: 181–195.
50. Hirsh J, Heddle N, Kelton JG. Treatment of heparin-induced thrombocytopenia. A critical review. *Arch Intern Med* 2004; 164: 361–369.
51. Casadevall N, Nataf J, Viron B, *et al*. Pure red-cell aplasia and antierythropoietin antibodies in patients treated with recombinant erythropoietin. *N Engl J Med* 2002; 346: 469–475.
52. Committee on Safety of Medicines. Epoetin alfa (Eprex): reports of pure red cell aplasia. *Curr Probl Pharmacovigilance* 2002; 28: 2.
53. Thompson DF, Gales MA. Drug-induced pure red cell aplasia. *Pharmacotherapy* 1996; 16: 1002–1008.
54. Gordon-Smith EC, Contreras M. Acquired haemolytic anaemia. In: Weatherall DJ, Ledingham JGG, Warrell DA, eds. *Oxford Textbook of Medicine*, 3rd edn. Oxford: Oxford Medical Publications, 1996: 3541–3551.
55. Hoffman R, Benz EJ, Shattil SJ, *et al*. Autoimmune hemolytic anemia. In: Hoffman R, ed. *Hematology: Basic Principles and Practice*, 4th edn. Orlando: Churchill Livingstone, 2005: 693–708.
56. Chang CH, Chen KY, Lai MY, *et al*. Meta-analysis: ribavirin-induced haemolytic anaemia in patients with chronic hepatitis C. *Aliment Pharmacol Ther* 2002; 16: 1623–1632.
57. Lee A, Rawlins MD. Adverse drug reactions. In: Walker R, Edwards C, eds. *Clinical Pharmacy and Therapeutics*. London: Churchill Livingstone, 1994: Chapter 3.
58. Hoffbrand V, Provan D. ABC of clinical haematology. Macrocytic anaemias. *Br Med J* 1997; 314: 430–433.
59. Hoffbrand AV. Megaloblastic anaemia and miscellaneous deficiency anaemias. In: Weatherall DJ, Ledingham JGG, Warrell DA, eds. *Oxford Textbook of Medicine*, 3rd edn. Oxford: Oxford Medical Publications, 1996: 3484–3500.
60. Steward WP. Granulocyte and granulocyte–macrophage colony stimulating factors. *Lancet* 1993; 342: 153–156.

Further reading

Anon. Drug-induced agranulocytosis. *Drug Ther Bull* 1997; 35: 49–52.
Carey PJ. Drug-induced myelosuppression: diagnosis and management. *Drug Safety* 2003; 26: 691–706.
Hirsh J, Heddle N, Kelton JG. Treatment of heparin-induced thrombocytopenia. A critical review. *Arch Intern Med* 2004; 164: 361–369.
Hoffbrand V, Provan D. ABC of clinical haematology. Macrocytic anaemias. *Br Med J* 1997; 314: 430–433.
Young NS. Acquired aplastic anemia. *Ann Intern Med* 2002; 136: 534–546.

13

Mental health disorders

Karen Fraser

Introduction

This chapter discusses drug-induced mental health problems, which are relatively common and include depression, psychosis, mania and confusion. The serious adverse effects of neuroleptic malignant syndrome, serotonin syndrome and the psychiatric manifestations of drug withdrawal reactions are reviewed briefly. The section on drug withdrawal reactions has been updated to reflect the latest UK Committee on Safety of Medicines (CSM) advice on selective serotonin reuptake inhibitors and other newer antidepressants. It is important to be aware that many of the psychiatric adverse effects of drugs do not meet the diagnostic criteria for recognised mental health disorders, and that there are many difficulties associated with their diagnosis, particularly in patients with underlying mental health problems.

Most adverse psychiatric effects of drugs are classified as type A reactions, being dose related or predictable, based on the drug's pharmacological profile, although some are idiosyncratic type B reactions. The relationship between the time the causative drug was started and the appearance of psychiatric symptoms can be unpredictable, occurring either insidiously or abruptly during drug use. Indeed, psychiatric symptoms are also a common feature of drug withdrawal reactions, occurring once the implicated drug has been stopped, particularly following sudden discontinuation.

In terms of predicting which patients may be susceptible to the psychiatric adverse of drugs, it is worth noting the following predisposing factors:[1]

- Presence of underlying mental health disorder, either current or in the past;
- Impaired cerebral function (e.g. elderly or patients with brain damage);
- Alcohol and drug misuse;

- Concurrent physical disease;
- Stressful environments (e.g. intensive treatment units).

The risk of developing a psychiatric adverse reaction to a drug may be especially high for patients with mental health disorders, as they may possess more than one predisposing factor: for example, there is evidence to suggest that this patient group are more likely to misuse alcohol and other substances.[2] Diagnosis of a drug-induced psychiatric problem is also understandably more difficult in this situation, as symptoms may be attributed to the underlying illness rather than drug therapy. The fact that many drugs used to treat mental health disorders can themselves cause psychiatric problems can be a further confounding factor.

The picture may be also be clouded by physical disorders causing or mimicking psychiatric problems (Table 13.1). Such disorders, for example dehydration or thyroid dysfunction, should be excluded and treated before confirming a drug-related adverse reaction.

Many medicines can cause more than one type of psychiatric adverse effect. Examples include levodopa, which has been implicated as a cause of psychotic symptoms, mania, depression and delirium, and corticosteroids, which can cause agitation, hyperactivity, irritability, euphoria and depressive symptoms.[3,4] Psychiatric adverse effects are usually considered to be serious reactions; the UK CSM classifies confusion, dependence, depression, hallucinations, psychosis and withdrawal syndrome among the central nervous system (CNS) serious reactions.

Table 13.1 Some conditions that may cause or mimic mental illness

Cushing's syndrome	Pernicious anaemia
Electrolyte imbalance	Renal dysfunction
Neurological disorders	Thyroid disease

Depression

Drug-induced depression is a cause for concern, representing around 1% of reported adverse drug reactions (ADRs). However, there has been a lack of consensus in the medical literature about the role of medicines in the aetiology of depression. In addition, published case reports often do not clearly distinguish between informal reporting of depressive symptoms and formal diagnosis of depression using validated rating scales. A recent systematic review attempted to address these issues and concluded that evidence is available to attribute depression to a small number of drugs.[5]

Table 13.2 Some drugs that may cause depression

Corticosteroids	Benzodiazepines
Interferon alfa	ACE inhibitors
Gonadotrophin-releasing hormone agonists	Calcium channel blockers
Mefloquine	Clonidine
Progestogens	Methyldopa
Oestrogens	Isotretinoin
Propranolol	Statins
Digoxin	

ACE, angiotensin-converting enzyme.

Of interest is the view that such depression caused by drugs appears to differ from classic major depressive disorder, with milder symptoms and atypical clinical features. It is important to remember that although depression has been reported as a possible side effect of all the drugs listed in Table 13.2, good evidence of causality is available only for a small minority.

There are consistent side-effect data available from clinical trials to demonstrate that some beta-blockers, in particular propranolol, are associated with reports of depression. However, studies using validated rating scales have only occasionally reported such an association. It has been suggested that misinterpretation of lethargy and fatigue – common side effects of beta-blockers – as depression, may offer a partial explanation.[6] It does seem clear that although there are neuropsychiatric side effects associated with beta-blockers, such effects are not symptomatic of classic major depressive disorder.

One randomised study comparing propranolol and atenolol using validated depression rating scales reported no difference between the groups in the incidence of depressive symptoms.[7] This is in contrast to another randomised study, where significantly higher depression scores were obtained in patients taking propranolol than in those taking metoprolol or placebo.[8] Depression has also been reported due to ophthalmic administration of beta-blockers, with one small crossover study indicating that higher levels of depressive symptoms occurred with ocular administration of timolol than with betaxolol.[9]

There is consistent evidence from published case reports of the psychiatric adverse effects of corticosteroids. Associated symptoms include agitation, hyperactivity, irritability, euphoria, and depressive symptoms such as sleep and appetite disturbance. Severe psychiatric reactions were reported in 1.3% of patients treated with prednisolone studied in the Boston Collaborative Drug Surveillance Program.[10] This is corroborated in the case series conducted by Wolkowitz,[4] where 75% of patients treated with prednisolone 80 mg for 5 days developed mood disorders.

Psychosis

Characteristic features of psychosis include distorted personality, delusions and hallucinations. Delusions are firmly sustained, false personal beliefs, which may occur with or without hallucinations. Paranoid delusions feature persecution. Hallucinations are uncontrolled false sensory perceptions which have no real external stimuli. Visual hallucinations are more commonly induced by drugs than auditory hallucinations.

The term 'drug-induced psychosis' has often been used in reference to the adverse effects of substance misuse, rather than of drugs used therapeutically. In the UK the misuse of drugs with the potential to cause psychosis is common, especially in people between the ages of 16 and 29 years. Indeed, substance misuse is always considered in the differential diagnosis of a patient presenting with psychotic symptoms. Although the literature on this subject is extensive, it is flawed and consists largely of case reports and uncontrolled studies. Diagnosis is extremely difficult, and it is important to remember that the consequences of misdiagnosis are potentially serious, whether a true functional psychosis is mistaken for a drug-induced state or vice versa. With these issues in mind, a classification system has been proposed, as detailed in Table 13.3.[11]

Amfetamines produce a hallucinogenic experience, often referred to as psychedelic. LSD, methylenedioxymethamfetamine (MDMA or 'Ecstasy') and other amfetamine-related substances stimulate dopamine-sensitive adenylcyclase, leading to increased dopamine activity, and are also serotonin antagonists. Acute intoxication can result in short-lived psychotic symptoms that resolve within a day. Usually delusions, hallucinations and panic last for 2 days or more. Making the decision that these symptoms are associated with amfetamine intoxication is often difficult because there can be a delay between taking the drug and the onset of psychosis. Long-term use of amfetamines may lead to the development of a chronic psychosis: paranoid ideas, bizarre thinking (often with religious content and grandiosity), disturbed memory, hallucinations and illusions.

Khat (also called qat or mirra) is a plant substance which is widely used, normally chewed, in some cultures. It contains cathionine, which has stimulant effects. Cathionine is controlled under the Misuse of Drugs Act (1971), but khat is not. A reaction similar to amfetamine psychosis has been reported. Other psychological reactions include sleep disturbance, anxiety and depression.[12]

Table 13.3 Interaction between psychosis and drug use

Interaction between psychosis and drug use	Definition
Intoxication mimicking functional psychosis	Direct pharmacological effect; occurs with stimulants and cannabis. Also probably occurs with solvents, Ecstasy and LSD. May persist for several days depending on half-life of drug
Pathoplastic reactions in functional psychosis	Psychotropic drugs can alter the clinical presentation in functional psychoses, e.g. worsening of schizophrenic symptoms after stimulant use
Chronic hallucinosis induced by substance abuse	Examples include alcoholic hallucinosis, LSD flashbacks and cannabis flashbacks. No other symptoms of psychosis are present
Drug-induced relapse of functional psychosis	Use of stimulants and cannabis in particular has been attributed to relapse of existing psychotic illness. However, issues around causality are controversial, e.g. patients may self-treat with such drugs in early relapse, so cause/effect unclear
Withdrawal states	Alcohol withdrawal can lead to delirium tremens; withdrawal states also reported with barbiturate and benzodiazepine withdrawal. Symptoms are distinct from major functional psychoses
True drug-induced psychosis	Refers to psychotic symptoms that arise during drug intoxication, but which persist following elimination of the drug. The reaction may be idiosyncratic or dose dependent, and recurs only if re-exposure to the drug occurs

LSD, lysergide.

Cannabis-induced psychosis is characterised differently, with symptoms of acute paranoid psychosis and feelings of panic. A further complication is that many people with schizophrenia may abuse substances as a form of 'self-medication' for distressing symptoms. Substance abuse is a common co-morbidity in as many as 50% of people with schizophrenia. Although substance abuse can precipitate relapse in a person predisposed to mental illness, it has not been conclusively shown to cause schizophrenia.[13] Table 13.4 summarises the psychiatric symptoms that may be induced by drugs of abuse.

Psychosis can, of course, be caused by several drugs used for therapeutic purposes, and Table 13.5 lists some that may be implicated.

Table 13.4 Psychiatric symptoms induced by drugs of abuse

Cannabis
Dysphoria, anxiety, agitation and suspicion, distortions of time and space, reduced vigilance and uncoordination, psychosis with confusion, hallucinations, delusions and emotional lability

CNS stimulants
High doses – agitation, panic attacks, impaired concentration. Transient or prolonged psychosis persisting for a few days after the drug is stopped

CNS depressants
Very high doses of benzodiazepines – amnesia, psychomotor impairment, aggressive and disinhibited behaviour

Hallucinogenic drugs
Alter perception, thoughts and feelings causing pseudohallucinations (illusions) and hallucinations

May uncover mental illness
Prolonged use of LSD may lead to prolonged psychosis resembling schizophrenia

Table 13.5 Some drugs that may cause psychosis

Amantadine	Ganciclovir
Amfetamines	Histamine H_2-receptor antagonists
Anticholinergics	Isoniazid
Antiepileptics	Levodopa
Bromocriptine	Mefloquine
Chloroquine	NSAIDs
Clonidine	Quinidine
Digoxin	Quinolone antibiotics
Disulfiram	Zolpidem

NSAIDs, non-steriodal anti-inflammatory drugs.

There is a high incidence (10–30%) of psychiatric effects with drugs used in the management of Parkinson's disease. Antimuscarinic agents such as trihexyphenidyl and procyclidine can cause disorientation, agitation and visual hallucinations. Levodopa has been associated with a much wider range of effects, including acute confusion, depression, delirium, delusions, euphoria, hallucinations, inappropriate sexual behaviour and mania.[3] Confusion, agitation, delusions and hallucinations are encountered more often in older patients. The overall incidence of hallucinations is believed to be about 20%. Psychoses, visual hallucinations and confusional states are serious enough to warrant drug discontinuation in about 10% of patients. With the exception of depression, the effects are usually dose related and resolve on discontinuation. These complications are more common in patients with a previous psychiatric history, and sometimes arise after many months of successful levodopa therapy. A withdrawal syndrome can develop on treatment discontinuation, featuring lethargy, anxiety, nightmares, depression and suicidal ideas. The diversity of levodopa-induced adverse effects illustrates how challenging the diagnosis of drug-induced mental health disorders can be.

Other dopaminergic drugs used in treating Parkinson's disease, such as bromocriptine, lysuride and pergolide, can cause hallucinations and other psychiatric effects.

Disulfiram is used as an aid to the management of alcohol misuse. It has been reported to cause psychosis and delirium.[13,14] These effects are postulated to be due to inhibition of the dopamine β-hydroxylase enzyme, leading to excess concentrations of dopamine. The rare delusion, Capgras syndrome, in which a relative or friend has been replaced by an identical double, has been reported.[13] Disulfiram should be discontinued if these effects occur; short-term use of benzodiazepines may be effective in their management.

An association between the acetylcholinesterase inhibitor donepezil, used to delay cognitive deterioration in Alzheimer's disease, and psychiatric disturbances, including hallucinations, agitation and aggressive behaviour, has been suggested.[15] As psychiatric disturbances may coexist with Alzheimer's disease these adverse effects may remain undetected.

For many years chloroquine has been known to cause psychosis and behavioural toxicity, especially in the higher doses used to treat malaria.[16] The link between mefloquine and neuropsychiatric reactions has attracted much debate on whether the risk of neuropsychiatric disorders is unacceptably high. Large observational studies suggest that severe neuropsychiatric reactions to prophylactic mefloquine occur at a frequency of around 1 in 10 000 to 1 in 20 000 patients.[17] Various reactions have been reported, including depression, anxiety, panic, confusion, hallucinations, paranoid delusions and convulsions. These reactions can be severe and protracted. Patients should be counselled about the risk of psychiatric symptoms with mefloquine and advised to seek medical advice promptly if they should develop. Prophylactic mefloquine is contraindicated in patients with a history of neuropsychiatric disturbance, including depression or convulsions.

Mania

Mania is characterised by the presentation of elevated mood. Associated symptoms are insomnia, rapid speech, grandiose ideas and disinhibition.

Less severe forms of mania are termed hypomania.[18] Drug-induced mania is rare but can occur by chance association, particularly in patients predisposed to mood disorders. This was illustrated in a small study examining the effect of donepezil in reversing memory loss induced by antidepressants and mood stabilisers. Mania was triggered in two patients with pre-existing, but stabilised, bipolar disorder.[19] Insomnia was also reported as an adverse effect of donepezil in this study. Studies with older cholinergic agonist drugs suggest that acetylcholine has a multifaceted neurophysiologic role in mood disorders, behaviour and sleep.[20] Although such case report evidence is of interest, more reliable information requires to be obtained from larger case series, particularly those with a matched control group.

Drugs with a clear propensity to cause manic symptoms include levodopa, corticosteroids and anabolic androgens (Table 13.6). The onset of manic symptoms usually occurs early in the course of treatment, or soon after a dose increase. Other drugs that may be capable of inducing mania, but for which the evidence is less robust, include other dopaminergic agents, levothyroxine, iproniazid and isoniazid, sympathomimetic drugs, chloroquine, baclofen, alprazolam, captopril, amfetamine and phencyclidine.[18]

There is evidence that antidepressants can induce mania, particularly in patients with pre-existing bipolar affective disorder. Mania may be precipitated by introducing an antidepressant or by increasing the dose. A switch from depression into mania has been reported in up to 10% of patients with bipolar disorder.[21] In a review of the literature, it has been demonstrated that in bipolar depressed patients tricyclic and monoamine oxidase inhibitor antidepressant drugs present a clear risk of switching, whereas the selective serotonin reuptake inhibitors (SSRIs) (at standard doses) do not appear to increase the risk.[22] The capacity of dual-action (serotonergic and noradrenergic) antidepressant agents such as venlafaxine to induce switching has not been established, but may be slight. However, caution is advised when treating any patient with a history of

Table 13.6 Some drugs that may cause mania

Antidepressants (particularly tricyclic and MAOI)
Baclofen
Chloroquine
Corticosteroids
Dopaminergic agents
Isoniazid
Levodopa

MAOI, monoamine oxidase inhibitor.

mania with an antidepressant. Cases of hypomania have been reported with all classes of antidepressants, including SSRI and dual-action agents. Rapid cycling disorder, where there is a short period between manic and depressive episodes, may also be triggered. If the symptoms are recognised early enough, reducing the antidepressant dose may be sufficient to stabilise mood. Management may require treatment of manic symptoms with antipsychotic drugs or a mood stabiliser such as lithium. On rare occasions, withdrawal of an antidepressant can cause mania.[23]

Manic episodes are among the most important manifestations of corticosteroid-induced psychiatric toxicity and there are many published case reports.[24] In one study, corticosteroid therapy was judged responsible for 54% of cases of mania seen by a psychiatric consultation service.[25] A prospective study investigated the neuropsychological effects of 8 days' treatment with oral methylprednisolone or fluocortolone (dose ranging between 50 and 150 mg daily) in 50 ophthalmologic patients.[26] The authors reported that 13 of 50 participants developed manic-like episodes and five developed a depressive syndrome. None of the episodes was severe and none associated with psychotic symptoms. Although this study was uncontrolled, the reported incidence of problems is much greater than expected. There are no clear predisposing factors for corticosteroid-induced psychiatric disturbances. However, there is good evidence of a dose–response relationship: prednisone doses above 40 mg daily (or equivalent) may be associated with an increased risk of problems.[24] Eight patients from a chest clinic who were interviewed about their experience of long-term corticosteroid therapy indicated that they would have preferred to have been warned about the possibility of psychiatric adverse effects.[27] Healthcare professionals should be more proactive in discussing the possibility of corticosteroid psychiatric adverse effects.

Behavioural toxicity

Drug-related disturbances in behaviour are common. Features include aggression, drowsiness, insomnia, vivid dreams, nightmares, restlessness, irritability and excitement. These symptoms may be the precursors of a more florid psychiatric disorder, such as delirium.

There is now a greater awareness of the behavioural effects of antiepileptic drugs. These adverse effects may be the result of their action on central gamma-aminobutyric acid (GABA) neurotransmission, producing inhibition, or on the excitatory glutamate system. Barbiturates can produce drowsiness, depression and delirium. Because the behavioural toxicity of the barbiturates has been recognised, particularly in children, they are seldom used in children with epilepsy.[28] Lamotrigine has been associated with sleep disturbance, agitation and confusion, irritability, and aggression. Aggressive behaviour was reported in a series of patients with learning disability who required dose reduction or discontinuation of treatment.

Vigabatrin is associated with drowsiness and fatigue, but in children excitation and agitation are more often seen. In addition, some patients have experienced confusion and memory disturbance. Postmarketing surveillance has identified more severe effects on mental health, including aggression, depression, psychosis and mania. Consequently, vigabatrin should be used with caution in people with a history of psychosis or behavioural problems. However, these effects can occur in patients with no history of mental illness.

Agitation and insomnia are recognised adverse effects of acetylcholinesterase inhibitors used in the management of Alzheimer's disease.[29,30]

New-generation antihistamines have fewer effects on behaviour than traditional agents. Diphenhydramine, for example, crosses the blood–brain barrier, causing drowsiness and impaired attention, memory and psychomotor functioning, and loratadine has similar effects to those of placebo on fatigue, cognitive functioning and driving performance.[31]

Atypical antipsychotics such as olanzapine and risperidone have fewer adverse effects on behaviour (insomnia, restlessness, bizarre dreams, social withdrawal and cognitive impairment) than conventional antipsychotics.[32]

Cognitive impairment

Drug-induced cognitive impairment may be divided into two types: delirium and dementia. Drug-induced delirium refers to the development of an acute confusional state, whereas drug-induced dementia refers to a more chronic alteration in mental function.[33] Drug-induced cognitive impairment is the most common reversible cause of confusion.[34] It can be either dose related or, particularly in some cases of delirium, idiosyncratic in nature. Cognitive impairment secondary to non-psychiatric medications may be more likely to result from an idiosyncratic mechanism. Compared with drug-induced delirium, the prevalence of drug-induced dementia is less well documented.[33] Elderly people are particularly sensitive to drug-induced cognitive impairment owing to age-related changes in pharmacokinetics and pharmacodynamics. Decreased functional reserve of the CNS and changes in brain perfusion may also increase the relative risk of this problem in the elderly compared with younger people. Additionally, dementia itself is a major predisposing factor for the development of drug-induced cognitive impairment. Polypharmacy, prevalent in older people, also increases the risk.

Delirium

Delirium has been defined by the American Psychiatric Association based on expert opinion and recent studies.[35] The following are the key features:

- Disturbance of consciousness (i.e. reduced clarity of awareness of the environment) with reduced ability to focus, sustain or shift attention.
- Change in cognition (such as memory deficit, disorientation or language disturbance) or the development of a perceptual disturbance that is not better accounted for by a pre-existing, established or evolving dementia.
- The disturbance develops over a short period of time (usually hours to days) and tends to fluctuate over the course of the day.
- There is evidence from the history, physical examination or laboratory findings that the disturbance is caused by the direct physiological consequences of a general medical condition, by an intoxicating substance, by medication use, or by more than one aetiology.

Drugs may be the most frequent single cause of delirium, and very often they are important where there are multiple contributing factors. In practice, patients with delirium are often taking several medications, many of which may be a possible cause. As the pathophysiology of delirium itself is poorly understood, the mechanisms of drug-induced delirium are also unclear. There is some evidence that cholinergic failure may occur in delirium, and anticholinergic intoxication causes a classic delirium syndrome that is reversible with cholinesterase inhibitors. Delirium is a possible consequence of toxicity due to lithium and digoxin. Postoperative delirium is common in the general surgical population (10–26%), with the complex range of drugs used in anaesthesia confounding the situation.

Epidemiological studies that have evaluated several drug classes as risk factors for delirium have shown inconsistent results. The drug classes that present a relatively high risk of delirium are documented in Table 13.7.

Table 13.7 Some drugs that may cause delirium or dementia

Antiarrhythmics
Antibacterials
Anticholinergics
Antidepressants (particularly anticholinergic agents)
Antiepileptics
Antiparkinsonian drugs (particularly anticholinergic agents)
Antipsychotics
Antituberculous drugs
Benzodiazepines
Corticosteroids
Disulfiram
Dopamine agonists
Histamine H$_2$-antagonists
Lithium
Opioid analgesics

Effective management of delirium involves early recognition of the condition, identification and withdrawal of the causative drug, management of agitation and disruptive behaviour, and supportive care. Drugs that may produce confusion should be stopped or the dosage reduced where possible. Supportive care such as ensuring adequate sleep, nutrition, hydration, and providing emotional reassurance is important for managing the patient with delirium.[33] If symptoms cannot be managed with supportive care, pharmacological treatment may be required.[36] Treatment may be required for aggression, risk of harm to self or others, hallucinations, distress or insomnia. Benzodiazepines (diazepam or lorazepam) and/or a short-acting antipsychotic may be used. The use of psychotropic medication can further complicate the assessment of mental state and diagnosis in delirious patients.[37]

The differential diagnosis of delirium is summarised in Table 13.8.

Dementia

Dementia presents as a deterioration of intellect, memory and personality. Consciousness is not impaired. Anxiety, lability of mood and depression may develop. The prevalence of dementia increases significantly with age, affecting 25–48% of those over 85 years of age.[33]

Drug-induced dementia (distinct from age-associated memory impairment) may be a cause of cognitive impairment in about 12% of patients with suspected dementia. In one study, ADR accounted for 5% of

Table 13.8 Differential diagnosis of delirium and dementia

Feature	Delirium	Dementia
Onset and course	Abrupt, acute/subacute, with an identifiable date. Fluctuates during day with worsening of symptoms at night	Gradual, chronic, insidious. Consistent pattern – no diurnal variation; may develop sundowning in later stages of disease
Duration	Hours to weeks/months in elderly (some permanent residual effects may remain)	Progressive, continuous
Memory	Immediate and recent memory impaired	Recent memory initially impaired; as it progresses, remote impaired
Sleep	Always disrupted with reversal of sleep–wake cycle	Fragmented sleep
Perception	Distorted with illusions, delusions, and hallucinations (visual and auditory) and difficulty distinguishing reality from misperceptions and psychomotor disturbances	Early stage minimally affected; later stages may be associated with delusions and hallucinations
Thought process and language	Disorganised, distorted, fragmented, incoherent speech, global cognitive impairment	Perseveration and confabulation, difficulty with abstraction, thoughts impoverished, judgment impaired
Mental status testing	Distracted, often unable to participate in testing	Usually tries hard; often tries to hide deficiencies
Interaction with environment	Reduced awareness. Fluctuating alertness. Impaired attention	In early stages, no problem with awareness. In early stages, normal alertness

Modified from ref. 37.

reversible dementias in patients aged 60 or older.[38] The prevalence of drug-induced dementia in the general population is unknown.

Possible mechanisms of drug-induced dementia include metabolic effects, such as hypoglycaemia, alteration of immunologic factors within the CNS, and effects on synaptic transmission. Drug classes most often implicated include benzodiazepines, antihypertensives and anticholinergic agents.

Symptoms of depression in the elderly are occasionally mistaken for dementia. This is known as pseudodementia, and this diagnosis should be excluded before considering a drug-related cause for dementia. There is considerable overlap between the features of dementia and delirium. Many drug classes can cause delirium/dementia in susceptible individuals, but several are associated with a greater risk. Drugs implicated as a cause of delirium or dementia are shown in Table 13.7, and the differential diagnosis of delirium and dementia is described in Table 13.8.

Psychiatric manifestations of drug withdrawal reactions

Recently there has been particular concern about withdrawal reactions associated with SSRIs and related antidepressants. It is very important to differentiate between withdrawal reactions and dependence syndromes, and this has been studied by an Expert Working Group of the UK Committee on Safety of Medicines (CSM) in relation to SSRI and related antidepressants following concerns about their dependence-producing potential.

The CSM review assessed the presence of symptoms of the 'dependence syndrome' in relation to SSRIs and related antidepressants, as defined by internationally recognised classification systems – DSM IV and ICD-10.[35,39] There was no clear evidence that the SSRIs and related antidepressants have a significant dependence liability or show the development of a dependence syndrome as defined by DSM IV or ICD-10. There have been isolated reports of abuse of certain SSRIs by patients with a history of substance misuse, but none in patients with no such background.

All SSRIs and related antidepressants may be associated with withdrawal reactions on stopping or reducing treatment. Reports of withdrawal reactions appear to be more frequently associated with paroxetine and venlafaxine. Withdrawal reactions can be severe and disabling. Features of the SSRI and related antidepressant withdrawal syndrome are shown in Table 13.9.

It is important that healthcare professionals are aware of the potential for such withdrawal reactions and discuss the risk with patients. Owing to the potential for withdrawal phenomena, antidepressants should not be stopped abruptly (unless a serious adverse effect has occurred). Instead, treatment should be tapered gradually. There is no fixed timescale for this, but if symptoms occur, restarting the antidepressant and subsequently withdrawing it more slowly should resolve the problem. It is also

Table 13.9 Features of withdrawal syndrome associated with SSRIs and related antidepressants

Dizziness
Numbness and tingling
Gastrointestinal disturbances (particularly nausea and vomiting)
Headache
Sweating
Anxiety
Sleep disturbances

Table 13.10 Some drugs implicated in withdrawal reactions

Alcohol	Barbiturates
Anticholinergic agents	Benzodiazepines
Antidepressants	Sympathomimetics
Baclofen	

important to reassure patients who experience these effects that antidepressants are not addictive.

A withdrawal syndrome can occur when tricyclic antidepressants are stopped suddenly. Symptoms include anxiety, nightmares, nausea and vomiting, dizziness, headache, muscular aches and akathisia.[40] In addition to these symptoms, abrupt withdrawal of monoamine oxidase inhibitors (MAOIs) can lead to delirium, auditory and visual hallucinations, and schizophreniform psychosis. The incidence of this syndrome has been reported to be as high as 32%.[41] Chronic administration of MAOIs leads to down-regulation and subsensitisation of alpha$_2$ and dopamine autoreceptors, which control the release of noradrenaline and dopamine. Sudden withdrawal of the MAOI leads to the release of noradrenaline and dopamine. This mechanism is thought to be similar to that underlying amfetamine withdrawal syndromes.[42–45] In contrast to the SSRIs, benzodiazepines have been established as drugs that may produce both dependence and withdrawal reactions. Rapid withdrawal after short-term use of benzodiazepines may cause rebound insomnia and anxiety. Withdrawal after chronic use (4–6 weeks or longer) gives rise to significant and often intolerable symptoms, including severe anxiety, perceptual changes, convulsions or delirium.[46] Up to 90% of long-term (more than 3 months) benzodiazepine users experience symptoms on discontinuation, especially if stopped abruptly. Gradual withdrawal over a period of weeks or months will reduce the risk of withdrawal reactions.

Delirium tremens, experienced within 48–72 hours of stopping chronic excessive alcohol intake, is characterised by disorientation, hallucinations, convulsions and increased psychomotor and autonomic activity.[47]

Use of SSRIs and venlafaxine in children and adolescents with major depressive disorder (MDD)

In 2003, an Expert Working Group of the UK CSM issued advice that the balance of risks and benefits for the treatment of MDD in children and adolescents under 18 years was unfavourable for venlafaxine and the SSRIs citalopram, paroxetine and sertraline. The advice was based on increased reporting rates of self-harm and suicidal thoughts in young people treated with these drugs compared with placebo. The advice also applies to escitalopram, based on an extrapolation of data from citalopram. Information for fluvoxamine was inaccessible.

Thus, the only SSRI with a favourable risk–benefit profile for treatment of MDD in under-18s is fluoxetine. This is in contrast to the adult population, where all SSRIs and venlafaxine have a favourable risk–benefit balance. It should be noted that fluoxetine is not licensed in this age group, and that it should only be recommended by specialists. The advice applies only to young people with MDD; sertraline and fluvoxamine may be used for paediatric obsessive–compulsive disorder under the terms of their UK marketing authorisations.

Serotonin syndrome and neuroleptic malignant syndrome

Serotonin syndrome and neuroleptic malignant syndrome are both rare but potentially life-threatening adverse effects.

Serotonin syndrome (SS) is associated with an excess of serotonin that results from therapeutic drug use, overdose or inadvertent interactions between drugs.[48] A case was first reported in the 1950s, but the term serotonin syndrome was not introduced until the 1990s.[49]

SS is associated with medications that affect serotonin systems. There are documented case reports where tricyclic antidepressants have been combined with a variety of drugs, including clonazepam, alprazolam, lithium, SSRIs, trazodone, nefazodone or thioridazine. The syndrome has also been described when MAOI antidepressants have been combined with L-tryptophan, dextromethorphan, SSRIs, pethidine, or clonazepam. Additionally, combinations between SSRIs and venlafaxine, dextromethorphan, buspirone, carbamazepine, mirtazapine, tramadol, nefazodone or sumatriptan have been implicated. Lastly, there are case reports of patients receiving monotherapy with venlafaxine, clomipramine, SSRIs, moclobemide, sumatriptan, and other serotonergic agents such as 'Ecstasy' who have developed serotonin syndrome.[49]

SS is characterised by a variety of symptoms, including confusion, disorientation, abnormal movements, exaggerated reflexes, fever, sweating, diarrhoea and hypotension or hypertension. Diagnosis is made when three or more of these symptoms are present and no other cause can be found. Drug-induced SS is generally mild and resolves when the implicated drugs are discontinued. However, it can be severe, and deaths have occurred.[50]

Neuroleptic malignant syndrome (NMS) has been associated with antipsychotic (neuroleptic) drugs and other drugs that affect dopamine neurotransmission.[51] It was first described during early studies of haloperidol in 1960.[52] The classic features include extreme rigidity, fever, autonomic instability, and mental status changes. The most important risk factors are a high antipsychotic dose, rapid dose titration and psychomotor agitation. Early recognition and treatment of NMS will minimise complications. The primary treatment relies on supportive measures combined with immediate discontinuation of the implicated drug. Specific drug treatments, such as bromocriptine or dantrolene, are frequently used. If possible, it is important to allow a period of 2 weeks after an episode of NMS has completely resolved before reinitiating antipsychotic treatment. Use of an antipsychotic from a different class may minimise the risk of recurrence.

Clozapine, an atypical antipsychotic that does not exhibit significant antagonism of D_2 dopamine receptors, has been thought to be less likely to cause NMS. However, a small number of cases have been reported.[53–55] There are also some case reports of NMS with other atypical antipsychotic drugs.[56,57] NMS has also been reported with other dopamine antagonists, such as metoclopramide, prochlorperazine and promethazine.[51] It is recommended that dopamine-blocking antiemetics should only be used long term in patients with a clear indication.

The abrupt withdrawal of dopaminergic drugs such as levodopa, bromocriptine and amantadine has also produced an NMS-like condition in patients with Huntington's disease and Parkinson's disease.[58]

The clinical and laboratory features of SS and NMS are described in Table 13.11.

From reviews of case reports, it appears that most cases of NMS occur within the first 1–2 weeks following the initiation of antipsychotic treatment or dose increase.[59–61] However, NMS may occur at any time during treatment.[59,60] NMS is a self-limiting condition once the impli-

Table 13.11 Comparison of the clinical and laboratory features of serotonin syndrome and neuroleptic malignant syndrome

Feature	Serotonin syndrome	Narcoleptic malignant syndrome
Temperature	Variable to hyperthermia	Hyperthermia
Mental status changes	Confusion Delirium Stupor Coma Anxiety Euphoria Irritability	Confusion Delirium Stupor
Neurologic	Variable muscle rigidity Hyperreflexia Tremor Myclonus Ankle clonus Incoordination	Muscle rigidity ('lead pipe rigidity') Hyperreflexia (uncommon) Tremor
Behavioural	Restlessness Agitation	Restlessness Agitation
Autonomic	HTN/HOTN Tachycardia Tachypnea Diaphoresis Mydriasis Incontinence Sialorrhoea Shivering	HTN/HOTN Tachycardia Tachypnea Diaphoresis Mydriasis Incontinence Sialorrhoea
Gastrointestinal	Diarrhoea Nausea Vomiting	
Laboratory	Elevated (uncommon): CPK WBC LFTs	Elevated (common): CPK WBC LFTs

Modified from ref.[49] HTN, hypertension. HOTN, hypotension. CPK, creatine phosphokinase. WBC, white blood cells. LFTs, liver function tests.

cated drug has been withdrawn. Most sources suggest that NMS will resolve with supportive care within 1–2 weeks unless the patient has been receiving depot antipsychotics,[59,62] in which case it may take up to 1 month for NMS to resolve.[59] Many NMS patients will continue to require an antipsychotic. Following the recommendations in Box 13.1 may help prevent recurrence.

Box 13.1 Rechallenge recommendations

- Reassess the indication for the antipsychotic
- Wait two weeks after resolution of NMS before rechallenge
- Rechallenge with a different chemical class antipsychotic and/or a different potency
- Use the lowest dose possible. Titrate slowly
- Consider alternative treatments such as benzodiazepines for agitation. Benzodiazepines may be effective alone for agitation, or, if given in combination with an antipsychotic, they will allow for a lower antipsychotic dose
- Avoid the long-acting depot antipsychotics, as patients with a history of NMS are at higher risk in the future and because episodes may last up to 1 month when associated with these dosage forms

---

Management of drug-induced psychiatric disturbances

Healthcare professionals have an important role in preventing psychiatric morbidity due to prescribed or over-the-counter medicines. The general principles of ensuring that drug therapy is needed, avoiding polypharmacy and using the minimum effective dose are important. In addition, drugs to be prescribed should be screened for their potential CNS effects. Drugs known or suspected to have psychiatric adverse effects should be introduced and withdrawn gradually where possible.

When a psychiatric reaction to a drug is suspected, the drug should be withdrawn wherever possible. There may be reluctance to do this when a patient is being treated with that drug for an existing mental health problem. Correspondingly, rechallenge may be more often attempted in such patients. Specialists (e.g. psychiatrists or clinical pharmacists) may be able to review previous drug treatment and advise on future treatment options and the risks of rechallenge. In addition, pharmacists may be able to give guidance on how to taper medication to minimise the risk of withdrawal reactions and how best to go about switching from one drug to another.

Most psychiatric adverse drug events resolve quickly. Short-term use of minor tranquillisers, or non-drug treatments, may be sufficient management options. If the symptoms persist and present a danger to the health of the patient or others, treatments such as electroconvulsive therapy for depressive symptoms or antipsychotics may be necessary.

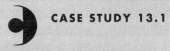

CASE STUDY 13.1

FS is a 28-year-old man with a 5-year history of schizophrenia, currently an inpatient in an acute adult mental health ward. He has recently been switched to quetiapine from olanzapine, which was discontinued because of weight gain. The dose of quetiapine has been titrated upwards to 300 mg daily according to the manufacturer's recommendation. Unfortunately FS's mental state has deteriorated and he has needed 'as required' intramuscular haloperidol 10 mg on at least one occasion per day.

Routine observations have shown that FS has been tachycardic on occasion and his blood pressure has been fluctuating. He appears confused and oversedated at times. Examination has revealed that his temperature is raised (39.5°C) and that he is exhibiting muscle rigidity. A preliminary diagnosis of neuroleptic malignant syndrome (NMS) is made, which is supported by laboratory findings of raised creatine kinase (CK).

What is the most likely cause of the NMS?

Risk factors for the development of NMS include a recent or rapid dose increase of an antipsychotic drug. FS has recently been switched from olanzapine to quetiapine, which has been titrated upwards according to the manufacturer's recommendations. Another risk factor is the use of high-potency typical antipsychotics, and FS has required daily haloperidol injections. It is likely that the combination of haloperidol and quetiapine has contributed to the development of NMS.

How should the symptoms of NMS be managed?

The antipsychotic drugs should be withdrawn, and FS's temperature, pulse and blood pressure regularly monitored. If his condition deteriorates, rehydration and treatment with bromocriptine and dantrolene should be initiated in an acute hospital setting. Sedation with benzodiazepines may be required.

Describe how antipsychotics should be selected and restarted following recovery from NMS

It is important to allow time for complete recovery from symptoms of NMS, and antipsychotics generally require to be withdrawn for 2 weeks. In a patient such as FS with a diagnosis of schizophrenia, antipsychotic treatment is going to be required and is associated with an acceptable risk. It is worth considering a drug which is structurally unrelated to the implicated agents and avoiding long-acting depot antipsychotics and high-potency conventional antipsychotics. When reintroducing an antipsychotic, very low doses should be used and increased cautiously. Temperature, pulse and blood pressure should continue to be monitored.

CASE STUDY 13.2

KR is a 33-year-old woman with a history of anxiety and depressive disorders, who has previously required treatment with sertraline. She was commenced on propranolol for symptoms of anxiety 3 weeks ago and is keen not to take any psychotropic medication. Over the past week she has started to feel that her mood is low and is worried that she may be becoming depressed again.

Could KR's lowering of mood be drug induced?

There is evidence that some beta-blockers, in particular propranolol, are associated with depression. However, studies using validated rating scales have only occasionally reported such an association. It has been suggested that misinterpretation of lethargy and fatigue – common side effects of beta-blockers – as depression may offer a partial explanation. It does seem clear that although there are neuropsychiatric side effects associated with beta-blockers, such effects are not symptomatic of classic major depressive disorder. The time to onset of KR's low mood does seem to relate to the introduction of propranolol.

What advice would you give?

KR should be referred back to her GP for discussion about the type of symptoms she has experienced following the introduction of propranolol. This will help the GP to decide whether the symptoms are due to beta-blocker-related fatigue or to the development of a depressive disorder.

What treatment options can be recommended?

In a patient who has a history of depression and has recently attended for treatment of anxiety, there is possibility of recurrence that will require treatment with an antidepressant. In this case, it may be prudent to discontinue propranolol and monitor symptoms. KR has been keen to avoid psychotropic medication – the reasons for this should be sensitively explored and consideration given to the choice of an appropriate antidepressant if indicated. She has previously responded to an SSRI (sertraline), which is a good indicator of future response. Consideration could also be given to treatment with paroxetine, an SSRI which is also licensed for generalised anxiety disorder.

References

1. Davison K, Hassanyeh F. Psychiatric disorders. In: Davies DM, ed. *Textbook of Adverse Drug Reactions*, 4th edn. Oxford: Oxford University Press, 1991: Chapter 21.

2. Hall W, Farrell M. Comorbidity of mental disorders with substance abuse. *Br J Psychiatry* 1997; 171: 4–5.

3. Saint-Cyr JA, Taylor AE, Lang AK. Neuropsychological and psychiatric side effects in the treatment of Parkinson's disease. *Neurology* 1993; 43(Suppl 6): S47–S52.

4. Wolkowitz OM. Prospective controlled studies of the behavioral and biological effects of exogenous corticosteroids. *Psychoneuroendocrinology* 1994; 19: 233–255.

5. Patten SB, Barbui C. Drug-induced depression: a systematic review to inform clinical practice. *Psychother Psychosom* 2004; 73: 207–215.

6. Goble AJ. Beta-blocker treatment and depression. *Arch Intern Med* 1992; 152: 649.

7. Adler L. CNS effects of beta blockade: a comparative study. *Psychopharmacol Bull* 1988; 24: 232–237.

8. Lorr M, McNair DM, Fisher SU. Evidence for bipolar mood states. *J Pers Assess* 1982; 46: 432–436.

9. Duch S, Duch C, Pasto L, Ferrer P. Changes in depressive status associated with topical betablockers. *Int Ophthamol* 1992; 16: 331–335.

10. Boston Collaborative Drug Surveillance Program. Psychiatric side effects of nonpsychiatric drugs. *Semin Psychiatry* 1971; 3: 406–420.

11. Poole R, Brabbins C. Drug induced psychosis. [Editorial] *Br J Psychiatry* 1996; 168: 135–138.

12. Griffiths P, Gossop M, Wickenden S, *et al*. A transcultural pattern of drug use: qat (khat) in the UK. *Br J Psychiatry* 1997; 170: 281–284.

13. Daniel DG, Swallows A, Wolff F. Capgras delusion and seizures in association with therapeutic dosages of disulfiram. *South Med J* 1987; 80: 1577–1579.

14. Murthy KK. Psychosis during disulfiram therapy for alcoholism. *J Indian Med Assoc* 1997; 95: 80–81.

15. Anon. Donepezil update. *Drug Ther Bull* 1998; 36: 60–61.

16. Philips–Howard PA, ter Kuile FO. CNS adverse events associated with anti-malarial agents. Fact or fiction? *Drug Safety* 1995; 12: 370–383.

17. Committee on Safety of Medicines. Mefloquine (Lariam) and neuropsychiatric reactions. *Curr Probl* 1996; 22: 6.

18. Peet M, Peters S. Drug–induced mania. *Drug Safety* 1995; 12: 146–153.

19. Jacobsen FM, Comas-Diaz L. Donepezil for psychotropic-induced memory loss. *J Clin Psychiatry* 1999; 60: 698–704.

20. Sunderland T, Tariot PN, Newhouse PA. Differential responsivity of mood behaviour and cognition to cholinergic agents in elderly neuropsychiatric population. *Brain Res* 1988; 13: 371–389.

21. Knight Laird L, Benefield WH. Mood disorders 1: Major depressive disorders. In: Young LY, Koda–Kimble MA. *Applied Therapeutics: the Clinical Use of Drugs*, 6th edn. Vancouver: Lippincott, Williams & Wilkins, 1995: Chapter 76.

22. Parker G, Parker K. Which antidepressants flick the switch? *Aust NZ J Psychiatry* 2003; 37: 464–468.

23. Goldstein TR, Frye MA. Antidepressant discontinuation-related mania: critical prospective observation and theoretical implications in bipolar disorder. *J Clin Psychiatry* 1999; 60: 563–567.

24. Patten SB, Neutel CI. Corticosteroid-induced adverse effects. *Drug Safety* 2000; 22: 111–122.
25. Rundell JR, Wise MG. Causes of organic mood disorder. *J Neuropsychiatry Clin Neurosci* 1989; 1: 398–400.
26. Naber D, Sand P, Heigl B. Psychopathological and neuropsychological effects of 8 days' corticosteroid treatment: a prospective study. *Psychoneuroendocrinology* 1996; 21: 25–31.
27. Reckart MD, Eisendrath SJ. Exogenous corticosteroid effects on mood and cognition: case presentation. *Int J Psychosom* 1990; 37: 57–61.
28. Ferrari M, Barabas G, Schempp Matthews W. Psychologic and behavioral disturbance among epileptic children treated with barbiturate anticonvulsants. *Am J Psychiatry* 1983; 140: 112–113.
29. Dooley M, Lamb HM. Donepezil: a review of its use in Alzheimer's disease. *Drugs Aging* 2000; 16: 199–226.
30. Greenberg SM, Tennis MK, Brown LB, *et al.* Donepezil therapy in clinical practice: a randomised crossover study. *Arch Neurol* 2000; 57: 94–99.
31. Kay GG, Berman B, Mockoviak SH, *et al.* Initial and steady state effects of diphenydramine and loratadine on sedation, cognition, mood and psychomotor performance. *Arch Intern Med* 1997; 157: 2350–2356.
32. Hollister LE. Current concepts in therapy. Complications from psychotherapeutic drugs. *N Engl J Med* 1961; 264: 291–293, 345–347, 399–400.
33. Gray SL, Lai KV, Larson EB. Drug-induced cognition disorders in the elderly: incidence, prevention and management. *Drug Safety* 1999; 21: 101–122.
34. Bowen JD, Larson ER. Drug-induced cognitive impairment – defining the problem and finding solutions. *Drugs Aging* 1993; 3: 349–357.
35. American Psychiatric Association. *Diagnostic and Statistical Manual of Mental Disorders*, 4th edn. Washington DC: American Psychiatric Association, 1994.
36. Carter GL, Dawson AH, Lopert R. Drug-induced delirium: incidence, management and prevention. *Drug Safety* 1996; 15: 291–301.
37. Lisi DM. Definition of drug-induced cognitive impairment in the elderly. *Medscape Pharmacother* 2000; 2: 2.
38. Larson EB, Kukull WA, Katzman RL. Adverse drug reactions associated with global cognitive impairment in elderly persons. *Ann Intern Med* 1987; 107: 169–173.
39. World Health Organization. *International Classification of Diseases*, 10th Revision. Geneva: World Health Organization, 1992.
40. Garner EM, Kelly MW, Thompson DF. Tricyclic antidepressant withdrawal syndrome. *Ann Pharmacother* 1993; 27: 1068–1072.
41. Tyrer P. Clinical effects of abrupt withdrawal from tricyclic antidepressants and monoamine oxidase inhibitors after long term treatment. *J Affect Disord* 1984; 6: 1–7.
42. Dilsaver SC. Monoamine oxidase inhibitor withdrawal phenomena: symptoms and pathophysiology. *Acta Psychiatr Scand* 1988; 78: 1–7.
43. Joyce PR, Walsh J. Nightmares during phenelzine withdrawal. *J Clin Psychopharmacol* 1983; 4: 121.
44. Liskin B, Roose SP, Walsh BT, Jackson WK. Acute psychosis following pheneizine discontinuation. *J Clin Psychopharmacol* 1985; 5: 46–47.

45. Naylor MW, Grunhaus I, Cameron O. Myoclonic seizures after abrupt withdrawal from phenelzine and alprazolam. *J Nerv Ment Dis* 1987; 175: 111–114.
46. Menkes DB, Laverty R. Hypnotics and sedatives. In: Davies DM, Ferner RE, de Glanville H, eds. *Davies's Textbook of Adverse Drug Reactions*, 5th edn. London: Chapman & Hall, 1999: Chapter 5.
47. Johns AR. Management of withdrawal syndromes. In: Weatherall DJ, Ledingham JGG, Warrell DA, eds. *Oxford Textbook of Medicine*, 3rd edn. Oxford: Oxford University Press, 1996: 4290–4294.
48. Boyer EW, Shannon M. Current concepts: the serotonin syndrome. *N Engl J Med* 2005; 352: 1112–1120.
49. Keck PE, Arnold L. The serotonin syndrome. *Psychiatr Ann* 2000; 30: 333–343.
50. Gravlin MA. Serotonin syndrome: What causes it, how to recognise it and ways to avoid it. *Hosp Pharm* 1997; 32: 570–575.
51. Carrof SN, Mann SC. Neuroleptic malignant syndrome (review). *Med Clin North Am* 1993; 77: 185–202.
52. Delay J, Pichot P, Lemperiere T, *et al.* Un neuroleptique majeur non-phenothiazine et non reserpinique, l'haloperidol, dans le traitement des psychoses. *Ann Med Psychol* 1960; 118: 145–152.
53. Reddig S, Minnema AM, Tandon R. Neuroleptic malignant syndrome and clozapine. *Ann Clin Psychiatry* 1993; 5: 25–27.
54. Sachdev P, Kruk J, Kneebone M, *et al.* Clozapine-induced neuroleptic malignant syndrome: review and report of new cases. *J Clin Psychopharmacol* 1995; 15: 365–371.
55. Thornberg SA, Ereshefsky L. Neuroleptic malignant syndrome associated with clozapine monotherapy. *Pharmacotherapy* 1993; 13: 510–514.
56. Webster P, Wijeratne C. Risperidone-induced neuroleptic malignant syndrome [Letter]. *Lancet* 1999; 344: 1228.
57. Raitasuo V, Vataja R, Elomaa E. Risperidone-induced neuroleptic malignant syndrome in young patient [Letter]. *Lancet* 1994; 344: 1705.
58. Ebadi M, Pfeiffer RF, Murrin LC. Pathogenesis and treatment of neuroleptic malignant syndrome [Review]. *Gen Pharmacol* 1990; 21: 367–386.
59. Addonizio G, Susman VL, Roth SD. Neuroleptic malignant syndrome: review and analysis of 115 cases. *Biol Psychiatry* 1987; 22: 1004–1020.
60. Caroff SN, Mann SC. Neuroleptic malignant syndrome. *Psychopharmacol Bull* 1988; 24: 25–29.
61. Shalev A, Munitz H. The neuroleptic malignant syndrome: agent and host interaction. *Acta Psychiatr Scand* 1986; 73: 337–347.
62. Rosenberg MR, Green M. Neuroleptic malignant syndrome: review of response to therapy. *Arch Intern Med* 1989; 149: 1927–1931.

Further reading

Bowen JD, Larson ER. Drug-induced cognitive impairment – defining the problem and finding solutions. *Drugs Aging* 1993; 3: 349–357.
Boyer EW, Shannon M. Current concepts: the serotonin syndrome. *N Engl J Med* 2005; 352: 1112–1120.

Caroff SN, Mann SC. Neuroleptic malignant syndrome. *Psychopharmacol Bull* 1988; 24: 25–29.

Carter GL, Dawson AH, Lopert R. Drug-induced delirium: incidence, management and prevention. *Drug Safety* 1996;15: 291–301.

Gray SL, Lai KV, Larson EB. Drug-induced cognition disorders in the elderly: incidence, prevention and management. *Drug Safety* 1999; 21: 101–122.

Lishman WA. Specific conditions giving rise to mental disorder. In: Weatherall DJ, Ledingham JGG, Warrell DA, eds. *Oxford Textbook of Medicine*, 3rd edn. Vol. 3. Oxford: Oxford Medical Publications, 1996; 4236–4243.

Patten SB, Barbui C. Drug-induced depression: a systematic review to inform clinical practice. *Psychotherapy and Psychosomatics* 2004; 73: 207–215.

Poole R, Brabbins C. Drug induced psychosis [Editorial]. *Br J Psychiatry* 1996; 168: 135–138.

Turjanski N, Lloyd GC. Psychiatric side-effects of medications: recent developments. *Adv Psychiatr Treat* 2005; 11: 58–70.

14

Cardiovascular effects

W. Stephen Waring

Introduction

Of the 1441 adverse drug reactions (ADRs) that lead to hospital admission annually, 173 (12%) involve the cardiovascular system. Of these, bradycardia is the most common, comprising around 5.7% of all serious ADRs. In the vast majority of cases patients who experience cardiovascular adverse drug effects have been receiving multiple medications. For example, 88% of such patients in one study had been receiving 3–10 different medications.[1]

Disorders of cardiac rhythm

Bradycardia

Bradycardia is a term used to denote a resting heart rate of less than 60 beats/minute (bpm). Bradycardia can be a physiological finding in physically fit young men and women, and is particularly common in healthy people during prolonged supine rest or sleep, during which the heart rate may fall as low as 40 bpm. However, bradycardia is less likely to be a normal finding in sedentary individuals and elderly patients, in whom an underlying cause should be sought. An isolated heart rate recording of less than 60 bpm, in the absence of other abnormal clinical signs, is unlikely to be of any significant clinical consequence. The potential hazards conferred by bradycardia are those associated with reduced cardiac output (cardiac output mL/min = heart rate/min $\times$ stroke volume mL) and, consequently, diminished tissue oxygen supply. Bradycardia can be accompanied by significant symptoms, for example fatigue, light-headedness, postural unsteadiness, vertigo, syncope or falls. These symptoms suggest that the heart rate is inappropriately low to maintain adequate tissue blood supply, and requires urgent attention. It should be remembered that in certain situations bradycardia might be detrimental, even in the absence of symptoms, for example in patients with severe ischaemic heart disease or critical renovascular function.

Bradycardia, as an ADR, arises as a result of suppression of cardiac tissue depolarisation and delayed action potential formation, and through the direct effect of drugs that delay intracardiac conduction. In many cases bradycardia is a predictable adverse effect of drugs that mediate therapeutic effects through cardiac deceleration, namely beta-blockers (nonselective or cardioselective), 'rate-limiting' calcium channel blockers (verapamil and diltiazem), digoxin and adenosine. A recent study has shown that bradycardia, as an ADR in hospitalised patients, was most commonly due to digoxin (35.8%), beta-blockers (27.2%), calcium channel blockers (26.0%) or antiarrhythmic drugs (1.7%). In this study, 31.2% of patients had been receiving more than one of these drugs.[1] A further recent study identified that those at greatest risk of developing drug-induced bradycardia were elderly women who had underlying atrial fibrillation (mean age 73 years, 75.9% females).[2] The coadministration of beta-blockers with verapamil or diltiazem is a potentially hazardous combination. Both beta-blockers and 'rate-limiting' calcium channel blockers suppress atrioventricular (AV) nodal conduction, and exert an additive effect in combination. Such a combination should only be initiated under specialist supervision in carefully selected patients because of the risks of severe bradycardia and complete heart block. Of note, profound bradycardia and AV nodal blockade (complete heart block) are recognised complications of combination therapy using verapamil and digoxin.[3] Verapamil and nifedipine have been shown to inhibit renal tubular clearance of digoxin, and can therefore potentiate the effect of digoxin on AV node conduction and increase the risk of digoxin toxicity.[4]

It is important to remember that the effects of beta-blockers to lower heart rate have also been observed in patients receiving topical treatment. For example, therapeutic doses of 0.25% timolol eye drops are associated with significant systemic drug absorption and have been found to cause bradycardia and even complete heart block.[5,6]

In a number of cases bradycardia has been described as an unpredictable adverse effect of drugs. In these cases, therapeutic drug use is not normally associated with a significant effect on resting heart rate, but idiosyncratic or toxic effects have been described. Examples are shown in Table 14.1.

The management of bradycardia will depend on the strength of the indication for the suspected causative drug, the severity of the adverse effect, and the premorbid clinical condition. In patients who are found to have mild bradycardia, and where there are no adverse symptoms or

Table 14.1 Some drugs that may cause bradycardia

Common	Less common
Beta-blockers	Lithium (especially in overdose)
Diltiazem, verapamil	Alpha-blockers
Digoxin	Histamine H_2-antagonists
Antiarrhythmics (amiodarone, procainamide)	Carbamazepine
	SSRI antidepressants
Adenosine	Prostaglandins
Opioids (particularly in overdose)	Centrally acting antihypertensives

SSRI, selective serotonin reuptake inhibitor.

findings suggesting tissue ischaemia, the causative drug may often be continued without significant consequence. This is often the case, for example, in the long-term use of beta-blockers to reduce cardiovascular risk in patients with hypertension or ischaemic heart disease.

Tachycardia

The definition of tachycardia is based arbitrarily on a resting heart rate of 100 bpm or more. Tachycardia is very commonly encountered in community and hospital practice and is often a non-specific sign of underlying disease, including heart failure, localised or systemic infection, asthma and many more. It is also commonly recognised as an adverse effect of several different groups of drug. In the majority of these situations the adverse effect is predictable and based on known interactions between the causative drug and mechanisms of cardiovascular regulation.

In health, the heart rate is influenced, at least in part, by autonomic activity such that sympathetic (adrenergic) stimulation increases heart rate, whereas parasympathetic (cholinergic) activation decreases it. Therefore, sympathomimetic drugs have the potential to cause tachycardia through sympathetic cardiac stimulation. A key example is pseudoephedrine hydrochloride, which is commonly included in cough linctus formulations and decongestant preparations. Similarly, drugs that interrupt cholinergic-mediated cardiac deceleration will also have the potential to cause increased heart rate. Tachycardia is a well recognised adverse effect of anticholinergic drugs used in the treatment of parkinsonism, such as benzatropine or trihexyphenidyl. In addition, tachycardia is a recognised feature of treatment with a wide range of other drugs that are known to have at least some anticholinergic properties, for example tricyclic antidepressants (TCAs), phenothiazine antipsychotics and antimuscarinic bronchodilators.[7,8] A case of supra-ventricular tachycardia (SVT) has been reported in a patient treated with therapeutic doses of ipratropium bromide.[9]

Normally, the baroreceptor reflex serves to maintain systemic blood pressure within physiological limits. Small decreases in blood pressure are detected by baroreceptors in the aortic arch and carotid bodies and stimulate increased sympathetic cardiovascular stimulation, so as to increase heart rate and cardiac output and hence restore blood pressure. Therefore, tachycardia is a recognised adverse effect of a number of drugs known to reduce systemic blood pressure. Among antihypertensive drugs, this effect is most characteristically observed during treatment with vasodilating dihydropyridine calcium channel blockers (for example nifedipine), diuretics and minoxidil.[10] Tachycardia is a recognised adverse effect of both standard and long-acting preparations. Reflex tachycardia is recognised as an early adverse effect after initiation of alpha-blockers (for example doxazosin), but does not occur with chronic administration.[11] Combination antihypertensive treatment with a rate-limiting drug, such as a beta-blocker, verapamil or diltiazem, offers the potential to abolish tachycardia while conferring better overall blood pressure control in this situation. Nitrate therapy (by sublingual, oral or parenteral routes) and sildenafil are other recognised causes of tachycardia secondary to arterial vasodilatation and baroreceptor reflex activation.[12] Withdrawal of clonidine is recognised as a precipitant of ventricular tachycardia (VT).[13]

Thyroxine normally enhances sympathetic autonomic activity. Thyroxine replacement to attain normal physiological levels should cause no effect on resting heart rate. However, tachycardia is one of the more consistent features of excessive thyroxine replacement therapy, and should prompt suspicion of overtreatment in this patient group.

Other recognised causes of drug-induced tachycardia are nicotine replacement therapy, digoxin, and beta$_2$-adrenoceptor agonists (e.g. salbutamol), beta$_1$-adrenoceptor partial agonists (e.g. pindolol), theophylline and caffeine (Table 14.2).

Atrial fibrillation

Atrial fibrillation is the commonest sustained disorder of heart rhythm and confers a significantly increased risk of stroke, thromboembolism and congestive heart failure. The prevalence of atrial fibrillation increases dramatically with advancing age, and the risk of complications is substantially increased in the presence of ischaemic heart disease, valvular heart disease and heart failure. In addition to these risk factors, a number of

Table 14.2 Some drugs that may cause tachycardia

Sympathomimetics
Anticholinergics
Tricyclic antidepressants
Beta$_2$-agonists
Theophylline
Nitrates
Vasodilating antihypertensives (minoxodil, hydralazine)
Dihydropyridine calcium antagonists
Nicotine
Amfetamines
Antipsychotics
Anaesthetic agents
Doxapram
Thyroid hormones
Caffeine

other factors are recognised as predisposing to atrial fibrillation. These include thyrotoxicosis, infection, pneumonia and pulmonary embolism. Drug therapy is rarely implicated as a cause of atrial fibrillation.

Alcohol excess is an important causal or contributory factor in the development of atrial fibrillation, particularly in men, and has been shown to play a significant role in as many as 15–35% of patients admitted to hospital with newly recognised atrial fibrillation.[14] Atrial fibrillation is frequently found in the presence of alcoholic cardiomyopathy, a potential consequence of chronic alcohol excess. In addition, new onset of atrial fibrillation is a recognised complication of acute alcohol ingestion. A recent retrospective study of the data gathered from the Framingham Study showed that chronic moderate ingestion of alcohol was not significantly related to the risk of atrial fibrillation, whereas consumption of more than 36 g/day (approximating three alcoholic drinks) was associated with substantially increased risk.[15]

A number of drugs have been implicated as potential causes of atrial fibrillation. Just as thyrotoxicosis is an established causal factor, so too is excess administration of levothyroxine in the treatment of hypothyroidism. In both cases patients are much more likely to be 'resistant' to digoxin, which will fail to control resting ventricular rate, than are patients with lone atrial fibrillation (the latter is a descriptive term used when recognisable precipitating factors are absent). Amiodarone is a recognised cause of deranged thyroid biochemistry (see Chapter 9), but does not appear to increase the risks of atrial fibrillation.

Caffeine is a recognised cause of drug-induced atrial fibrillation. Caffeine is an important constituent of a number of drugs, particularly simple analgesic preparations, and its use as an additive in foods and beverages has become increasingly widespread. A number of different non-alcoholic energy drinks containing large quantities of caffeine are now available, and their use has seen an increased occurrence of atrial fibrillation in otherwise healthy individuals. Symptoms attributable to sinus tachycardia or atrial fibrillation can include intermittent palpitations or breathlessness. Caffeine is metabolised by acetylation, and slow acetylators might be more prone to its potentially adverse cardiovascular effects. The half-life of caffeine is comparatively short, and therefore pharmacodynamic tolerance to the cardiovascular effects does not occur.[16]

Digoxin is a recognised cause of arrhythmia and should be avoided in patients who experience episodic (paroxysmal) atrial fibrillation, because it does not appear effective for reducing the frequency or duration of recurrent episodes.[17,18] Digoxin should only be used to control resting ventricular rate in patients with persistent atrial fibrillation, particularly those with concomitant heart failure, in view of its positively inotropic properties.[18] Other recognised causes of drug-induced atrial fibrillation include tricyclic antidepressants, trazodone, fluoxetine and high-dose corticosteroids.

Management of suspected drug-induced atrial fibrillation will consist of withdrawal of the offending drug, if possible. Advice related to modifying alcohol and caffeine intake should be offered, if appropriate. In some patients, avoiding excess alcohol and caffeine can prevent further atrial fibrillation episodes. In patients receiving thyroxine replacement therapy a new onset of atrial fibrillation should prompt suspicion of treatment excess, which can be confirmed by measurement of thyroid-stimulating hormone (TSH) concentrations. As in situations of non-drug related atrial fibrillation, consideration must be given to long-term anticoagulation, cardioversion to restore sinus rhythm (e.g. direct current or amiodarone), and control of heart rate at rest (digoxin) and during ambulation (beta-blocker, verapamil or diltiazem).

Prolonged QT interval and *torsades de pointes*

The term '*torsades de pointes*' was first coined by Francois Dessertenne in 1966 to describe a specific form of polymorphic ventricular tachycardia.[19] The term can be translated as 'twisting of the points', and refers to the characteristic undulating cardiac axis seen on an electrocardiogram that distinguishes this arrhythmia from conventional ventricular tachycardia.

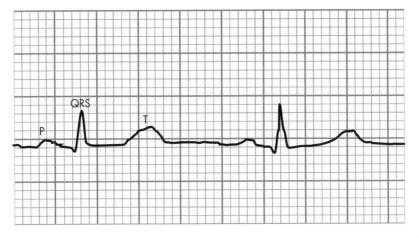

Figure 14.1 ECG in a 24-year-old man taking erythromycin, showing prolongation of the QT interval (455 ms).

Myocyte repolarisation depends on cellular potassium efflux, which is mediated via a number of channels, including the rapid current (I_{Kr}) and slow current (I_{Ks}). Rapid channel conductance appears most susceptible to pharmacological influence, but blockade of either potassium efflux channel causes a number of electrocardiograph (ECG) abnormalities, including QT prolongation, aberrant T-wave morphology and the emergence of U waves. The QT interval is measured from the beginning of the QRS complex to the end of the subsequent T wave (Figure 14.1), and this has been conventionally measured from ECG lead II recordings. QT interval normally varies with heart rate. Although the relationship between QT interval and heart rate differs between individuals, a number of formulae have been derived to reduce the effects of heart rate as a confounding factor. The 'corrected' QT interval (QTc) is most widely obtained using Bazett's formula (QTcB = $QT/RR^{1/2}$). In general, automated 12-lead ECG recordings calculate QTc using the mean QT and mean RR interval over a 10-s recording. Less commonly, QTc can be calculated as the mean of $QT/RR^{1/2}$ of successive beats during the recording. Fredericia's formula ($QT/RR^{1/3}$) is less commonly used, but may be more appropriate at physiological extremes of heart rate. Normal QTc values are considered to be less than 430 ms in men and less than 450 ms in women. The QT interval is regarded as prolonged in excess of 440 ms in men and 460 ms in women, and the risk of arrhythmia increases significantly beyond 500 ms.[20]

The arrhythmia risk associated with any given QTc interval varies significantly between patients and between drugs. Recently, there has

Table 14.3 Some drugs that may cause prolonged QT interval and *torsades de pointes*

Antiarrhythmics:	*Quinidine, procainamide, disopyramide, amiodarone, sotalol*
Antihistamines:	*Astemizole, diphenhydramine*
Antidepressants:	*Lithium, tricyclics*
Antipsychotics:	*Phenothiazines, haloperidol, droperidol, doxepin, pimozide*
Macrolide antibiotics:	*Clarithromycin, erythromycin*
Azole antifungals:	*Ketoconazole, fluconazole*
Digitalis toxicity	
Probucol	
Tacrolimus	

been increasing interest in QT dispersion (maximum QT – minimum QT on a standard 12-lead ECG recording), which appears to be more closely associated with arrhythmia risk than QTc prolongation.[21] However, the clinical implications of QT dispersion, and its utility as a marker of arrhythmia risk, require further evaluation.

An extensive number of drugs have been implicated as causes of QT prolongation (Table 14.3 lists those most frequently implicated). Often, these have been administered in doses at or beyond the upper part of the normal dose range. Hepatic enzyme inhibition, by certain drugs or by grapefruit juice, may increase the risk of QT prolongation or *torsades de pointes* owing to higher circulating drug concentrations. Several drugs have been withdrawn from the UK market in recent years because of QT prolongation and *torsades de pointes*, which have been fatal in certain cases. These including terodiline (an antispasmodic used to treat urinary incontinence), cisapride (a prokinetic agent used to treat gastroparesis), terfenadine (an antihistamine) and pimozide (an antipsychotic agent). Patients with hypomagnesaemia, hypocalcaemia and bradycardia with atrioventricular (AV) block may be predisposed to the development of *torsades de pointes*.

Disorders of systemic blood pressure

Hypertension

Optimal blood pressure is regarded as systolic pressure of 120 mmHg and diastolic 80 mmHg, whereas hypertension is defined by persistent systolic or diastolic pressures of more than 140 mmg and 90 mmHg, respectively. Erythropoietin is used as a treatment for anaemia in patients with end-stage renal impairment, who characteristically have coexistent hypertension. Erythropoietin is a recognised cause of systemic hypertension, and occurs during treatment with alpha and beta preparations of epoetin (recombinant human erythropoietin), and the glycosylated epoetin derivative darbepoetin. Treatment causes a dose-dependent increase in blood pressure in both normotensive and hypertensive individuals. In most cases the increase in blood pressure is modest, and occurs in around 25–35% of patients, particularly during the first 3 months of treatment.[22] To minimise the risk of hypertension, the dose of erythropoietin should be carefully titrated so as to allow haemoglobin concentration to increase no more rapidly than 1 g/dL per month. Blood pressure should be closely monitored, and might require intervention to maintain target blood pressure. If hypertension develops, fluid overload should be treated with diuretic therapy or dialysis as appropriate. In the absence of fluid overload, arterial vasodilator antihypertensive treatment should be considered. In rare situations, severe hypertension and hypertensive encephalopathy have been reported, even in the setting of normal baseline blood pressure. If severe hypertension occurs, with or without encephalopathy, treatment should be discontinued; thereafter, haemoglobin concentrations will typically decrease by around 0.5 g/dL per week. In extreme situations phlebotomy may be considered, especially for individuals in whom the haemoglobin (Hb) concentration is greater than 12 g/dL, or has risen by more than 2 g/dL per month. Erythropoietin should be reintroduced cautiously, only with close monitoring of Hb and blood pressure until the Hb is stabilised in the range of 10–12 g/dL.

Ciclosporin is a powerful immunosuppressant that is used to prevent graft rejection and graft-versus-host disease after tissue transplantation, and in selected patients with rheumatoid arthritis, atopic dermatitis and psoriasis. Its major complication is nephrotoxicity, but other recognised adverse effects are hypertension, alopecia, hepatotoxicity and an increased risk of future malignant disease. Hypertension is commonly seen shortly after the initiation of treatment, but often resolves over time, and is most commonly observed after heart transplantation.[23] A number of mechanisms have been implicated, including endothelial dysfunction, such that systemic vascular resistance is increased, and renal impairment. Blood pressure should be carefully monitored and antihypertensive treatment initiated as appropriate. Ciclosporin is contraindicated in patients with severe hypertension, and therefore blood pressure should be adequately controlled before treatment is initiated.

Monoamine oxidase inhibitor (MAOI) antidepressants are a recognised cause of hypertension, because they inhibit the breakdown of noradrenal and thereby promote its pressor effects. By this mechanism, MAOIs are subject to particularly important drug interactions with food-stuffs containing tyramine (the precursor to noradrenaline) and sympathomimetic agents, including adrenaline, noradrenaline, dobutamine, dopamine and phenylephrine. Such interactions can cause severe increases in blood pressure – so-called hypertensive crises – and patients should be given adequate counselling about these risks and carry a treatment card.[24] The risk of severe hypertension is greatest with unselective MAOI treatment, such as phenelzine, rather than $MAOI_B$-selective agents, such as selegiline. It should be remembered that the potential for MAOI-induced hypertensive crises persists for up to 3 weeks after drug discontinuation.

The oestrogen component of the oral contraceptive pill is a very important cause of secondary hypertension, and treatment causes a small but detectable increase in both systolic and diastolic blood pressures in most women. The prevalence of hypertension is around two to three times that of age-matched women not taking the oral contraceptive pill, and the risk increases with advancing age, duration of treatment, baseline blood pressure and increased body mass. The rise in blood pressure and the corresponding risk of hypertension associated with current low oestrogen content contraceptive pills is less than that of earlier preparations.[25] There are a number of mechanisms by which oestrogen can increase blood pressure, including increased body mass, circulating fluid volume and peripheral insulin resistance, and activation of the renin–angiotensin–aldosterone system.[26]

Although it is advisable to avoid using the oral contraceptive pill in women with pre-existing hypertension, this is not always practical. Other means of contraception should be explored, and this modality should only be considered for carefully selected patients in whom the potential risks of pregnancy outweigh the risks of mild hypertension. Only preparations with low oestrogen content should be used, if possible, and blood pressure closely monitored. Progestogen-only preparations do not appear to cause elevation of blood pressure and may therefore be a suitable alternative means of contraception for those women in whom hypertension occurs.[27] Blood pressure should be checked at least every 6 months for the duration of treatment, which is facilitated by dispensing no more than 6 months' supply between medical appointments.[28]

If blood pressure rises, then the decision to discontinue treatment should be based on the degree of hypertension, the overall cardiovascular risk profile and the potential risks of pregnancy. In most cases, withdrawal of treatment will allow gradual restoration of normal blood pressure over 2–6 weeks.

Table 14.4 Some drugs that can cause or worsen
hypertension

Erythropoietin
Ergotamine
Oestrogens
Ciclosporin
NSAIDs
Corticosteroids
Carbenoxolone
Liquorice
Monoamine oxidase inhibitors
Sympathomimetics
Anticholinergics
Alcohol excess
Cocaine

Drugs that cause fluid retention and increase circulating fluid load
can increase blood pressure and aggravate pre-existing hypertension. The
most important drugs in this group are non-steroidal anti-inflammatory
drugs (NSAIDs), corticosteroids, carbenoxolone, liquorice and substances
with a high sodium content, such as antacids. Similarly, regular alcohol
intake and excess salt intake are associated with sustained increases in
systemic blood pressure, characterised by structural arteriolar wall
changes. Avoidance of drugs that promote fluid retention, and abstinence
from alcohol and excess dietary salt intake allows a modest reduction in
systemic blood pressure and significantly enhances the potential effectiveness of antihypertensive drugs. Some drugs that may cause hypertension are shown in Table 14.4.

Hypotension

Unlike the situation where blood pressure is abnormally high, there is no
clear definition of abnormally low blood pressure. Across populations
there is a linear relationship between blood pressure and cardiovascular
risk, such that no lower threshold for normality has been identified.
However, hypotension can become apparent due to inadequate tissue
perfusion, and most commonly manifests in the setting of postural
hypotension. Symptoms are usually transient and may occur on standing; these include headache, blurred vision, dizziness and syncope.

Postural hypotension is a characteristic adverse effect of treatment
with alpha-blockers, which can be used to treat symptoms attributable to
benign prostatic hypertrophy. In view of this, treatment is often introduced

at low dosages that are gradually titrated up towards an optimal therapeutic dose. The risk of significant first-dose hypotension can be minimised by initiating treatment at night before bedtime, or where the patient remains recumbent, such as might be encountered in a hospital setting. Postural hypotension is also a characteristic adverse effect of angiotensin-converting enzyme (ACE) inhibitors and angiotensin-II receptor antagonists, which are widely used in patients with diabetes, ischaemic heart disease and cardiac failure. Similarly, these agents should be initiated using a low dose followed by gradual dose titration and patient monitoring.

As with alpha-blockers and drugs inhibiting the renin–angiotensin–aldosterone system, other existing treatments for hypertension are more correctly blood-pressure-lowering agents, rather than true antihypertensives. They do not specifically target the underlying mechanisms that result in abnormally high blood pressure, and generally cause a similar effect on blood-pressure in both normotensive and hypertensive individuals. In view of this, all current blood pressure lowering agents have the potential to cause hypotension, and this adverse effect is particularly important when they are used in combination. To minimise the risks of symptomatic hypotension, implementation of antihypertensive treatment should aim to cause a gradual and progressive reduction in blood pressure toward target values over a period of weeks and months.

Levodopa and, to a lesser extent, other dopaminergic agents are a recognised cause of postural hypotension. This may contribute to falls and postural instability in patients with parkinsonism, and erect and supine blood pressure measurements should be monitored closely. In some cases, significant postural hypotension can be avoided by increasing the frequency of levodopa administration so that the individual dosages can be reduced. Some drugs that may cause hypotension are shown in Table 14.5.

Table 14.5 Some drugs that can cause hypotension

Dopaminergic agents
Nitrates
Alpha-blockers
Centrally acting antihypertensives
ACE inhibitors
Angiotensin II receptor antagonists
Opioids
Diuretics (especially high-dose loop diuretics)
Acetylcysteine
Phenytoin
Antipsychotics
Benzodiazepines (especially in high dose)
Lithium

Congestive heart failure

Heart failure is characterised by inability of the heart to supply sufficient blood to meet the metabolic demands of the body. This can occur in situations where the metabolic rate is significantly enhanced, for example severe thyrotoxicosis or sepsis syndrome. However, in the vast majority of cases congestive heart failure is usually indicative of reduced cardiac output due to myocardial inadequacy. The diagnosis of heart failure is based on clinical history and physical examination. Symptoms include reduced exercise tolerance, breathlessness on exertion, orthopnoea, cough and muscle weakness. Clinical signs include the presence of a third heart sound, respiratory crackles, hepatomegaly and peripheral oedema. Investigations in isolation, including echocardiography, cannot be used to make a diagnosis of heart failure, and are generally used to establish the severity of left ventricular impairment. Drugs can cause or worsen heart failure via two principal mechanisms, namely by reducing cardiac output or by causing excess fluid retention and circulating volume overload (Table 14.6).

Negatively inotropic drugs that directly impair myocardial function, and thereby reduce cardiac output, are an important cause of heart failure. These include calcium channel blockers, of which verapamil has the greatest cardiodepressant effects, and to a lesser extent diltiazem. Vasodilating calcium channel blockers, including nifedipine, have negative inotropic effects *in vitro* but do not appear to significantly impair cardiac output *in vivo*. More recently introduced calcium channel blockers, such as felodipine and isradipine, are highly selective for vascular smooth muscle and have minimal cardiodepressant effects.[29]

Beta-blockers impair myocardial contractility and reduce heart rate. Furthermore, they increase peripheral vascular resistance and cardiac afterload, which additionally impairs cardiac output.[30] In view of these potentially deleterious haemodynamic effects, beta-blockers are a recognised cause of congestive heart failure and have conventionally been contraindicated in this patient group. However, arrhythmia is a major cause of death in severe heart failure owing, at least in part, to a characteristic increase in sympathetic cardiac activation. Recent clinical trials have shown that beta-blockers can significantly reduce mortality in severe heart

Table 14.6 Some drugs that can cause or worsen congestive heart failure

Antacids (high salt content)	NSAIDs
Beta-blockers	Corticosteroids
Verapamil	Class I antiarrhythmic drugs
Diltiazem	Carbenoxolone
Alpha-blockers	

failure, probably because of their sympatholytic action.[31] Trial evidence most strongly advocates the use of metoprolol, carvedilol and bisoprolol, but the beneficial properties appear to be due to cardiac beta-adrenoceptor antagonism, rather than any other ancillary property, and are likely to also be conferred by other beta-blockers. Beta-blockers have not yet been found to reduce mortality in patients with mild to moderate heart failure, in whom beneficial antiarrhythmic effects might be outweighed by potentially harmful negatively inotropic haemodynamic effects. Therefore, consideration should still be given to discontinuation of beta-blockers in patients who present with mild or moderate heart failure, in whom their use might aggravate symptoms. In general, the initiation of beta-blocker treatment in patients with severe heart failure should be undertaken only under specialist supervision, with careful titration and optimisation of dose.

Other negatively inotropic drugs include amiodarone and antiarrhythmic agents, and these should be used with particular caution in patients with severe heart failure. The recent Antihypertensive and Lipid-Lowering Treatment to Prevent Heart Attack Trial (ALLHAT) found that alpha-blockers were equally effective in reducing cardiovascular mortality in patients with hypertension compared to other types of blood pressure lowering treatment, but were associated with a significantly increased incidence of congestive heart failure.[32] The mechanisms underlying this finding are not yet entirely clear, but it is possible that the diagnosis of heart failure might have been more readily apparent in those patients who were receiving alpha-blockers owing to the occurrence of peripheral oedema, a recognised adverse effect.

A number of drugs are known to cause excess fluid retention and, as a consequence of increased circulating fluid volume, can precipitate heart failure. Principal among these are non-steroidal anti-inflammatory agents (NSAIDs), which cause increased salt and water reabsorption by the kidney.[33] This effect is observed with both non-selective NSAIDs and those that selectively inhibit type 2 cyclooxygenase (COX-2). Corticosteroids exert a similar effect and, like NSAIDs, antagonise the effects of diuretic treatment in congestive heart failure.[34]

Myocardial toxicity

A number of drugs exert direct injurious effects on the heart that result in cardiomyopathy, abnormalities of contractile function, conduction defects and arrhythmia (Table 14.7). Morphological changes can evolve over a prolonged period after drug exposure, and the clinical diagnosis is often delayed, so that establishing causality is often difficult.

Table 14.7 Some cytotoxic drugs that may cause cardiac toxicity

Busulfan	Etoposide
Carmustine	Ifosfamide
Cisplatin	Mitomycin
Cyclophosphamide	Mitoxantrone
Cytarabine	Paclitaxel
Daunorubicin	Trastuzumab
Doxorubicin	Vinca alkaloids
Epirubicin	

Anthracycline cytotoxics, for example doxorubicin, are a recognised cause of direct myocardial damage that manifests as acute or subacute toxicity, early-onset progressive cardiotoxicity and late-onset chronic progressive cardiotoxicity.[35] The mechanism underlying cardiotoxicity is thought due to local free-radical-mediated myocardial injury, catalysed by doxorubicin–iron complexes. Morbidity and mortality due to anthracycline cardiotoxicity are high, and predisposing factors are mediastinal radiotherapy, female gender, pre-existing heart disease, hypertension and high doxorubicin exposure. Acute or subacute anthracycline toxicity presents with features resembling acute heart failure, or as a pericarditis–myocarditis syndrome with accompanying electrocardiogram abnormalities. Early-onset chronic progressive cardiotoxicity is a more typical manifestation, which usually occurs within 1 year after commencing treatment. The clinical course is persistence or progression of heart failure despite discontinuation of the drug, and often evolves into a chronic dilated cardiomyopathy in adults or a restrictive cardiomyopathy in children. Less commonly, anthracycline-induced myocardial injury manifests as late-onset progressive cardiotoxicity. This can present many years after treatment, and usually the clinical features are those of a progressively declining dilated cardiomyopathy.

To minimise risk, the cumulative lifetime dose of doxorubicin should not exceed 450–550 mg/m^2. Patients should be carefully monitored for evidence of cardiotoxicity during treatment and in long-term follow-up, to include physical examination, chest radiograph, electrocardiograph and echocardiograph. Dexrazoxane prevents the formation of doxorubicin–iron complexes by binding to intracellular iron.[36] When given to patients who would have received a cumulative doxorubicin dose of more than 300 mg/kg, dexrazoxane appears to reduce the risks of cardiotoxicity. However, there is debate over whether dextrazoxane might diminish the antitumour efficacy of anthracycline-based regimens, and it is not yet established in routine clinical use.[37] Melatonin has also been shown to demonstrate protective effects against anthracycline-induced cardiotoxicity, and appears to work by minimising oxidative free radical activity.[38]

Interferon alfa is used in the treatment of lymphoma and certain solid tumours, and as an adjunctive treatment in chronic hepatitis B and hepatitis C. Common adverse effects include flu-like symptoms, nausea and depression. Cardiovascular toxicity has been reported in as many as 5–15% of patients, and usually occurs within the first few days of treatment.[39] Clinical features include hypertension, hypotension, arrhythmia and, rarely, severe and reversible cardiomyopathy has been reported in patients with no previous history of heart disease; in some cases cardiac failure can be irreversible.[40] Interferon alfa should be used with caution in patients with pre-existing heart failure or ischaemic heart disease.

Fluorouracil is a rare but recognised cause of significant myocardial toxicity, typically due to vasospasm and myocardial ischaemia.[41] Toxicity can present with clinical features that range from mild angina to massive myocardial infarction. The mechanism underlying this adverse effect is unclear, but the risks appear greatest in those with pre-existing ischaemic heart disease.

Clozapine, an atypical antipsychotic, has been reported to cause myocarditis as a rare idiosyncratic adverse effect.[42]

Pulmonary hypertension

Pulmonary hypertension is a rare lung disorder in which the blood pressure in the pulmonary circulation is abnormally high. The pulmonary arteries, unaccustomed to high pressures, become hypertrophic and narrowed such that the opportunities for restoration of normal pressures are limited. Pulmonary hypertension can be associated with a number of symptoms, including breathlessness, dizziness, syncope, palpitations and lethargy. In most cases of this rare condition an underlying cause is not identified. In some cases there is an underlying collagen vascular disease, for example scleroderma. Since the 1970s, amfetamines and their derivatives have been researched as a potentially effective pharmacological adjunct to weight loss attempts in overweight and obese patients. In 1997, the anorexigens fenfluramine (AH Robins) and dexfenfluramine (Wyeth–Ayerst) were reported to increase the risk of cardiac valvulopathy and pulmonary hypertension.[43] These findings attracted worldwide interest and resulted in large class-action compensation claims that are still being pursued through the courts. Other amfetamines and cocaine are also recognised as causes of pulmonary hypertension.[44]

Stroke and heart attack risk

A number of studies have recently shown that selective COX-2 inhibitors appear to increase the risk of heart attacks and strokes. In 2004, Merck voluntarily withdrew rofecoxib from the market because of unfavourable interim data from the Adenomatous Polyp Prevention on Vioxx (APPROVe) study, which had enrolled around 2600 patients. After 18 months of treatment, myocardial infarction and stroke had occurred in 3.5% of patients who had received rofecoxib 25 mg daily, compared to 1.9% of those who had received placebo.[45] Rofecoxib had received regulatory approval for use in 1999, and the original safety database (incorporating around 5000 patients) had not shown any indication of increased risk. A retrospective meta-analysis of data from 18 randomised controlled trials and 11 observational studies (not including data from the APPROVe study) confirmed a significant increase in cardiovascular risk. This analysis included more than 20 000 patients and showed that rofecoxib conferred an overall relative risk of 2.3 (95% CI 1.22–4.33) for myocardial infarction, 1.02 (0.54–1.93) for stroke, and 1.55 (1.05–2.29) for all serious cardiovascular events.[46]

The Adenoma Prevention with Celecoxib (APC) study involved around 2000 patients treated with placebo, celecoxib 200 mg twice daily or celecoxib 400 mg twice daily. An independent Data Safety Monitoring Board showed a significant 2.5-fold increased risk of major fatal and non-fatal cardiovascular events for participants taking the drug compared to those on a placebo, and the trial was halted prematurely by the National Cancer Institute in December 2004. After a mean treatment duration of 33 months, the incidence of serious cardiovascular event was 0.9% in the placebo arm, 2.2% in the celecoxib 400 mg daily arm, and 3.0% in the celecoxib 800 mg daily arm. A similar clinical trial, the Prevention of Spontaneous Adenomatous Polyps (PreSAP) study, did not find any association between celecoxib treatment and cardiovascular risk. Fatal cardiovascular events occurred in 1.7% of patients treated with celecoxib 400 mg daily, and 1.8% of those treated with placebo. The trial was suspended on the basis of findings from the APC safety committee.[46]

No study of the gastrointestinal effects of valdecoxib treatment has been reported. However, in patients undergoing coronary artery bypass grafting, treatment with parecoxib (a prodrug of valdecoxib) was associated with increased cardiovascular events, and the drug licence application was rejected by the Food and Drug Administration (FDA). Approval of valdecoxib was based on studies in patients at low cardiovascular risk. However, there are persisting concerns about a possible relationship between valdecoxib and cardiovascular risk based, at least in part, on the association between its prodrug and cardiovascular disease.[47]

The Therapeutic Arthritis Research and Gastrointestinal Event Trial (TARGET) compared lumiracoxib with naproxen or ibuprofen and showed a significantly lower incidence of serious gastrointestinal events in patients receiving lumiracoxib. This difference was observed only in patients not taking aspirin. Among non-aspirin users, cardiovascular events were much more frequent in the lumiracoxib group than in other patients (0.26 vs 0.18 per 100 patient-years; hazard ratio 1.47), although the difference was not statistically significant.[48,49]

The emergence of safety concerns about the use of COX-2-selective NSAIDs has raised interest in the potential mechanisms by which they could exert detrimental cardiovascular effects. In healthy volunteers, rofecoxib and celecoxib had been shown to suppress the formation of prostaglandin I_2 (PGI_2), which is the predominant cyclooxygenase product in endothelium that inhibits platelet aggregation and causes vasodilatation.[47] It is possible that COX-2 inhibitors exert detrimental effects on cardiovascular function through the loss of potentially beneficial actions mediated by PGI_2. However, at present the exact pathogenic link between COX-2 inhibitors and increased cardiovascular risk remains uncertain.

Recent guidance issued by the Medicines and Healthcare products Regulatory Agency (MHRA) indicates that patients who have established ischaemic heart disease or cerebrovascular disease should be switched from a COX-2-selective NSAID to an alternative treatments as soon as is convenient. Furthermore, careful consideration should be given to cardiovascular, gastrointestinal and other risk factors when judging the risks and benefits of COX-2 inhibitors, and alternative treatments should be considered for all patients. In keeping with good prescribing practice, all NSAIDs (including COX-2-selective inhibitors) should be used in the lowest effective dose and for the shortest duration necessary. For patients switched to chronic non-selective NSAIDs, consideration should be given to gastroprotective treatments.[50]

CASE STUDY 14.1

A 69-year-old man has been treated for atrial fibrillation and angina for the past 2 years and is taking aspirin 75 mg daily, digoxin 125 μg daily, atenolol 50 mg

→

◖ CASE STUDY 14.1 (continued)

daily and 3–4 mg warfarin daily. He attends his GP complaining of indigestion for the past 3 weeks, which has failed to respond adequately to over-the-counter antacid preparations. His GP refers him to the gastroenterology outpatient department and prescribes a course of omeprazole 20 mg daily.

Five days later, the patient is rushed to the Accident and Emergency department after collapsing suddenly. On examination he is pale, with marked bruising over his limbs and trunk, and dipstick urinalysis strongly indicates haematuria. His International Normalised Ratio (INR) is found to be 5.8, having been normal during his recent GP attendance, and he is treated with intravenous vitamin K.

What is the most likely explanation for the sudden increase in INR?

This is most likely a drug interaction between omeprazole and warfarin. Proton pump inhibitors are subject to pharmacokinetic interactions with a number of drugs metabolised by the cytochrome P450 (CYP450) system, including warfarin. Proton pump inhibitors are significantly metabolised by CYP2C19, whereas warfarin is mainly metabolised by the CYP2C9 isoenzyme. Certain individuals will have reduced or absent expression of these respective isoforms, so that proton pump inhibitors may compete with warfarin for alternative enzyme pathways, for example the CYP3A4 pathway.

Proton pump inhibitor interactions with warfarin are comparatively rare, but the consequences can be serious and potentially fatal. The worldwide incidence of warfarin interactions that resulted in significant haemorrhage (within 19 months of drug availability) have been reported as 0.08 per million packs for omeprazole, 0.23 per million packs for lansoprazole and 0.11 per million packs pantoprazole.[51]

Will regular low-dose aspirin therapy increase INR?

No, but aspirin will increase the risk of bleeding, particularly that due to gastrointestinal haemorrhage, even when taken in low doses. Aspirin inhibits cyclooxygenase and exerts an antiplatelet effect, which reduces the risks of atherothrombosis in patients with established vascular disease. The potential benefits of regular aspirin therapy must be considered in the context of increased bleeding risk, and its use should be confined to those patients at greatest cardiovascular risk. This is particularly important where there is a clear indication for anticoagulation therapy, and the combination with antiplatelet therapy is usually initiated only under specialist guidance.

CASE STUDY 14.2

A 65-year-old woman is referred to the general medical outpatient department of your local hospital. She has regularly attended her GP for treatment of hypertension, and has been taking atenolol 50 mg daily and Adalat LA 20 mg daily for the past 8 years. Over the past 3 months she has been aware of progressively worsening breathlessness on exertion, accompanied by increasing ankle swelling. She is found to have a resting heart rate of 58 bpm, blood pressure 156/88 mmHg and peripheral oedema to mid-calf level. She is thought to have developed congestive heart failure, and her usual medicines are withdrawn. Instead, she is commenced on spironolactone 25 mg twice daily and losartan 50 mg daily, and arrangements are made for a follow-up clinical appointment in 8 weeks' time.

Why has she developed heart failure?

Congestive heart failure is the natural consequence of untreated hypertension. Not surprisingly, it is very common in patients with longstanding hypertension, particularly where blood pressure has not been treated adequately to target levels. Treatment targets are usually 140 mmHg or lower for systolic blood pressure and 90 mmHg or lower for diastolic, and lower in certain high-risk patient subgroups. Blood pressure measurement in this patient suggests that her existing therapy might be inadequate. Bradycardia in this case is presumably due to beta-blocker treatment.

Why might her antihypertensive medications have been withdrawn?

Atenolol reduces heart rate and myocardial contractility and stroke volume, so that cardiac output is significantly lowered. In some patients, these potentially deleterious haemodynamic actions can precipitate or exacerbate the symptoms and signs of congestive heart failure. In most cases, gradual withdrawal of the beta-blocker results in improved haemodynamics and enhanced cardiac function. The decision to withdraw therapy needs to be offset against the clinical need for beta-blocker treatment. For example, the indication for continued beta-blocker treatment might be more pressing in patients with myocardial ischaemia or arrhythmia rather than hypertension alone.

Dihydropyridine calcium channel blockers, for example nifedipine, cause peripheral oedema in up to around 30% of patients owing to peripheral arterial vasodilatation. This adverse effect is often well tolerated, and in many cases does not necessitate withdrawal of the offending drug.

→

> **CASE STUDY 14.2** (continued)
>
> ### Why might treatment with an angiotensin receptor antagonist be helpful?
>
> Angiotensin receptor antagonists, for example losartan, block the effects of the renin–angiotensin–aldosterone system. Their therapeutic and adverse-effect profiles are very similar to those of ACE inhibitors, and both of these groups are widely used in the treatment of hypertension and heart failure. Recent evidence suggests that angiotensin receptor antagonists may be highly effective when used to treat hypertension in patients with established left ventricular hypertrophy or coexistent diabetes. A number of recent studies have suggested that, in patients with congestive heart failure, the combination of an ACE inhibitor and an angiotensin receptor antagonist might offer a small benefit over either treatment alone, but this is currently not established as routine practice.
>
> ### What potential adverse interaction might arise from her new medication?
>
> The combination of spironolactone with an ACE inhibitor or angiotensin receptor antagonist significantly increases the risk of hyperkalaemia in patients with heart failure, especially in the setting of diabetes or renal impairment. Hyperkalaemia is generally asymptomatic but predisposes to arrhythmia, and in most cases requires urgent treatment. Spironolactone, when prescribed in addition to conventional heart failure therapy, results in around 50 hospital admissions for hyperkalaemia for every 1000 patients treated.[52]

References

1. Haase G, Pietzsch M, Fahnrich A, Voss W, Riethling AK. Results of a systematic adverse drug reaction (ADR)-screening concerning bradycardia caused by drug interactions in departments of internal medicine in Rostock. *Int J Clin Pharmacol Ther* 2002; 40: 116–119.
2. Cabezon Ruiz S, Moran Risco JE, Pedrote Martinez A, *et al*. Drug brady-arrhythmias as a cause of hospital admission: study of 83 cases. *Med Clin* 2003; 120: 574–575.
3. Anderson JR, Nawarskas JJ. Cardiovascular drug–drug interactions. *Cardiol Clin* 2001; 19: 215–234.
4. Suematsu F, Yukawa E, Yukawa M, *et al*. Pharmacoepidemiologic detection of calcium channel blocker-induced change on digoxin clearance using multiple trough screen analysis. *Biopharm Drug Dispos* 2002; 23: 173–181.
5. Zhang WY, Po AL, Dua HS, Azuara-Blanco A. Meta-analysis of randomised controlled trials comparing latanoprost with timolol in the treatment of patients with open angle glaucoma or ocular hypertension. *Br J Ophthalmol* 2001; 85: 983–990.

6. Sharifi M, Koch JM, Steele RJ, *et al*. Third degree AC block due to ophthalmic timolol solution. *Int J Cardiol* 2001; 80: 257–259.

7. Rudorfer MV, Manji HK, Potter WZ. Comparative tolerability profiles of the newer versus older antidepressants. *Drug Safety* 1994; 10: 18–46.

8. Buckley NA, Sanders P. Cardiovascular adverse effects of antipsychotic drugs. *Drug Safety* 2000; 23: 215–228.

9. O'Driscoll BR. Supraventricular tachycardia caused by nebulised ipratropium bromide. *Thorax* 1989; 44: 312.

10. Sica DA. Minoxidil: an underused vasodilator for resistant or severe hypertension. *J Clin Hypertens* 2004; 6: 283–287.

11. Jacobs MC, Lenders JW, Willemsen JJ, Thien T. Chronic alpha-1-adrenergic blockade increases sympathoneural but not adrenomedullary activity in patients with essential hypertension. *J Hypertens* 1995; 13: 1837–1841.

12. Steers W, Guay AT, Leriche A, *et al*. Assessment of the efficacy and safety of Viagra (sildenafil citrate) in men with erectile dysfunction during long-term treatment. *Int J Impotence Res* 2001; 13: 261–267.

13. Nakagawa S, Yamamoto Y, Koiwaya Y. Ventricular tachycardia induced by clonidine withdrawal. *Br Heart J* 1985; 53: 654–658.

14. Frost L, Vestergaard P. Alcohol and risk of atrial fibrillation or flutter: a cohort study. *Arch Intern Med* 2004; 164: 1993–1998.

15. Djousse L, Levy D, Benjamin EJ, *et al*. Long-term alcohol consumption and the risk of atrial fibrillation in the Framingham Study. *Am J Cardiol* 2004; 93: 710–713.

16. Waring WS, Goudsmit J, Marwick J, Webb DJ, Maxwell SR. Acute caffeine intake influences central more than peripheral blood pressure in young adults. *Am J Hypertens* 2003; 16: 919–924.

17. Valent S, Kelly P. Images in clinical medicine. Digoxin-induced bidirectional ventricular tachycardia. *N Engl J Med* 1997; 336: 550.

18. Robles de Medina EO, Algra A. Digoxin in the treatment of paroxysmal atrial fibrillation. *Lancet* 1999; 354: 882–883.

19. Dessertenne F. La tachycardre ventriculaire a deux foyers opposes variables. *Arch Mal Coeur Vaiss* 1966; 59: 263–272.

20. Gowda RM, Khan IA, Wilbur SL, Vasavada BC, Sacchi TJ. Torsades de pointes: the clinical considerations. *Int J Cardiol* 2004; 96: 1–6.

21. Sheehan J, Perry IJ, Reilly M, *et al*. QT dispersion, QT maximum and risk of cardiac death in the Caerphilly Heart Study. *Eur J Cardiovasc Prev Rehab* 2004; 11: 63–68.

22. Miyashita K, Tojo A, Kimura K, *et al*. Blood pressure response to erythropoietin injection in hemodialysis and predialysis patients. *Hypertens Res* 2004; 27: 79–84.

23. Texter SC, Canzanello VJ, Tate SJ, *et al*. Cyclosporin-induced hypertension after transplantation. *Mayo Clin Proc* 1994; 69: 1182–1193.

24. Lavin MR, Mendelowitz A, Kronig MH. Spontaneous hypertensive reactions with monoamine oxidase inhibitors. *Biol Psychiatry* 1993; 34: 146–151.

25. WHO Task Force on Oral Contraceptives. The WHO Multicentre Trial of the Vasopressor Effects of Combined Oral Contraceptives. I. Comparisons with IUD. *Contraception* 1989; 40: 129–145.

26. Byrne KP, Geraghty DP, Stewart BJ, Burcher E. Effect of contraceptive steroid and enalapril treatment of systolic blood pressure and plasma renin–angiotensin in the rat. *Clin Exp Hypertens* 1994; 16: 627–657.

27. Bigrigg A, Evans M, Gbolade B, *et al*. Depo Provera. Position paper on clinical use, effectiveness and side effects. *Br J Fam Plann* 1999; 25: 69–76.
28. Chasan-Taber L, Willett WC, Manson JE, *et al*. Prospective study of oral contraceptives and hypertension among women in the United States. *Circulation* 1996; 94: 483–489.
29. Mahe I, Chassany O, Grenard AS, Caulin C, Bergmann JF. Defining the role of calcium channel antagonists in heart failure due to systolic dysfunction. *Am J Cardiovasc Drugs* 2003; 3: 33–41.
30. Roberts DH, Tsao Y, Grimmer SF, *et al*. Haemodynamic effects of atenolol, labetalol, pindolol and captopril: a comparison in hypertensive patients with special reference to changes in limb blood flow, heart rate and left ventricular function. *Br J Clin Pharmacol* 1987; 24: 163–172.
31. Bauman JL, Talbert RL. Pharmacodynamics of beta-blockers in heart failure: lessons from the carvedilol or metoprolol European trial. *J Cardiovasc Pharmacol Ther* 2004; 9: 117–128.
32. ALLHAT Officers and Coordinators for the ALLHAT Collaborative Research Group. Major cardiovascular events in hypertensive patients randomized to doxazosin vs chlorthalidone: the antihypertensive and lipid-lowering treatment to prevent heart attack trial (ALLHAT). ALLHAT Collaborative Research Group. *JAMA* 2000; 283: 1967–1975.
33. Whelton A, Hamilton CW. Nonsteroidal anti-inflammatory drugs: effects on kidney function. *J Clin Pharmacol* 1991; 31: 588–598.
34. Swartz SL, Dluhy RG. Corticosteroids: clinical pharmacology and therapeutic use. *Drugs* 1978; 16: 238–255.
35. Minotti G, Menna P, Salvatorelli E, Cairo G, Gianni L. Anthracyclines: molecular advances and pharmacologic developments in antitumor activity and cardiotoxicity. *Pharmacol Rev* 2004; 56: 185–229.
36. Pouillart P. Evaluating the role of dexrazoxane as a cardioprotectant in cancer patients receiving anthracyclines. *Cancer Treat Rev* 2004; 30: 643–650.
37. Dalen E, Caron H, Dickinson H, Kremer L. Cardioprotective interventions for cancer patients receiving anthracyclines. *Cochrane Database Syst Rev* 2005; 1: CD003917.
38. Ahmed HH, Mannaa F, Elmegeed GA, Doss SH. Cardioprotective activity of melatonin and its novel synthesized derivatives on doxorubicin-induced cardiotoxicity. *Bioorg Med Chem* 2005; 13: 1847–1857.
39. Kruit WH, Punt KJ, Goey SH, *et al*. Cardiotoxicity as a dose-limiting factor in a schedule of high dose bolus therapy with interleukin-2 and alpha-interferon. An unexpectedly frequent complication. *Cancer* 1994; 74: 2850–2856.
40. Zimmerman S, Adkins D, Graham M, *et al*. Irreversible, severe congestive cardiomyopathy occurring in association with interferon alpha therapy. *Cancer Biother* 1994; 9: 291–299.
41. Sudhoff T, Enderle MD, Pahlke M, *et al*. 5-Fluorouracil induces arterial vasocontractions. *Ann Oncol* 2004; 15: 661–664.
42. Wehmeier PM, Heiser P, Remschmidt H. Myocarditis, pericarditis and cardiomyopathy in patients treated with clozapine. *J Clin Pharmacol Ther* 2005; 30: 91–96.
43. Naqvi TZ, Gross SB. Anorexigen-induced cardiac valvulopathy and female gender. *Curr Womens Health Rep* 2003; 3: 116–125.
44. Albertson TE, Walby WF, Derlet RW. Stimulant-induced pulmonary toxicity. *Chest* 1995; 108: 1140–1149.

45. Merck. Merck announces voluntary worldwide withdrawal of VIOXX®. http://www.vioxx.com/vioxx/documents/english/vioxx_press_release.pdf
46. Juni P, Nartey L, Reichenbach S, *et al*. Risk of cardiovascular events and rofecoxib: cumulative meta-analysis. *Lancet* 2004; 364: 2021–2029.
46. http: //www.nci.nih.gov/newscenter/COXInhibitorsFactSheet
47. FitzGerald GA. COX-2 and beyond: approaches to prostaglandin inhibition in human disease. *Nature Rev Drug Discov* 2003; 2: 879–890.
48. Schnitzer TJ, Burmester GR, Mysler E, *et al*. Comparison of lumiracoxib with naproxen and ibuprofen in the Therapeutic Arthritis Research and Gastrointestinal Event Trial (TARGET), reduction in ulcer complications: randomised controlled trial. *Lancet* 2004; 364: 665–674.
49. Farkouh ME, Kirshner H, Harrington RA, *et al*. Comparison of lumiracoxib with naproxen and ibuprofen in the Therapeutic Arthritis Research and Gastrointestinal Event Trial (TARGET), cardiovascular outcomes: randomised controlled trial. *Lancet* 2004; 364: 675–684.
50. http: //www.mhra.gov.uk/news/2004/celecoxibhealthlink201204doc.pdf
51. Labenz J, Petersen KU, Rosch W, Koelz HR. A summary of Food and Drug Administration-reported adverse events and drug interactions occurring during therapy with omeprazole, lansoprazole and pantoprazole. *Aliment Pharmacol Ther* 2003; 17: 1015–1019.
52. Juurlink DN, Mamdani MM, Lee DS, *et al*. Rates of hyperkalemia after publication of the Randomized Aldactone Evaluation Study. *N Engl J Med*. 2004; 351: 543–551.

Further reading

Anderson JR, Nawarskas JJ. Cardiovascular drug–drug interactions. *Cardiol Clin* 2001; 19: 215–234.
Buckley NA, Sanders P. Cardiovascular adverse effects of antipsychotic drugs. *Drug Safety* 2000; 23: 215–228.
Fitzgerald GA. Coxibs and cardiovascular disease. *N Engl J Med* 2004; 351: 1709–1711.
Juni P, Nartey L, Reichenbach S, *et al*. Risk of cardiovascular events and rofecoxib: cumulative meta-analysis. *Lancet* 2004; 364: 2021–2029.
Kearney MT, Wright DJ, Tan L-B. Cardiac disorders. In: Davies DM, Ferner RE, de Glanville H, eds. *Davies's Textbook of Adverse Drug Reactions*, 5th edn. London: Chapman & Hall, 1998: 119–168.
Maxwell SRJ. Webb DJ. COX-2 selective inhibitors – important lessons learned. *Lancet* 2005; 365: 449–451.
Roden DM. Drug therapy: Drug-induced prolongation of the QT interval. *N Engl J Med* 2004; 350: 1013–1022.

15

Neurological disorders

Fiona Needleman and Donald Grosset

Introduction

This chapter discusses drug-induced neurological adverse effects in the central and peripheral nervous systems; drug-induced psychiatric effects are considered in Chapter 13. Some common disorders and the drugs implicated are discussed, along with prevention and management strategies.

Neurological drug effects may mimic disease, making it difficult to establish a drug's causative role. Certain drugs tend to cause dose-related adverse effects in the central nervous system (CNS). Often the risks and benefits of medicines need to be closely balanced: for example, in epilepsy doses are titrated upwards to maximise therapeutic effect but reduced if side effects such as ataxia occur. In some cases neurological toxicity is not dose related but due, for example, to an immunological mechanism.

In a number of conditions drugs may predictably exacerbate a pre-existing neurological disorder.[1] Examples include (i) the precipitation of seizures in epilepsy through a lowering of the seizure threshold; (ii) worsening or precipitation of Parkinson's disease through dopamine blockade or antagonism; and (iii) precipitation or exacerbation of myasthenia gravis through interruption of neuromuscular transmission. Patient education and vigilance by healthcare professionals are needed in such settings to minimise the risk of inappropriate prescription.

Dose-related neurological side effects are increased, as in other disease areas, by coexistent impairment of hepatic or renal function, leading to drug accumulation through decreased metabolism or excretion.[2] Penicillin-induced neurotoxicity is associated with high-dose therapy in patients with reduced renal function.[3] Recognising such risk factors for neurotoxicity can reduce complications. Another example is the careful selection of an atypical antipsychotic drug at low dose to treat neuropsychiatric features in Parkinson's disease.

Perhaps because of the chronic nature of neurological disease, and the limitations of prescription therapies, many patients add over-the-counter

(OTC) or complementary medicines, and their effects should also be considered. Ingredients sometimes found in herbal medicines (e.g. mercury, lead and arsenic) can cause seizures.[4]

New drug classes such as the anti-tumour-necrosis-factor-alpha agents are associated with a range of neurological effects, including demyelination.[5] The causality, mechanism and overlap with the underlying condition (for example rheumatoid arthritis) are not yet certain. A further example is natalizumab, a monoclonal antibody whose research programme for multiple sclerosis was suspended in light of serious neurological effects, including cases of progressive multifocal leuko-encephalopathy, a rare and frequently fatal demyelinating CNS disease that occurred in patients co-treated with interferon beta.[6]

Neurologic side effects of drugs used to treat cancer are numerous, but as cancer is frequently associated with neurological manifestations other causes, such as direct effects of the cancer itself, for example nerve compression or paraneoplastic syndromes, need to be excluded before drug-induced neurotoxicity is presumed.[7]

Drug-induced neurological disorders may be minimised by:

- Identifying drugs that may be contributing to a patient's neurological symptoms, through either dose-related or idiosyncratic mechanisms;
- Avoiding drugs that may exacerbate pre-existing neurological disorders;
- Identifying patients at specific risk of drug-induced neurological disorders and managing appropriately.

Headache

Headache is a common symptom. The condition may be primary (e.g. migraine, tension headache) or secondary to factors such as systemic infection, head injury or drugs.[8] Drugs should always be worth considering as a possible cause, as many can cause headache and 8% of headaches may be drug-induced.[9] Headache may also be a symptom of other neurological disease, for example aseptic meningitis, idiopathic intracranial hypertension or serotonin syndrome (discussed in Chapter 13).[10,11] It is also a feature of the hypertensive crisis induced by monoamine oxidase (type A) inhibitors when taken in combination with sympathetic agonists such as ephedrine, tricyclic antidepressants, or foods containing tyramine.

Drug-induced headache may occur by various mechanisms, including (i) direct pharmacological effects, such as stretching of pain-sensitive cerebral blood vessel walls through vasodilatation or vasoconstriction;

(ii) chemical irritation of the meninges;[9,12] or (iii) as a secondary effect of other neurological disorders, such as drug-induced intracranial hypertension.

Calcium channel blockers, nitrates or hydralazine may precipitate headache due to vasodilation. Patients complaining of headache after starting treatment with these drugs should persevere, as tolerance usually develops with continued use.

Medication overuse headache

Medication overuse headache (MOH) is a term that describes chronic daily headache associated with overuse of analgesics or other medicines used to treat headache. MOH is rare when such medication is taken for conditions other than headache, such as rheumatoid arthritis, even with chronic use, although it is more likely where there is a past history of migraine.[13] Often there is a mixed picture of overlapping headache types. The International Headache Society Classification, which has extended the list of implicated substances to include triptans, defines overuse in terms of treatment days/month. Criteria are fulfilled when therapy is both regular and frequent, for example use of triptans, ergotamine, opioids or compound analgesics on 10 days or more per month, and simple analgesics on more than 15 days per month.[8] Concurrent caffeine intake in drinks or analgesic preparations may contribute. People with frequent headache often do not realise that excessive self-treatment can perpetuate the problem, and OTC analgesics as well as prescribed medicines should be considered.[10]

Medication overuse headache is difficult to manage because patients become dependent on symptomatic medication, and the headache initially rebounds on stopping the treatment. Gradual drug withdrawal supported by prophylactic use of non-steroidal anti-inflammatory drugs, amitriptyline, selective serotonin reuptake inhibitors, verapamil, beta-blockers or sodium valproate is helpful, particularly when appropriate for the primary headache. There may be only a partial response to prophylactic treatment while overuse of antiheadache drugs continues, and a better response is achieved after withdrawal. As well as headache, additional withdrawal symptoms include nausea, vomiting, arterial hypotension, tachycardia, sleep disturbances, restlessness, anxiety and nervousness, which can last for several days.[13] There is potentially a high relapse rate after successful drug withdrawal.

To minimise the problem, patients with frequent headaches should be advised about the possibility of MOH and guided on the most appropriate analgesic choice (avoiding or limiting codeine-containing compounds, in particular), the maximum frequency of use, and the preference of simple rather than combination analgesics. Monitoring the prescribing frequency of ergot derivatives and triptan medications helps identify patients using these treatments excessively. Headache diaries can usefully supplement prescription data.

Idiopathic intracranial hypertension (pseudotumour cerebri)

Drugs may cause benign intracranial hypertension (pseudotumour cerebri), an uncommon but potentially serious disorder that may lead to blindness as a result of optic nerve damage.[14] The underlying mechanism is unclear. Headache and visual disturbance are the cardinal features (headache is present in 92–98% of patients) and papilloedema (oedema of the optic nerve head) is usually detected. The diagnosis is confirmed by lumbar puncture where cerebrospinal fluid pressure is elevated. Nausea, vomiting and tinnitus may also be present.

The incidence is highest in women of childbearing age who are obese or who have recent weight gain. Drug-related causes are shown in Table 15.1.[15–17] Onset occurs days to months after initiating therapy, and withdrawing the causative agent encourages resolution. Patients prescribed drugs with a strong association, such as tetracyclines, should be informed of warning symptoms such as visual disturbance and headache, especially where other risk factors are present. Treatment is directed at preventing visual loss and symptomatic management of headache, by correcting precipitating factors (drugs, obesity) as well as pharmacologic treatments with acetazolamide or furosemide, repeat lumbar punctures and occasionally surgery. It is essential that any implicated drugs are identified and withdrawn.

Table 15.1 Drugs associated with benign intracranial hypertension

Amiodarone	Lithium
Anabolic steroids	Nalidixic acid
Corticosteroid (withdrawal)	Nitrofurantoin
Danazol	Nitrous oxide
Etretinate	Oral contraceptives
Ketamine	Tetracyclines
Leuprorelin	Valproate
Levothyroxine	Vitamin A (high doses and deficiency)

Patients with a history of benign intracranial hypertension should generally avoid drugs with a well-established association (e.g. combined oral contraceptives (COC), retinoids and vitamin A derivatives, tetracyclines). Specific risk is not clearly defined, however, nor is the interaction of other risk factors such as obesity. A history of benign intracranial hypertension is usually a contraindication to starting or continuing the COC.[17]

Aseptic meningitis

In aseptic meningitis patients develop classic symptoms of meningitis with fever, headache and meningeal signs, but an infective cause cannot be demonstrated. In severe cases, coma and hypotension may occur. Symptoms reverse rapidly on drug withdrawal. Sometimes aseptic meningitis is drug induced.[18] Because this syndrome is difficult to distinguish from infective meningitis it should be always be considered, but empirical antibiotics are required initially until the diagnosis is confirmed.[19] The two main mechanisms are thought to be direct chemical 'irritation' of the meninges by drugs entering the cerebral fluid (either through direct administration or by systemic administration followed by passage across the blood–brain barrier) or a hypersensitivity reaction involving the meninges. Some drugs associated with aseptic meningitis are listed in Table 15.2. The effect is well documented with conventional non-steroidal anti-inflammatory drugs (NSAIDs), and there are also case reports implicating cyclooxygenase-2 (COX-2) inhibitors.[20–22] Patients with a history of drug-induced aseptic meningitis should be advised to avoid NSAIDs, including OTC ibuprofen.[23] Intrathecal drug administration may directly irritate the meninges up to several weeks after drug administration, but other factors such as pre-existing CNS disease or injection of contaminants should be considered when assessing causality.[18]

The underlying conditions most commonly associated with drug-induced aseptic meningitis are systemic lupus erythematosus (SLE) or other connective tissue disorders. The mechanism for this possible predisposition is unclear; SLE may itself rarely be associated with aseptic

Table 15.2 Drugs that may cause aseptic meningitis

Azathioprine	Infliximab
Ciprofloxacin	Isoniazid
Co-trimoxazole	Monoclonal antibodies
Cytarabine (intrathecal)	Penicillin/clavulanic acid
Immunoglobulins	Vaccines

meningitis. Over 80% of patients with SLE require NSAIDs and this association should not preclude their use, but patients and prescribers should be aware of possible symptoms of this adverse effect.[24]

Effects on the neuromuscular junction and myasthenia gravis

Drugs affecting neuromuscular transmission are shown in Table 15.3.[25–27] Possible consequences include postoperative respiratory depression, the unmasking or exacerbation of myasthenia gravis, and a drug-induced myasthenic syndrome. Contributory factors include electrolyte disturbances (e.g. hyperkalaemia, hypocalcaemia) leading to muscle weakness, high drug plasma concentrations due to impaired elimination, physiologic stress such as infection or surgery, or concomitant medications.

Some drugs with neuromuscular-blocking effects, if used during the perioperative period, may prevent the re-establishment of spontaneous respiration after the procedure.[28] This problem, known as myasthenic crisis, may occur with aminoglycoside antibiotics, tetracyclines and iodinated contrast media. Features include generalised weakness and paralysis of respiratory muscles. Treatment usually involves assisted respiration and use of anticholinesterase drugs, e.g. neostigmine or pyridostigmine. Patients with myasthenia gravis usually have relative resistance to succinylcholine, whereas sensitivity to non-depolarising muscle relaxants is greatly increased.

Table 15.3 Drugs that may affect the neuromuscular junction

Aminoglycoside antibiotics – gentamicin, neomycin, clindamycin, amikacin, streptomycin	Lithium
	Macrolide antibiotics, e.g. erythromycin, clarithromcyin, azithromycin, telithromycin
Beta-blockers (including eye drops)	Magnesium
Botulinum toxin	Muscle relaxants
Calcium channel blockers	Penicillamine
Carnitine	Phenytoin
Chloroquine	Polymixins
Chlorpromazine and other antipsychotics	Procainamide
Cocaine	Quinidine
Colomycin	Quinine
Hydroxychloroquine	Quinolone antibiotics, e.g. ofloxacin, ciprofloxacin
Interferon alfa	
Interleukin-2	Tetracyclines
Iodinated radiographic contrast media	

Activation or exacerbation of myasthenia gravis

In myasthenia gravis normal transmission at the neuromuscular junction is impaired, leading to weakness and fatiguability of voluntary muscles. Characteristic features include generalised muscle weakness, ptosis, dysphonia, dysphagia, difficulty chewing, dyspnoea and respiratory failure.

Several classes of drug may worsen existing myasthenia gravis, and a small number may cause a specific variant of the condition.[25-27] Various mechanisms are proposed, including interference with neural transmission by inducing the development of acetylcholine (ACh) receptor antibodies, and inhibition of ACh synthesis or release. Other drugs may have indirect effects, for example barbiturates or benzodiazepines may exacerbate some myasthenia symptoms through their CNS depressant effects, diuretics may exacerbate muscle weakness by causing hypokalaemia, and laxatives may impair absorption of myasthenia gravis therapy, particularly pyridostigmine.

Drugs used to treat myasthenia should also be considered. Corticosteroids are a key component of management and are often used with adjunctive immunosuppressants in an attempt to achieve remission. Corticosteroids themselves may initially worsen myasthenia, usually around a week after starting treatment, requiring close patient monitoring. Pyridostigmine, a cholinesterase inhibitor, is used for symptomatic management, but excess dosing can lead to cholinergic symptoms and potentially cholinergic crisis, in which weakness is worsened.

Because of the potentially serious consequences myasthenia patients need guidance to avoid drugs such as aminoglycosides, which are strongly associated with exacerbations. Even small amounts of quinine in tonic water should be avoided. Where the drug association is less well established, or there is a clear indication for use, an individual risk–benefit assessment is required. A patient whose myasthenia is well controlled or in remission is less likely to experience adverse effects than one who has a severe chest infection associated with severe myasthenia requiring antibiotic treatment. Some drugs whose product information lists myasthenia as a caution or contraindication have been used safely in selected patients. An example is propantheline, an anticholinergic drug which is flagged as potentially problematic but which has an established role in managing peripheral cholinergic side effects associated with pyridostigmine. Although a number of case reports link interferon alfa, used to treat hepatitis C, with myasthenia gravis, myasthenia may be independently associated with hepatitis C.[29-31]

Myasthenia gravis is relatively rare, with a prevalence of 0.005–0.01%, so prescribers may not be entirely familiar with medicines that may exacerbate the condition. Patient guidance is essential, using, for example, lists produced by the Myasthenia Gravis Association and a medical card to highlight the need for cautious prescribing.[25]

There is no evidence that vaccines worsen myasthenia. Indeed, for those patients on immunosuppressants for this and other neurological diseases with an immune basis, vaccines are specifically indicated where appropriate (except live vaccines). Influenza and pneumococcal vaccinations are usually indicated, as patients are at higher risk of infection.

Drug-induced myasthenic syndrome

In this uncommon syndrome the patient rapidly develops features of myasthenia gravis that remit promptly on drug withdrawal. In some cases, drug exposure unmasks myasthenia in predisposed patients. Again, factors such as electrolyte disturbances or impaired drug elimination may contribute. This syndrome can be distinguished from true myasthenia gravis by the absence of acetylcholine receptor antibodies. Drugs implicated include aminoglycoside antibiotics, polymixins, beta-blockers and phenytoin.

Penicillamine may cause a syndrome almost identical to myasthenia gravis, mainly in patients with other autoimmune diseases such as rheumatoid arthritis, but also in Wilson's disease. In some cases respiratory deterioration is wrongly attributed to chronic pulmonary disease. Nearly all such patients have acetylcholine receptor antibodies, but the condition usually remits within a year of discontinuing penicillamine. Although the exact mechanism has not been determined, an immunological basis is likely.[32]

Seizures

Drugs may precipitate seizures, although the incidence is low. Risk factors include pre-existing epilepsy or a history of seizures, cerebral or systemic disease (e.g. cerebrovascular disease or infection), or treatment with drugs known to reduce the seizure threshold.[33–35] Mechanisms include (i) a direct epileptogenic effect, related to either taking the drug or withdrawal; or (ii) a secondary effect as a consequence of another problem, e.g. metabolic effects such as hypoglycaemia, hyponatraemia, or syndrome of inappropriate secretion of antidiuretic hormone (SIADH), hyperpyrexia or hypoxia; or (iii) a drug interaction leading to reduced efficacy of antiepileptic drugs. Risk factors include patient factors such as structural brain abnormalities, altered pharmacokinetics (as a result of renal impairment or drug interactions); excessive drug dosing or rate of dose escalation. The risk of seizure may vary between individual drugs within the same or similar classes. Thus there has been interest in, for example, comparing the newer atypical antipsychotics such as clozapine with conventional agents such as chlorpromazine and haloperidol.[36–38]

Loss of seizure control has potentially serious implications in established epilepsy. As well as the morbidity and mortality from seizures, a single medication-induced seizure has consequences such as loss of driving licence. Patients with epilepsy should be encouraged to check new treatments (prescriptions, OTC and complementary medicines).[34] St John's Wort is a key example of a complementary medicine that interacts with antiepileptics via the induction of cytochrome P450 isoenzymes.[39]

Antiepileptic drugs can themselves provoke or aggravate seizures and trigger new seizure types, as well as aggravate pre-existing seizures. Carbamazepine may precipitate or exacerbate absence, atonic or myoclonic seizures in patients with generalised epilepsies, and both phenytoin and vigabatrin have been implicated in worsening particularly generalised seizures. Although well documented in the context of antiepileptic drug toxicity, therapeutic doses are sometimes considered proconvulsant. Distinguishing from other causes is difficult: for example, seizures attributed to antiepileptics but actually due to porphyria have been described. Risk factors include antiepileptic-drug-induced encephalopathy or hepatotoxicity (e.g. with valproate), polypharmacy, or inappropriate choice of drug to treat the seizure type, especially in children. At least two separate mechanisms operate: first, a syndrome of drug toxicity, which may be reversible with dose reduction or removal of polypharmacy; and second, a distinct adverse primary action of the drug in specific seizure types due to incorrect diagnosis of the seizure type or epilepsy syndrome, use of a drug contraindicated in the specific type of epilepsy, or prescription of excessive drug dosages or combinations.[40]

Seizures have been attributed to co-prescription of ciprofloxacin and theophylline, and although this appears rare the combination should be avoided if possible. Presumed risk factors include seizure history, hypokalaemia, alkalosis, renal failure, and concomitant NSAID treatment.[41]

Withdrawal seizures usually occur soon after stopping a drug and are well documented with barbiturates, benzodiazepines and alcohol, but may also occur with other antiepileptics, even when used for other medical conditions, such as neuropathic pain.[33,42]

Table 15.4 Drugs that may cause seizures

Anaesthetics, e.g. enflurane, isoflurane, ketamine, propofol, bupivacaine
Antibiotics, e.g. penicillins, carbapenems, cephalosporins, quinolones
Antidepressants, e.g. tricyclics, SSRIs
Antiepileptic drugs or their withdrawal
Antimalarials, e.g. chloroquine, mefloquine
Antipsychotics
Antiretrovirals, e.g. zidovudine, efavirenz
Baclofen or its withdrawal
Cholinesterase inhibitors, e.g. donepezil
Ciclosporin
Drugs of abuse, e.g. cocaine, amfetamines, methylenedioxymethamfetamine
    (MDMA or Ecstasy)
Isoniazid
Ketamine
Lidocaine
Lithium
Non-steroidal anti-inflammatory drugs
Oral contraceptives
Pethidine and other opioids
Theophylline
Tramadol
Tricyclic antidepressants
Vaccines
Vincristine

Table 15.4 shows some drugs that may cause seizures. Postmarketing surveillance has played a key role in recognising these effects.[35] Although evidence of causality is variable in several areas, there are well-recognised associations that should inform the choice of drug for particular indications in patients with epilepsy. The treatment of choice for depression, for example, is usually an SSRI such as paroxetine or citalopram.[43] Malaria prophylaxis for overseas travel requires an assessment of local risk, but mefloquine and chloroquine are usually avoided.[34] The incidence of seizures with psychotropic medications is generally low. The UK Committee on Safety of Medicines has warned against using tramadol unless essential in patients with epilepsy or risk factors for seizures.[44]

Coma and encephalopathy

The clinical features of drug-induced coma are similar regardless of the drug involved. Coma involves depressed cortical and cerebral function and is a profound state of unconsciousness from which the individual cannot be aroused. It features loss of brainstem reflexes, generalised flaccidity, and depressed or absent tendon reflexes. Encephalopathy is a general term for cerebral dysfunction with a spectrum of symptoms, including tremor, myoclonus, confusion, lethargy, agitation, hallucinations and seizures. Drug-induced coma can arise through a primary neurotoxic effect on the CNS, through indirect effects on cerebral metabolism, or through alterations in cerebral blood flow. Primary neurotoxic effects are usually dose related. Most cases of drug-induced coma are caused by poisoning or overdose with drugs acting on the CNS, including benzodiazepines, antipsychotics, antidepressants and opioids (including those in OTC cough medicines).[45] Patient factors affecting metabolism or elimination may contribute to neurotoxicity as a result of drug accumulation.

Ciclosporin may cause coma among other neurological adverse effects, including encephalopathy with seizures and movement disorders.[46,47] A direct toxic effect on vascular endothelial cells in the nervous system is suggested, resulting in uncontrolled cerebral vasospasm. Neurotoxicity may be independent of plasma ciclosporin concentrations. Possible risk factors include high-dose steroid therapy, hypocholesterolaemia, hypomagnesaemia and systemic hypertension. Ciclosporin encephalopathy is a form of posterior leukoencephalopathy which requires removal of the offending drug to prevent irreversible brain damage.

Aciclovir, ganciclovir and valaciclovir may cause neurotoxicity. Symptoms usually occur within the first few days of treatment. Risk factors include intravenous administration, the use of high doses, renal impairment and old age.[48] Acute renal failure and neurotoxicity has been associated with oral aciclovir administration even in mild pre-existing renal impairment.[49] Aciclovir is frequently used at high intravenous doses for herpes simplex encephalitis, and distinguishing adverse drug effects from the primary condition is challenging.[50]

Coma and seizures are described with the immunosuppressants tacrolimus and muromonab-CD3.[51]

A number of cytotoxic drugs, including cisplatin, ifosfamide and high-dose methotrexate, may cause direct neurotoxicity.[7,52] Encephalopathy, coma and blindness suggesting posterior leukoencephalopathy are reported with vincristine. Inadvertent intrathecal administration of vincristine into the cerebrospinal fluid (CSF) causes an encephalopathy that is usually fatal even with rapid CSF drainage. Adherence to strict government recommendations on the intrathecal use of cytotoxic drugs should prevent such cases.[53]

Antiepileptics may cause encephalopathy, which is usually dose related. Prevention strategies include plasma concentration monitoring where appropriate, and patient education in the signs of toxicity. Valproate may cause coma in association with hyperammonaemia, especially when given intravenously, at high doses, or in association with hepatic impairment.[54]

Severe and prolonged hypoglycaemia can cause coma. Drugs with metabolic effects (discussed in Chapter 9) can therefore lead to this. Risk factors that contribute substantially to the morbidity and mortality of diabetic patients with drug-induced hypoglycaemic coma are age over 60 years, renal impairment, decreased energy intake and infection.[55] Glibenclamide in some herbal medicines may cause coma and death.[4]

Neuropathies

Drugs may have toxic effects on cranial and peripheral nerves.

Cranial neuropathies

Symptoms of cranial nerve toxicity depend on the nerve affected. These nerves are involved in vision and eye movements, smell, taste, hearing and balance. Toxicity, probably due to damage to the third (oculomotor) cranial nerve, affects 1–10% of patients receiving vinca alkaloids. The main features are ptosis (drooping eyelids) and ophthalmoplegia (paralysis of the eye muscles). Other cytotoxics causing cranial neuropathy include ifosfamide, platinum compounds and fluorouracil.[7,52]

Ethambutol may cause optic neuropathy, with loss of visual acuity, colour blindness and reduced visual fields. Visual acuity should be tested before starting ethambutol and patients should have regular eye examinations and asked to report changes in vision. If visual complications develop, early treatment cessation is important for recovery of normal eyesight. Risk factors include high drug dose and poor renal function. Other drugs associated with optic neuritis include amiodarone, hydroxychloroquine, infliximab and linezolid. Some drugs associated with primary retinopathy, such as vigabatrin and desferrioxamine, also cause optic neuropathy.[56–58]

Peripheral neuropathies

Peripheral neuropathy is a general term encompassing several disorders of peripheral nerves, i.e. nerves distal to the spinal cord and spinal nerve roots. Drug-induced peripheral neuropathy is uncommon but usually reversible on early drug withdrawal.[59,60] Depending on the type of nerve damage, different features arise. Patients often complain of symmetrical numbness and tingling (paraesthesia) in the hands and feet, which is referred to as 'glove and stocking' neuropathy. There may be muscle weakness and wasting and sensory loss. Nerve conduction studies ascertain the type of neuropathy and nerves affected, and can reveal axonal degeneration or breakdown of the myelin sheath (demyelination). Neuropathies may be predominantly sensory, motor, or a mixture of both.

Possible risk factors for drug-induced neuropathy are shown in Table 15.5 and drugs known to cause peripheral neuropathy in Table 15.6.

Alcohol is a common cause of neuropathy, arising mainly from nutritional deficiency and a reduced capacity to absorb thiamine, although a direct toxic effect on peripheral nerves may also be involved. The clinical features are similar to those of beri-beri, but there may be associated problems such as Wernicke–Korsakoff encephalopathy. Thiamine is widely used to prevent and treat this problem in alcohol-dependent patients. Thiamine should never be given acutely with glucose initially, as this may cause severe metabolic encephalopathy and neurologic sequelae.[61]

Table 15.5 Risk factors for drug-induced neuropathy

Diabetes mellitus
Alcoholism
Vitamin deficiency/poor nutrition
Impaired renal/hepatic function (leading to drug accumulation)
Slow acetylator status (isoniazid, hydralazine)

Table 15.6 Drugs that may cause peripheral neuropathy

Alcohol	Metronidazole
Amiodarone	Nitrofurantoin
Antiretrovirals, e.g. nucleosides	Phenytoin
Chloramphenicol	Platinum compounds (cisplatin, carboplatin)
Colchicine	Pyridoxine (vitamin B_6)
Dapsone	Quinolones
Disulfiram	Stavudine
Ethambutol	Taxanes (paclitaxel, docetaxel)
Hydralazine	Thalidomide
Interferon alfa	Vinca alkaloids (vincristine)
Isoniazid	Zalcitabine
Linezolid	Zidovudine

Peripheral neuropathies are well-established side effects of cytotoxic agents, such as the vinca alkaloids, platinum-containing compounds, etoposide and taxanes.[7,52,60] The problem is dose related and of
particular relevance now that the bone marrow suppression associated
with high-intensity regimens can be managed with growth factors or
even bone marrow transplant. Mild sensory symptoms are often tolerated
to achieve a therapeutic response, but progression from wrist and finger
weakness may necessitate adjustment of the cytotoxic regimen.
Peripheral neuropathies caused by cytotoxics need to be distinguished
from neuropathies due to paraneoplastic mechanisms or caused by
direct effects of cancer, such as nerve compression.

Isoniazid is one of the best-recognised causes, leading to a mixed sen-
sorimotor neuropathy, especially in slow acetylators. Interference with
pyridoxine metabolism can be prevented by prophylaxis with pyridoxine, ensuring a sufficient dose to take account of other risk factors. Slow
acetylators also have increased susceptibility to peripheral neuropathy
caused by hydralazine and dapsone (see Chapter 3).

Paradoxically, pyridoxine itself may cause neuropathy at high doses.
Pyridoxine is widely available and patients should be advised to take no
more than 10 mg/day as a vitamin supplement, although higher doses
are prescribed in those at risk of deficiency, for example patients taking
isoniazid with other risk factors.

Peripheral neuropathy is a well-documented adverse effect of antiretroviral drugs, particularly the nucleoside reverse transcriptase inhibitors,
including didanosine, stavudine, zidovudine and zalcitabine.[62] It may
resolve with dose reduction, but may require discontinuation. The temporal relationship may help distinguish drug-induced peripheral neuropathy from that associated with human immunodeficiency virus (HIV)
itself. As well as the recognised risk factors for drug-induced peripheral
neuropathy, patients at particular risk include those with a low CD4 count,
a prior history of an AIDS-defining illness or neoplasm, or a previous
history of peripheral neuropathy. This complication may be prevented to
some extent by choosing lower-risk agents and by close monitoring
during treatment.

Peripheral neuropathy (and associated myopathy) with lipid-lowering
drugs such as simvastatin is well established, and to minimise this risk the
manufacturers' recommended doses should not be exceeded. The risk of
toxicity may increase through concomitant use of cytochrome P450
isoenzyme inhibitors, which may affect metabolism.[63]

Thalidomide is a well-documented cause of neuropathy, which can
be irreversible. Testing nerve conduction before treatment and at regular

intervals thereafter, educating about early symptoms and risk factors, and keeping doses low may minimise this effect. The effect is sometimes reversible, but stopping the drug requires a risk–benefit assessment and depends on the disease being treated.[64]

Guillain–Barré syndrome

Guillain–Barré syndrome is a rare immune-mediated acute symmetrical polyneuropathy which presents as rapidly progressive paralysis with areflexia and variable sensory involvement. It can be life-threatening if paralysis of the respiratory muscles ensues, and a quarter to a third of all patients with Guillain–Barré syndrome require ventilatory support. Weakness progresses rapidly, starting with paraesthesia of the toes and fingertips, followed by upper and lower limb and then total body weakness, and involves cranial as well as respiratory muscles. Guillain–Barré syndrome may be associated with drugs, but the interval from treatment has varied between days and 14 months.[59] Immunoglobulins or plasmapheresis are used in all but the mildest cases. Guillain–Barré syndrome frequently follows an infection (e.g. *Campylobacter* enteritis, viral infections), but vaccines have not been shown to have a causal effect. Table 15.7 lists drugs that are associated with causing Guillain–Barré syndrome.

Drug-induced movement disorders

Drug-induced movement disorders include parkinsonism (tremor, rigidity, akinesia), neuroleptic malignant syndrome, acute dystonia, acute akathisia and tardive dyskinesia.[65–75] Neuroleptic malignant syndrome is discussed in Chapter 13.

Table 15.7 Drugs associated with Guillain–Barré syndrome

Captopril
Corticosteroids
Gold
Penicillamine
Streptokinase
Vaccines, e.g. hepatitis B, influenza, MMR

MMR, measles, mumps and rubella.

Parkinsonism

Drugs may precipitate parkinsonism or exacerbate pre-existing parkinsonism. This is a frequent problem with drugs that affect dopaminergic neurotransmission in the basal ganglia. The mechanism may be depletion of presynaptic dopamine or blockage of postsynaptic dopamine receptors. Drug-induced parkinsonism is often clinically indistinguishable from Parkinson's disease (i.e. primary parkinsonism), although in drug-induced cases postural tremor is more frequent and other movement disorders such as tardive dyskinesia or akathisia are sometimes present. In most patients (90%) parkinsonism develops within 3 months of starting the causative drug. It is usually reversible within weeks or months of drug withdrawal, although in some cases this may be longer, which may reflect unmasking of subclinical idiopathic Parkinson's disease. Usually antiparkinsonian therapy is delayed for at least 3 months after drug withdrawal, but functional imaging using single photon emission computerised tomography (CT), a measure of the presynaptic dopamine transporter system, may be used to differentiate drug-induced parkinsonism from idiopathic Parkinson's disease, enabling earlier diagnosis and management.[10]

A number of commonly prescribed drugs, for example metoclopramide, prochlorperazine or antipsychotics, are likely to induce or exacerbate parkinsonism. These should be withdrawn where possible, and avoided in patients who already have Parkinson's disease. A detailed drug history is necessary in patients presenting with parkinsonism, as many other drugs have also been implicated. Where the causality is less clear or other therapeutic options are not available, the risk–benefit ratio of continuing (or starting) treatment should be considered. Patients with parkinsonism should be monitored for worsened symptoms when new medication is started, but this can be difficult against a background of fluctuating and progressing disease. Table 15.8 lists some drugs associated with parkinsonism.

Neuropsychiatric features such as hallucinations and cognitive impairment are associated with Parkinson's disease and can be particularly

Table 15.8 Drugs that may induce or exacerbate parkinsonism

Antidepressants
Antiemetics, e.g. prochlorperazine, metoclopramide
Antipsychotics (including atypical antipsychotics)
Calcium channel blockers – flunarizine, cinnarizine
Tetrabenazine

difficult to treat. Drugs with neuropsychiatric effects should be used with caution, and these are discussed in Chapter 13. Elderly patients with dementia are particularly susceptible to extrapyramidal reactions, especially if the parkinsonism is due to Lewy body dementia.[69] In some cases low-dose antipsychotic treatment may be helpful. Cholinesterase inhibitors may be beneficial but are not licensed for this indication.[70]

Tardive dyskinesia

Tardive dyskinesia (TD) is a chronic involuntary movement disorder associated with use of antipsychotic drugs.[67] Symptoms include choreiform (i.e. rapid and jerky), athetoid (slow and sinuous) or rhythmic stereotyped movements involving the tongue, jaw, trunk or extremities. The most common form involves orofacial movements (buccolinguomasticatory syndrome). It is variable in severity and persistence but can be socially disabling, and can be severe enough to compromise functional capacity (e.g. speaking, eating and walking). TD occurs during or within a few weeks of stopping long-term treatment (at least a month in patients older than 60 years, and at least 3 months in younger patients) with a dopamine antagonist. Estimates of prevalence are hampered by difficulty in distinguishing TD from spontaneous dyskinesias, which may occur as a disease-associated effect in schizophrenia. However, around 10–20% of patients taking long-term conventional antipsychotics may exhibit this reaction.

The atypical antipsychotics are less likely to cause TD because they impair extrapyramidal function less. Although many case reports implicate clozapine, previous conventional antipsychotic use is frequent and it is difficult to distinguish between drug-induced TD and spontaneous dyskinesia. With other atypical antipsychotics, such as risperidone and olanzapine, there is evidence of a substantially lower risk of TD than with conventional antipsychotics.

Although increased use of atypical antipsychotics will reduce tardive dyskinesia rates, the condition remains important in clinical practice. Many patients remain on conventional antipsychotics for whom risk factors and prevention need to be considered, and patients with this condition require appropriate management. Risk factors include age, co-morbidities, coadministration of anticholinergic agents (which is no longer recommended for the prevention of parkinsonism because of the risk of unmasking or worsening tardive dyskinesia), and predominant negative or cognitive symptoms in schizophrenic patients. Because there is no effective treatment, preventive strategies are important such as using the lowest dose of antipsychotic required, using atypical agents, informing patients of the risk, and monitoring. Approaches to treatment have variable response, but include withdrawal or reduction of the antipsychotic, switching to an atypical antipsychotic, and stopping concomitant anticholinergic medication if appropriate. Off-label use of benzodiazepines, vitamin E or cholinesterase inhibitors is unproven. Any antipsychotic agent may mask TD if given in sufficient doses, but conventional antipsychotics are thought to inhibit recovery whereas atypical agents may enhance recovery, and there is some evidence that clozapine may improve the condition or even achieve remission.

Tardive dyskinesia needs to be differentiated from other neurological movement disorders, such as Huntington's chorea, and from other drug-induced movement disorders due to agents such as phenytoin, oestrogens, antidepressants or levodopa.[71]

Acute dystonia

Acute dystonia is characterised by abnormal postures or muscle spasms. These may manifest as abnormal movements of the head and neck (e.g. torticollis), spasms of the jaw muscles (e.g. trismus), grimacing, dysphonia, or tongue spasms leading to problems with speech, oculogyric crisis and opisthotonus.[72] Dystonia is described as acute or chronic (tardive), depending on onset, but the symptoms are practically identical. Acute drug-induced dystonia is most commonly associated with antipsychotics, particularly high-potency drugs such as the butyrophenones, fluphenazine and pimozide. Lower-potency agents such as chlorpromazine and the atypical antipsychotics such as olanzapine and quetiapine are associated with a low incidence of acute dystonia. It may also occur with antiemetics such as metoclopramide (which should be avoided or used at low doses in patients at high risk), SSRIs and antiparkinsonian agents. Other agents implicated, with varying evidence of causality, are shown in Table 15.9.

Acute dystonia with antipsychotic drugs generally develops within 7 days of starting treatment, after a dose change, or after reducing

Table 15.9 Some drugs that may cause dystonia

5-HT$_1$ antagonists, e.g. sumatriptan
Antiepileptic drugs, e.g. carbamazepine, phenytoin
Antipsychotics (especially high potency)
Antiparkinsonian drugs
Calcium channel blockers, e.g. verapamil, diltiazem, cinnarizine
SSRI antidepressants
Metoclopramide and related drugs

medication given to prevent or treat extrapyramidal effects (e.g. anticholinergics). In most cases it will resolve within 24 hours. Tardive dystonia is much less frequent and occurs only after months or years of treatment.

Acute dystonia is very frightening for the patient. Awareness of risk factors is helpful: younger age, female gender (with metoclopramide), previous instance of acute dystonia and recent cocaine use.

Acute akathisia

Akathisia is a subjective sensation of restlessness, with an incidence of 20–75% in patients treated with antipsychotics.[73] Patients find it highly disturbing and it often leads to rocking, pacing and an inability to keep still, which may be mistaken for psychotic agitation leading to further antipsychotic treatment which worsens or prolongs the condition.[68]

Myoclonus

Myoclonus is a sudden abrupt 'shock-like' involuntary movement caused by muscular contractions or sudden brief lapses in muscle contraction in active postural muscles. It has various causes, such as neurodegenerative and systemic metabolic disorders and CNS infections. It can also be caused by drugs such as levodopa, tricylic antidepressants and bismuth salts, and multiple other agents are implicated anecdotally. The mechanism is not fully understood, but may be partly due to increased serotonergic transmission. It usually resolves on drug withdrawal, but may sometimes require specific treatment with clonazepam or tetrabenazine.[76]

Sudden sleep onset with dopaminergic drugs

Somolence is common in Parkinson's disease and may be aggravated by dopaminergic drugs, including levodopa and dopamine agonists.[77–80] 'Sudden onset of sleep' is associated with the non-ergot dopamine agonists (ropinirole and pramipexole), and patients developing this complication need to refrain from driving. Dopamine agonists may unmask severe sleepiness causing a 'sleep attack' similar to a narcoleptic event. Increasing evidence supports the early use of dopamine agonists in Parkinson's disease to delay levodopa therapy and motor complications, and many such patients may be driving. Ergot-based dopamine agonists are an alternative but cause cardiopulmonary fibrotic reactions. Changing between dopamine agonists is an option, but often the agent needs to be stopped.[81] Slower titration may be helpful. Enquiry about sleepiness and scoring such as on the Epworth Sleep Scale may help assess the risk.[80] Concurrent sedative drugs should only be used only with caution.

CASE STUDY 15.1

Mr A is a 65-year-old man with Parkinson's disease, diagnosed 7 years ago. Over the last few months he has experienced a deterioration in symptom control, and although various treatment changes have reduced 'off' time he has become confused and has difficulty sleeping. His wife reports that he has flailing movements suggesting dyskinesias, especially in the late afternoon and early evening. Mr A is currently prescribed:

Half Sinemet CR (100/25) half a tablet four times a day
Sinemet Plus 100/25 four times a day
Pergolide 1 mg five times a day
Selegiline 5 mg twice a day
Atenolol 25 mg once a day
Temazepam 10 mg at night.

What are dyskinesias, and which drugs are they associated with?

Dyskinesias are severe levodopa-induced involuntary movements. Dyskinesia sometimes shows a temporal relationship with the dose, perhaps associated with high plasma concentrations (peak-dose dyskinesia), but often a diphasic pattern may follow where the patient switches 'on' and 'off' less predictably in relation to dose. This may necessitate using smaller and more frequent doses of levodopa, but although this may give a more constant level in the plasma this in itself does not generally solve the problem of dyskinesias. Motor fluctuations can also result from erratic absorption and accumulation of levodopa during the day, leading to dyskinesia in the evening ('time-bomb effect').

Dopamine agonists are increasingly selected as first-line therapy in Parkinson's disease. They are associated with lower rates of motor complications, including dyskinesia. Levodopa remains the gold standard of treatment in terms of motor benefit, and all Parkinson's patients ultimately require levodopa treatment. In later disease stages dyskinesias may be even more troublesome than impaired motor function. However, most patients tolerate dyskinesia rather than suffer immobility.

→

CASE STUDY 15.1 (continued)

How can dyskinesias be managed?

There are various options for the management of dyskinesia. The trade-off between improvement of dyskinesias and potential motor impairment needs to be considered, depending on patient preference. Simplifying the levodopa regimen to one formulation (standard rather than controlled release) may produce benefits. An alternative dopamine agonist may be tried, such as ropinirole or pramipexole. Amantadine may provide some benefit in patients with dyskinesia. Subcutaneous apomorphine infusion may be beneficial in patients with dyskinesia where other options are ineffective, as it enables more continuous dopaminergic stimulation.

What other drug safety issues does this case raise?

The pergolide dose is above the normal recommended maximum. Because it may cause ergot-related side effects such as cardiac valvulopathy and other fibrotic reactions, reducing to 4.5 mg daily or conversion to another dopamine agonist is appropriate. If pergolide is maintained, episodic screening for ergot side effects is necessary (blood tests, chest X-ray, echocardiogram, and possibly respiratory function tests). If Mr A is changed to a non-ergot derivative he should be warned about excess daytime sleepiness and sudden onset of sleep, especially if he drives.

The prescribed dose of Half Sinemet CR is unusual and is probably meant to be Half Sinemet CR one tablet. The name of this preparation often causes confusion. Accurate drug history taking is important in people with Parkinson's disease, many of whom are likely to be on complex therapy, to prevent further adverse effects or treatment failure.

Benzodiazepines may exacerbate cognitive impairment and contribute to the risk of falls. Many patients with advanced Parkinson's disease are sedentary, and the disease and its treatment contribute to fatigue. Guidance to both patient and carer to limit daytime sleep may be helpful. Selegiline may also cause insomnia due to amfetamine metabolites, and for this reason both doses should be given before early afternoon.

Is Mr A's confusion likely to be drug induced?

Confusion may be related to drugs or to the underlying disease process. Assessment of cognitive function, and excluding causes such as intercurrent infection or metabolic derangement, may be useful. Discontinuation of adjunctive therapy (dopamine agonist or selegiline) may become appropriate if Parkinson's-related dementia supervenes.

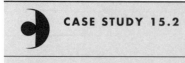

Mrs J, a 45-year-old woman, was admitted to hospital with worsening symptoms of tiredness and muscle weakness that were diagnosed as myasthenia gravis. Her previous medical history included hypertension, and she was taking bendroflumethiazide 2.5 mg daily and amlodipine 5 mg daily.

Mrs J was started on a combination of pyridostigmine 30 mg four times a day, prednisolone 60 mg once a day and azathioprine 50 mg daily.

Is it likely that myasthenia gravis is drug induced in this patient?

This depends on other factors, such as the temporal relationship. The possibility of an iatrogenic component should always be explored. Neither medication currently taken is strongly associated with precipitating myasthenia gravis, although calcium channel blockers theoretically affect neuromuscular transmission, and electrolyte imbalances from diuretics may contribute. Enquiry should be made about OTC and complementary medicines being taken. Even if these drugs have contributed it is likely that myasthenia treatment will be required.

What neurological adverse effects should Mrs J be warned about, and how can these be minimised?

Pyridostigmine needs to be closely tailored to the patient's symptoms, as too-high doses may cause cholinergic crisis, which has similar symptoms to myasthenia gravis. Patients with myasthenia can often judge when their next pyridostigmine dose is due by symptoms that worsen over the dosing period.

Prednisolone and azathioprine have been started to induce remission through immunosuppression. Azathioprine is titrated slowly and takes weeks to months to reach full therapeutic effect. High starting doses of prednisolone often paradoxically worsen the myasthenia gravis at week 1, and is therefore usually started as an inpatient treatment. An alternative prednisolone strategy – low dose titrated upwards – is sometimes suitable in an outpatient setting.

Consideration of non-neurological side effects, such as osteoporosis, hypertension or infection, is important.

What other information does Mrs J require?

Mrs J should be given a list of medicines that may worsen myasthenia and advised to discuss with a healthcare professional every time a new medicine is prescribed or purchased. Because her condition is relatively rare she should be given contact details for further advice. Special mention should be made of

→

> **CASE STUDY 15.2** (continued)
>
> infection, such as chest and urinary infections, which require prompt treatment in people with myasthenia (because infection may precipitate myasthenic crisis) where a number of antibiotics are contraindicated. Agents such as macrolides, tetracyclines or quinolone antibiotics may worsen myasthenia, but are sometimes used cautiously with appropriate monitoring if other options are unsuitable after careful risk–benefit assessment. Penicillins or cephalosporins or other beta-lactams such as meropenem or imipenem are generally considered safer in myasthenia gravis, and would normally be preferred as first-line treatment depending on the suspected causative organisms. Other agents that appear to be safe in myasthenia include vancomycin, teicoplanin, rifampicin and metronidazole.

References

1. Wittbrodt ET. Drugs and myasthenia gravis. *Arch Intern Med* 1997; 157: 399–407.
2. Blain PG, Lane JM. Neurological disorders. In: Davies DM, ed. *Textbook of Adverse Drug Reactions*, 5th edn. Oxford: Oxford Medical Publications, 1998: 585–629.
3. Schliamser SE, Cars O, Norrby SR. Neurotoxicity of beta-lactam antibiotics: predisposing factors and pathogenesis. *J Antimicrob Chemother* 1991; 27: 405–425.
4. Committee on Safety of Medicines. Reminder: safety of traditional Chinese medicines and herbal remedies. *Curr Probl Pharmacovigilance* 2004; 30: 10–11.
5. Khanna D, McMahon M, Furst DE. Safety of tumour necrosis factor-alpha antagonists. *Drug Safety* 2004; 27: 307–324.
6. Sheridan C. Tysabri raises alarm bells on drug class. *Nature Biotechnol* 2005; 23: 397–398.
7. Verstappen CC, Heimans JJ, Hoekman K, *et al.* Neurotoxic complications of chemotherapy in patients with cancer: clinical signs and optimal management *Drugs* 2003; 63: 1549–1563.
8. Headache Classification Subcommittee of the International Headache Society. The International Classification of Headache Disorders, 2nd edn. *Cephalalgia* 2004; 24(Suppl 1): 1–151.
9. Toth C. Medications and substances as a cause of headache: a systematic review of the literature. *Clin Neuropharmacol* 2003; 26: 122–136.
10. Grosset KA, Grosset DG. Prescribed drugs and neurological complications. *J Neurol Neurosurg Psychiatry* 2004; 75(Suppl III): iii2–iii8.
11. Ener RA, Meglathery SB, Van Decker WA, Gallacher RM. Serotonin syndrome and other serotonergic disorders. *Pain Med* 2003; 4: 63–74.

12. Levin M. The many causes of headache. Migraine, vascular, drug-induced and more. *Postgrad Med* 2002; 112: 67–82.

13. Katsarava A, Diener H-C, Limmroth V. Medication overuse headache. A focus on analgesics, ergot alkaloids and triptans. *Drug Safety* 2001; 24: 921–927.

14. Uddin ABMS. Drug-induced pseudotumour cerebri. *Clin Neuropharmacol* 2003; 26: 236–238.

15. Friedman DJ. Medication-induced intracranial hypertension in dermatology. *Am J Clin Dermatol* 2005; 6: 29–37.

16. Digre KB. Not so benign intracranial hypertension [Editorial]. *Br Med J* 2003; 326: 613–614.

17. Guillebaud J. *Contraception: Your Questions Answered*, 4th edn. London: Churchill Livingstone, 2004.

18. Jolles S, Sewell WA, Leighton C. Drug-induced aseptic meningitis: diagnosis and management. *Drug Safety* 2000; 22: 215–226.

19. Moris G, Garcia-Monco JC. The challenge of drug-induced aseptic meningitis. *Arch Intern Med* 1999; 159: 1185–1194.

20. Ashwath ML, Katner HP. Recurrent aseptic meningitis due to different non-steroidal anti-inflammatory drugs including rofecoxib. *Postgrad Med J* 2003; 79: 295–296.

21. Papaioannides DH, Korantzopoulos PG, Giotis CH. Aseptic meningitis possibly associated with celecoxib. *Ann Pharmacother* 2004; 38: 172.

22. Nguyen HT, Juurlink DN. Recurrent ibuprofen-induced aseptic meningitis. *Ann Pharmacother* 2004; 38: 408–410.

23. Olin JL, Gugliotta JL. Possible valaciclovir-related neurotoxicity and aseptic meningitis. *Ann Pharmacother* 2003; 37: 1814–1817.

24. Horizon AA, Wallace DJ. Risk:benefit ratio of nonsteroidal anti-inflammatory drugs in systemic lupus erythematosus. *Expert Opin Drug Safety* 2004; 3: 273–278.

25. Freedman S. Drugs which may exacerbate myasthenia gravis. Myasthenia Gravis Association, accessed 28 February 2005. http://www.mgauk.org/main/mgdrugs1.htm

26. Wittbrodt ET. Drugs and myasthenia gravis: an update. *Arch Intern Med* 1997; 157: 399–408.

27. Saleh FG, Seidman RJ. Drug-induced myopathy and neuropathy. *J Clin Neuromusc Dis* 2003; 5: 81–92.

28. Stevens RD. Neuromuscular disorders and anaesthesia. *Curr Opin Anaesthesiol* 2001; 14: 693–698.

29. Redig PJ, Newman PK. Untreated hepatitis C may provoke myasthenia gravis. *J Neurol Neurosurg Psychiatry* 1998; 64: 820.

30. Battochi AP, Evoli A, Servidei S, *et al.* Myasthenia gravis during interferon alfa therapy. *Neurology* 1995; 45: 382–383.

31. Bori I, Karli N, Bakar M, *et al.* Myasthenia gravis following IFN-alpha-2a treatment. *Eur Neurol* 1997; 38: 68.

32. Adelman HM, Winters PR, Mahan SC, *et al.* D-Penicillamine-induced myasthenia gravis: diagnosis obscured by co-existing chronic obstructive pulmonary disease. *Am J Med Sci* 1995; 309: 191–193.

33. Coleman JJ. Drug-induced seizures. *Adv Drug React Bull* 2004; 227: 1–4.

34. Scottish Intercollegiate Guidelines Network. *Diagnosis and Management of Epilepsy in Adults*. SIGN Guideline number 70, 2003.

35. Murphy K, Delanty N. Drug-induced seizures: general principles in assessment, management and prevention. *CNS Drugs* 2000; 14: 135–146.

36. Lee KC, Finley PR, Alldredge BK. Risk of seizures associated with psychotropic medications: emphasis on new drugs and new findings. *Expert Opin Drug Safety* 2003; 2: 233–247.

37. Pisani F, Oteri G, Costa C, Di Raimondo G, Di Perri R. Effects of psychotropic drugs on seizure threshold. *Drug Safety* 2002; 25: 91–110.

38. Alldredge BK. Seizure risk associated with psychotropic drugs: Clinical and pharmacokinetic considerations. *Neurology* 1999; 53(Suppl 2): S68–S75.

39. Committee on Safety of Medicines. Reminder. St John's Wort (*Hypericum perforatum*) interactions. *Curr Probl Pharmacovigilance* 2000; 26: 6–7.

40. Perucca E. Gram L, Avanzini G, Dulac O. Antiepileptic drugs as a cause of worsening seizures. *Epilepsia* 1998; 39: 5–17.

41. Committee on Safety of Medicines. Convulsions due to quinolone antimicrobial agents. *Curr Probl Pharmacovigilance* 1991; 32: 3.

42. Committee on Safety of Medicines. Withdrawal reactions with paroxetine. *Curr Probl Pharmacovigilance* 2003; 29: 4.

43. Harden CL, Goldstein MA. Mood disorders in people with epilepsy: recognition and management. *CNS Drugs* 2002; 16: 291–301.

44. Committee on Safety of Medicines. Tramadol (Zydol, Tramake and Zamadol). *Curr Probl Pharmacovigilance* 1996; 22: 11.

45. Cartlidge NEF. Drug-induced coma. *Adv Drug React Bull* 1981; 88: 320–333.

46. Hauben M. Cyclosporin neurotoxicity. *Pharmacotherapy* 1996; 16: 576–583.

47. Madan B, Schey SA. Reversible cortical blindness and convulsions with cyclosporin A toxicity in a patient undergoing allogenic peripheral stem cell transplantation. *Bone Marrow Transplant* 1997; 20: 793–795.

48. Ernst ME, Franey RJ. Acyclovir- and ganciclovir-induced neurotoxicity. *Ann Pharmacother* 1998; 32: 111–113.

49. Johnson GL, Limon L, Trikha G, Wall H. Acute renal failure and neurotoxicity following oral aciclovir. *Ann Pharmacother* 1994; 28: 460–463.

50. Rashiq S, Briewa L, Mooney M, *et al.* Distinguishing aciclovir neurotoxicity from encephalomyelitis. *J Intern Med* 1993; 234: 507–511.

51. Kiemeneij IM, de Leeuw FE, Ramos LMP, van Gijn J. Acute headache as a presenting symptom of tacrolimus encephalopathy. *J Neurol Neurosurg Psychiatry* 2003; 74: 1126–1127.

52. Visovsky C. Chemotherapy-induced peripheral neuropathy. *Cancer Invest* 2003; 21: 439–451.

53. Department of Health HSC 2003/010 – *Updated National Guidance on the Safe Administration of Intrathecal Chemotherapy*. London: Department of Health, 2003.

54. Verrotti A, Trotta D, Morgese G, Chiarelli F. Valproate-induced hyperammonemic encephalopathy. *Metabol Brain Dis* 2002; 17: 367–373.

55. Ben-Ami H, Nagachandran P, Mendelson A, *et al.* Drug-induced hypoglycaemic coma in 102 diabetic patients. *Arch Intern Med* 1999; 159: 281.

56. McKinley SH, Foroozan R. Optic neuropathy associated with linezolid treatment. *J Neuro-ophthalmol* 2005; 25: 18–21.

57. Johnson LN, Krohel GB, Thomas ER. The clinical spectrum of amiodarone-associated optic neuropathy. *J Natl Med Assoc* 2004; 96: 1477–1491.

58. Kerrison JB. Optic neuropathies caused by toxins and adverse drug reactions. *Ophthalmol Clin North Am* 2004; 17: 481–488.
59. England JD, Asbury AK. Peripheral neuropathy. *Lancet* 2004; 363: 2151–2161.
60. Weimer LH. Medication-induced peripheral neuropathy. *Curr Neurol Neurosci Rep* 2003; 3: 86–92.
61. Hack JB, Hoffman RS. Thiamine before glucose to prevent Wernicke encephalopathy: examining the conventional wisdom. *JAMA* 1998; 279: 583–584.
62. Treisman GJ, Kaplin AI. Neurologic and psychiatric complications of antiretroviral agents. *AIDS* 2002; 16: 1201–1215.
63. Committee on Safety of Medicines. Statins and cytochrome P450 interactions. *Curr Probl Pharmacovigilance* 2004; 30: 1–2.
64. Apfel SC, Zochodne DW. Thalidomide neuropathy. Too much or too long? *Neurology* 2004; 62: 2158–2159.
65. Van Gerpen JA. Drug-induced parkinsonism. *Neurologist* 2002; 8: 363–370.
66. Pierre JM. Extrapyramidal symptoms with atypical antipsychotics. Incidence, prevention and management. *Drug Safety* 2005; 28: 191–208.
67. Caroff SN, Mann S, Sullivan KA, Campbell EC. Tardive dyskinesia. *Adv Drug React Bull* 2004; 224: 1–4.
68. Pierre JM. Extrapyramidal symptoms with atypical antipsychotics. Incidence, prevention and management. *Drug Safety* 2005; 28: 191–208.
69. Committee on Safety of Medicines. Drug-induced extrapyramidal reactions. *Curr Probl Pharmacovigilance* 1994; 20: 6.
70. Boeve BF. Evidence for cholinesterase-inhibitor therapy for dementia associated with Parkinson's disease. *Lancet Neurol* 2005; 4: 137–138.
71. Egan MF, Apud J, Wyatt RJ. Treatment of tardive dyskinesia. *Schizophrenia Bull* 1997; 23: 583–609.
72. van Harten PN, Hoek HW, Kahn RS. Acute dystonia induced by drug treatment. *Br Med J* 1999; 319: 623–626.
73. Halstead SM, Barnes TR, Speller JC. Akathisia: prevalence and associated dysphoria in an in-patient population with chronic schizophrenia. *Br J Psychiatry* 1994; 164: 177–183.
74. Kipps CM, Fung VSC, Grattan-Smith P, de Moore GM, Morris JGL. Movement disorder emergencies. *Mov Disord* 2005; 20: 322–334.
75. Jiminez-Jiminez FJ, Garcia-Ruiz PJ, Molina JA. Drug-induced movement disorders. *Drug Safety* 1997; 16: 180–204.
76. Jiminez-Jiminez FJ, Puertas I, De Toledo-Heras M. Drug-induced myoclonus: frequency, mechanisms and management. *CNS Drugs* 2004; 18: 93–104.
77. Committee on Safety of Medicines. Dopaminergic drugs and sudden sleep onset. *Curr Probl Pharmacovigilance* 2003; 29: 9.
78. CPMP Position statement on dopaminergic substances and sudden sleep onset. European Agency for the Evaluation of Medicinal Products CPMP/578/02 Rev 1.
79. Homann CN, Wenzel K, Suppan K, et al. Sleep attacks in patients taking dopamine agonists; review. *Br Med J* 2003; 324: 1483–1487.
80. Chaudhuri KR, Pal S, Brefel-Courbon C. 'Sleep attacks' or 'Unintended sleep episodes' occur with dopamine agonists. Is this a class effect? *Drug Safety* 2002; 25: 473–483.
81. Stewart D, Morgan E, Burn D, et al. Dopamine agonist switching in Parkinson's disease. *Hosp Med (Lond)* 2004; 65: 215–219.

16

Sexual dysfunction and infertility

Fiona MacLean

Introduction

The issue of sexual health has been better recognised recently, among both healthcare professionals and the public, largely as a consequence of the introduction of sildenafil, the first licensed oral treatment for male erectile dysfunction. It is now generally accepted that good sexual health is an important aspect of physical wellbeing, and the possibility that drug therapy can cause sexual dysfunction is increasingly recognised.[1,2] Although sexual dysfunction is sometimes trivialised, it can have a major impact on personal relationships, quality of life and the ability to conceive. It is also an important factor in non-compliance: studies have confirmed that many patients with hypertension, depression and schizophrenia discontinue their medication because of sexual side effects.[3,4] Patient information leaflets may alert patients to the possibility that their sexual function may be affected by a medicine. Healthcare professionals should have some knowledge of the types of problem that can occur in case questions arise. Pharmacists are well placed to identify non-compliance, and if sensitive questioning indicates that diminished sexual function may be a contributing factor this should be discussed with the prescriber.

The overall incidence of drug-induced sexual dysfunction is difficult to quantify. Patients are often unwilling to raise the issue of sexual health with healthcare professionals, leading to underreporting of problems. In addition, many diseases can affect sexual function, making it difficult to establish a causal link with a medicine rather than concurrent illness. Antihypertensive medication, for example, is associated with erectile dysfunction but it is often prescribed for patients with diabetes, which itself may cause impotence. Other factors that can influence sexual function in men and women are age, alcohol consumption, smoking, drugs of abuse, over-the-counter medicines, and exposure to environmental or occupational toxins.[4] Most of the published literature relates to the adverse effects of drugs on male sexual function. It is more difficult to assess these effects in women, and this aspect of drug safety is not well studied.

Sexual dysfunction as a consequence of drug therapy has been reported with a range of medicines, notably antihypertensives, antipsychotics and antidepressants. Some types of reproductive dysfunction should be regarded as serious (e.g. infertility, congenital abnormalities and some pregnancy complications), and if these problems are suspected to be due to drug therapy they should always be reported to the appropriate regulatory authority. This chapter reviews the most frequently reported drug-induced sexual problems, including infertility. The effects of environmental toxins and drugs of abuse will not be discussed.

Infertility

Infertility is one element of a spectrum of reproductive disorders that includes miscarriage, congenital abnormality, premature delivery and stillbirth. Infertility, defined as the failure to conceive after 1 year of unprotected intercourse, is fairly common, affecting one in six couples at some time during their reproductive lives. It is generally only detected when a couple is actively trying to conceive. It can be difficult to draw firm conclusions about trends in infertility rates, but the number of couples seeking treatment for infertility is increasing each year as awareness that effective treatments are available increases.[5,6] Although the prevalence of infertility does not seem to be increasing the spectrum of disorders is changing, and there is good evidence that sperm quality is falling throughout the developed world.[7]

Causes of infertility in women include failure of ovulation, tubal damage, endometriosis and hostile cervical mucus. In men, sperm defects, coital factors such as impotence or retrograde ejaculation, and hypogonadism may be implicated.[6,8] Drug-induced male infertility arises through four basic mechanisms. There may be a direct toxic effect on the gonads, the hypothalamic–pituitary–gonadal axis may be altered, drugs may impair ejaculation and erectile function, or may adversely affect libido.[9] In about 20% of couples who have difficulty conceiving, the cause of the problem cannot be found. Drugs and environmental toxins may be responsible in a small proportion of cases, but in general the effects of drugs on fertility have been poorly studied.

The activity of the gonads (testes or ovaries) is regulated by the pituitary gonadotrophins follicle-stimulating hormone (FSH) and luteinising hormone (LH). Secretion of both hormones is controlled by gonadotrophin-releasing hormone (GnRH) from the hypothalamus. FSH regulates the development of Sertoli cells (which are involved in

Table 16.1 Some drugs that may cause primary infertility

Alkylating agents (e.g. chlorambucil, cyclophosphamide, melphalan)
Anabolic steroids
Antiandrogens (e.g. cyproterone)
Antimetabolites (e.g. cytarabine, methotrexate)
Cisplatin
Colchicine
Diethylstilbestrol
Non-steroidal anti-inflammatory drugs (women)
Procarbazine
Sulfasalazine (men)
Vincristine

---

sperm maturation) in the testes, and the Graafian follicle in females.[2,10] LH controls formation of the corpus luteum in females and testosterone production by the Leydig cells in males. Both FSH and LH regulate oestrogen production and ovulation. Reduced amounts of FSH and/or LH reaching the testes can inhibit spermatogenesis.[2,5] Gonadotoxic drugs affect sperm by directly damaging testicular germ cells or inhibiting Sertoli cell function. This may result in reduced or absent sperm production, suboptimal sperm maturation, motility or morphology.[9]

Primary drug-induced infertility results from a direct toxic effect of the drug on the gonads or an indirect effect on pituitary gonadotrophin secretion (Table 16.1). Secondary drug-induced infertility results from drug effects on erection, libido or performance, which may compromise the ability to conceive.

Cytotoxic chemotherapy

Cytotoxic chemotherapy can cause infertility by a direct effect on the gonads. Ovarian failure was described in the 1940s and 1950s with busulfan and cyclophosphamide, and in the 1970s following combination chemotherapy for lymphoma.[11,12] The effects differ in men, women and children, and depend on the patient's stage of reproductive life at the time of treatment. Resumption of menses post chemotherapy is age dependent, with permanent amenorrhoea occurring in more than 90% of women over 40 years of age who received a cyclophosphamide-containing regimen, but in less than 10% of women under the age of 30 treated with the same regimen.[11] In men, cytotoxic drugs damage differentiating spermatogonia. Leydig cells may also be affected, resulting in a raised LH and low to normal testosterone levels. Following chemotherapy, the most commonly detected hormonal abnormality is an elevated serum FSH. This can be used in the clinical setting to assist in predicting the return of spermatogenesis.[9] The potential effect of chemotherapy on reproductive function is therefore an important consideration in cancer treatment, particularly of young patients. The effects are influenced by the treatment regimen, dose, and duration of drug exposure.[4,13] An estimated 20–25% of female patients are of premenopausal age when breast cancer is diagnosed.[14] Now that a number of cancers are curable, the long-term effects of chemotherapy on fertility may influence the choice of therapy. Men may be offered sperm banking before treatment is begun, but for many reasons this may not be possible or successful. It must also be remembered that cytotoxic drugs are used in non-malignant conditions where life expectancy is not reduced, such as autoimmune diseases, and azoospermia (absence of sperm) may result. As cryopreservation of ova is not yet established, women may be faced with the prospect of premature menopause and/or drug-induced infertility. Advances in the techniques used to preserve ovarian and testicular tissue have recently been reported, but more research is required before these are adopted into practice.[15]

Alkylating agents are highly toxic to the testes. They are cell-cycle non-specific and have the ability to cause damage to dividing and resting cells.[14] Cyclophosphamide and chlorambucil have been most extensively studied. The extent of gonadal damage depends on the dose and duration of treatment. The risk of permanent male sterility is associated with cyclophosphamide doses greater than 7.5 g/m^2.[16] Typically there is a progressive decline in sperm numbers, leading to azoospermia within several months, which may be irreversible. Damage may be avoided if low doses are used, as the cumulative dose administered is an important factor.[17,18] Ifosfamide also exhibits dose-dependent reproductive toxicity. There is often partial recovery of spermatogenesis after cyclophosphamide treatment, and with chlorambucil recovery can occur even after many years. Cyclophosphamide has also been associated with gonadal failure in women.[18] It has been suggested that women given alkylating agents have a higher risk of primary ovarian failure if they are older than 30 years at diagnosis.[19] Premenarchal ovaries appear to be more resistant than postmenarchal ovaries to the toxicity of chemotherapy owing to the greater oocyte reserves.[18] This may be reassuring to parents of young females diagnosed with cancer.

Methotrexate is thought to be less toxic than the alkylating agents but it does cause a reduction in sperm count. Reversible reductions in sperm count have been reported with the use of low doses of methotrexate in the treatment of psoriasis.[20] Vincristine and cisplatin have been reported to cause azoospermia.[21,22] Irreversible impairment of spermatogenesis can occur with cisplatin and is determined by the cumulative dose. Long-lasting effects on sperm production are unlikely at doses below 400 mg/m^2.[23] The anthracyclines, antimetabolites and etoposide have been reported to have detrimental effects on female fertility.[14]

In general, combination chemotherapy, at least in males, appears to produce more persistent effects on reproductive function than single-agent treatment.

It is more difficult to determine how chemotherapy affects female reproductive function, as there is no direct way of monitoring toxic effects on the ovaries. Gonadal damage is often manifest by amenorrhoea, low oestrogen levels and increased concentrations of FSH and LH, which resemble the hormonal changes seen at menopause. As in men, alkylating agents appear to be the most toxic. Primary ovarian failure has been reported with both melphalan and cyclophosphamide.[17]

Other drugs

Sulfasalazine was reported 20 years ago to cause oligospermia (subnormal concentration of sperm) and infertility in men with inflammatory bowel disease.[24] The effects on sperm become apparent within 2 months of starting treatment. Sperm motility is reduced, abnormal forms develop and sperm density is decreased.[25,26] These effects are reversible within 2–3 months of stopping treatment. The effects on sperm function are probably due to the sulfapyridine component of sulfasalazine; slow acetylators of the drug are more likely to be affected. Return to normal fertility has been reported when treatment was changed to mesalazine.[27,28]

Diethylstilbestrol (DES) is a synthetic oestrogen that was given to some pregnant women between the years 1940 and 1970; it was used to prevent threatened and recurrent abortion. An estimated 5–10 million American women received DES in pregnancy or were exposed to it *in utero*.[29] Prescriptions for DES in pregnancy were banned in 1971 by the US Food and Drug Administration after it was linked to a number of reproductive tract abnormalities in the offspring of exposed women.[2,30] These include clear-cell adenocarcinoma of the vagina, anatomical abnormalities of the uterus, and increased risk of ectopic pregnancy, miscarriage and premature delivery. Fertility rates appear to be reduced in the daughters, but not the sons, of exposed women.[31] A collaborative follow-up study of adult women who had been exposed to DES *in utero* provided information on difficulties in conceiving, and the reasons for this. A greater proportion of women exposed to DES were nulligravid and a greater proportion had tried unsuccessfully to become pregnant for at least 12 months. DES exposure appeared to be associated with infertility due to uterine and tubal problems.[32]

The fertility rate is significantly lower in men treated for epilepsy than in the general population. Although few studies have carried out a detailed analysis of semen from men with epilepsy, some antiepileptics have been associated with infertility, abnormal sperm morphology, reduced motility and sperm count. Most reports implicate phenytoin and valproate.[33]

Anovulation and amenorrhoea

About 30% of infertile women have anovulatory infertility. They may present with amenorrhoea (primary or secondary), oligomenorrhoea (infrequent or irregular periods), or occasionally with regular menstrual cycles but low or undetectable serum progesterone concentrations in the putative luteal phase.[34] Secondary amenorrhoea is defined as the absence of menstruation for at least 6 months in a woman with previously normal and regular menses.[35] Hyperprolactinaemia is a common finding in women with amenorrhoea or oligomenorrhoea; occasionally this is drug induced (see Chapter 9). Drugs known to increase prolactin include methyldopa, metoclopramide, cimetidine and oestrogens (see Chapter 9). All traditional neuroleptics and risperidone, amisulpride and zotepine are capable of elevating serum prolactin by blocking dopamine receptors.[36–38] The true incidence of antipsychotic-induced sexual dysfunction is probably underestimated, as women in particular are reluctant to report these events. Antipsychotic-induced hyperprolactinaemia affects gonadotrophin production and the secretion of FSH and LH. This may result in impaired ovulation, infertility, spontaneous abortion, pseudo-pregnancy and sex-organ atrophy.[39] It has also been suggested that prolonged hyperprolactinaemia may incur an increased risk of breast cancer. Although there are wide interpatient variations, the magnitude of increase in prolactin is generally proportional to the drug dose.[38] Of the newer atypical antipsychotics, sertindole, quetiapine, ziprasidone, aripiprazole and clozapine have no important effect on prolactin (see Chapter 9).[36] Olanzapine may produce a transient increase in prolactin level, which decreases within days or weeks of commencing treatment.[39]

Amenorrhoea has been associated with high-dose corticosteroids, danazol and isoniazid therapy.[2] Oestrogens promote synthesis and storage of prolactin. There has in the past been concern about a high incidence of amenorrhoea shortly after stopping combined oral contraceptives. Current oral contraceptives have low doses of oestrogen and less than 1%

of women actually show hyperprolactinaemia.[38] Furthermore, studies have shown that the incidence of amenorrhoea in such women is no greater than in the general population, and that the use of oral contraceptives does not impair subsequent fertility.[40] Spironolactone has been reported to cause amenorrhoea at daily doses of 100–200 mg. Normal menstrual periods usually return within 2 months of its being stopped. The mechanism is believed to involve inhibition of dihydrotestosterone binding to androgen receptors.[41]

Evidence is accumulating that non-steroidal anti-inflammatory drugs (NSAIDs) taken in the middle of the menstrual cycle may inhibit ovulation.[42–45] There are increasing numbers of case reports of unexplained fertility associated with chronic NSAID use, but it is difficult to establish a causal relationship as the underlying inflammatory or connective tissue disorders may be the cause of the reproductive problem, and not drug therapy. Cyclooxygenase-2 (COX-2) has a role in the reproductive system, being implicated in ovulation, fertilisation, implantation and maintenance of pregnancy. Prostaglandins are essential mediators of ovulation, and COX-2-dependent prostaglandins may be indirectly responsible for follicle rupture. It has been suggested that the inhibition of prostaglandins by NSAIDs prevents rupture of the developed ovarian follicle, known as luteinised unruptured follicle syndrome.[46] Progesterone levels measured in the second half of the menstrual cycle may be compatible with ovulation having occurred, which can obscure the diagnosis.

This problem has been reported with indometacin, diclofenac, piroxicam and naproxen. The reports suggest that conception often occurs within a short time of discontinuing NSAID medication.[47,48]

Large clinical studies are needed to establish causality and to determine the prevalence of this problem. The evidence to date suggests that NSAID withdrawal should be considered in women undergoing investigation for infertility. The selective COX-2 inhibitors rofecoxib and celecoxib are not recommended in women attempting to conceive. All NSAIDs should preferably be avoided around the time of ovulation in women trying to conceive. Table 16.2 lists some drugs that may cause anovulation or amenorrhoea.

Sexual dysfunction

Sexual function may be divided into three categories, reflecting the sexual response cycle: (1) libido or sexual desire; (2) arousal, including erectile function in men and lubrication in women; and (3) release (orgasm in

Table 16.2 Some drugs that may cause anovulation or amenorrhoea

---

Anabolic steroids
Danazol
Dopamine antagonists (e.g. chlorpromazine, prochlorperazine)
Isoniazid
Levonorgestrel-releasing intrauterine system
Risperidone
Sodium valproate
Spironolactone

---

women and ejaculation in men).[4,49] Drugs can affect one or more areas of the response cycle. Understanding of the sexual response remains incomplete, but there is evidence of dopaminergic, adrenergic, muscarinic and serotonergic involvement. In general, dopamine increases sexual behaviour and serotonin inhibits it. Libido is influenced by reproductive hormones and the emotional and physical health of the individual. Testosterone is necessary for normal sexual arousal, probably in both men and women, and in men testosterone deficiency is associated with impotence.

Erectile dysfunction and ejaculatory disorders

Erectile dysfunction, or impotence, is the inability to achieve or maintain an erection sufficient for satisfactory sexual performance. It is the most common form of male sexual dysfunction. The prevalence of erectile dysfunction is up to 10% across all ages, rising to over 50% in men between 50 and 70 years old.[50–52] The aetiology is often vascular, but other contributory factors include drug therapy, endocrine disease and neurological dysfunction. Erectile dysfunction often occurs with diabetes, heart disease, hypertension and peripheral vascular disease. It may also be a consequence of spinal cord injuries and pelvic or perineal radiotherapy or surgery.[53] Smoking and alcohol intake are important contributing factors.[54,55]

Male sexual function depends on the coordination of neurogenic, hormonal and psychological mechanisms; disruption of one or more of these may result in erectile dysfunction. The penile blood vessels and smooth muscle receive both sympathetic and parasympathetic innervation, and erection is primarily a parasympathetic function.[56] In the flaccid state the smooth muscle is contracted, preventing inflow of blood. Parasympathetic nerve stimuli, mediated by nitric oxide, relax the smooth muscle of the arterioles in the corpora cavernosa, allowing blood to flow rapidly

Table 16.3 Some drugs that may cause erectile dysfunction

ACE inhibitors	Digoxin
Anabolic steroids	Gabapentin
Antiandrogens (e.g. finasteride)	Methyldopa
Anticholinergics	Metoclopramide
Antidepressants (tricyclics, monoamine	Omeprazole
oxidase inhibitors, selective serotonin	Phenothiazines
reuptake inhibitors)	Phenytoin
Benzodiazepines	Prazosin
Beta-blockers	Spironolactone
Carbamazepine	Thiazide diuretics
Cimetidine	

ACE, angiotensin-converting enzyme.

into the penis. Venous outflow from the penis is reduced, blood is trapped within the corpora cavernosa, and rigid erection ensues.[50]

About 25% of cases of erectile dysfunction are believed to be drug induced.[54,57] The classes of drug most frequently implicated are antihypertensives, antidepressants, antipsychotics and antiepileptics (Table 16.3).

Ejaculation is the expulsion of seminal fluid from the posterior urethra. This is achieved via stimulation of alpha-adrenergic receptors, leading to contraction of the smooth muscle of the prostate, seminal vesicles and vas deferens.[58] Disorders of ejaculation comprise ejaculatory failure and retrograde ejaculation, in which semen passes into the bladder. A number of drugs have been implicated in these disorders.

Antihypertensives

The prevalence of both erectile dysfunction and ejaculatory disorders is significantly greater in untreated hypertensive men than in matched normotensive controls, so caution is needed when assessing whether medication is likely to be the cause of such problems. Most epidemiological studies addressing this issue were carried out over 10 years ago, when the types of drugs used did not reflect those in use today. More recent studies confirm that the rate of erectile dysfunction depends on the class of antihypertensive.[4,59] The effects of treatment on quality of life are particularly important in the management of hypertension, which can require lifelong therapy despite being asymptomatic. Evidence suggests that many hypertensive patients experiencing sexual side effects will stop taking their medication.

Most classes of antihypertensive agent have been reported as causing erectile dysfunction, with centrally acting agents, non-selective beta-blockers, potassium-sparing and thiazide diuretics most often implicated. High rates of erectile dysfunction and ejaculatory failure are associated with the older adrenergic blockers reserpine and guanethidine, which are no longer used. Clonidine and methyldopa have also caused loss of libido, erectile dysfunction and ejaculatory failure. The alpha-adrenergic blockers indoramin and prazosin can cause ejaculatory failure and retrograde ejaculation.

The incidence of sexual dysfunction in men taking diuretics is between two and six times higher than in men taking placebo.[60] Thiazides may cause reduced libido, erectile dysfunction and problems with ejaculation. The underlying mechanism is unclear, as thiazides lack significant hormonal, autonomic or central nervous system effects; a direct effect on smooth muscle decreasing penile blood flow is thought to be responsible.

Erectile dysfunction is well documented with propranolol and can occur with other beta-blockers. The problem is more likely with lipid-soluble beta-blockers, but has also been reported with atenolol and with ophthalmic timolol.[61,62] Reduced perfusion pressure caused by a drop in blood pressure or a direct effect on smooth muscle may be responsible.

In a study comparing five different antihypertensive classes (the Treatment of Mild Hypertension Study, TOMHS) most problems were associated with the thiazide chlortalidone.[63] The rate of erectile failure in patients taking chlortalidone was 17% versus 8% in controls. The incidence with amlodipine, acebutolol and enalapril was similar to that in controls, and doxazosin was associated with the lowest rate of erectile dysfunction.

Although there are several published case reports of erectile dysfunction with calcium channel blockers and ACE inhibitors, these classes of antihypertensive seem to cause fewer problems with sexual function than diuretics or beta-blockers.[57]

Psychotropic drugs

There is a paucity of research about sexual function in patients with mental illness, and it can be extremely difficult to assess the relative contributions of the underlying condition and the drug therapy. Both depression and the drugs used to treat it can cause disorders of desire, arousal and orgasm.[64,65]

Antidepressants have a range of pharmacological effects, including sedation, hormonal changes, disturbance of cholinergic/adrenergic balance and increased serotonin neurotransmission, all of which can result in sexual dysfunction. Sexual dysfunction has been reported as a side effect of all antidepressants, although the frequency between individual drugs and drug classes is variable.

Erectile dysfunction has been described with all classes of antidepressant. Numerous case reports have implicated tricyclic antidepressants (TCAs), but the association has not been confirmed in the few published controlled trials.[66] There is consistent evidence that serotonergic antidepressants (e.g. selective serotonin reuptake inhibitors [SSRIs], monoamine oxidase inhibitors [MAOIs] and clomipramine) are associated with high rates of decreased libido, ejaculatory disturbance, delayed orgasm and anorgasmia.[49,67] Serotonin appears to have a mainly inhibitory effect on sexual function. The mechanism of orgasm has not been confirmed, but it is thought to be regulated by a balance of cholinergic and adrenergic influences, and that serotonin receptor stimulation inhibits adrenergically mediated ejaculation.[66]

Evidence that SSRIs cause sexual dysfunction is accumulating as their use increases. The reported incidence varies widely, mainly because of differences in methodology between studies, but is probably at least 20%.[66,67] Problems may occur with all SSRIs. Delayed orgasm or ejaculation appears to be the most frequent problem, and this has been observed in controlled studies. As a consequence of this effect, the SSRIs are now used in the treatment of premature ejaculation.[49,65] Newer antidepressants such as mirtazapine may be less likely to interfere with sexual function, perhaps because of its postsynaptic $5HT_2$ blocking properties.[68,69] MAOIs, although seldom used now, are a recognised cause of cause delayed ejaculation.[65]

Sexual dysfunction has been reported as a side effect of all antipsychotics, and up to 45% of people taking typical antipsychotics experience sexual dysfunction. However, people with psychosis are less able to develop good psychosexual relationships, and for some treatment with an antipsychotic can improve sexual functioning. Antipsychotics decrease dopaminergic transmission, which in itself can decrease libido but may also increase prolactin levels via negative feedback. This can cause amenorrhoea in women, and a lack of libido, breast enlargement and galactorrhoea in both men and women. Anticholinergic effects can cause disorders of arousal, and drugs that block peripheral $alpha_1$ receptors cause particular problems with erection and ejaculation in men. The phenothiazines, particularly thioridazine, have caused changes in ejaculation (no ejaculate or a reduced volume) and pain on orgasm. Chlorpromazine is also associated with dose-related ejaculatory failure. Newer atypical antipsychotics, such as olanzapine, may be less likely to cause these problems.

Table 16.4 Some drugs that may cause priapism

Anticoagulants	Phenothiazines
Haloperidol	Phentolamine
Hydralazine	Prazosin
Nifedipine	Risperidone
Olanzapine	Trazodone
Papaverine	

Priapism

Priapism is a prolonged penile erection that is usually unrelated to sexual stimulation. The problem occurs when the regulatory mechanisms that initiate and maintain penile flaccidity are disturbed and venous drainage from the corpora cavernosa is obstructed.[70] It is a medical emergency requiring immediate treatment to prevent fibrosis or even gangrene. Management involves the aspiration of blood and administration of a vasoconstrictor sympathomimetic such as phenylephrine or metaraminol. Drug therapy is an important cause of priapism, accounting for up to 40% of cases (Table 16.4).[71] Alpha-adrenoceptor antagonism is the most likely mechanism: constriction of the blood vessels supplying erectile tissue is prevented and detumescence does not occur. Prazosin is the drug most frequently associated with the problem.[65,72] Among psychotropic drugs, the phenothiazines and the antidepressant trazodone are most commonly implicated. Trazodone-induced priapism may affect patients at any age, and is most likely to occur in the first month of treatment. Priapism has also been attributed to hydralazine, nifedipine, anticoagulants, risperidone and olanzapine. In most reported cases priapism occurs as a result of a rebound hypercoagulable state which results after stopping anticoagulant therapy.[73] This is seen with both the oral coumarins and heparin. Drugs given by intracavernosal injection in the treatment of erectile dysfunction (e.g. papaverine, phentolamine, alprostadil) may cause priapism, and patients should be warned of this and advised to seek prompt medical attention should it occur. Sildenafil and other phosphodiesterase type-5 inhibitors have been implicated in priapism, in association with the smooth muscle relaxatory effect of these drugs.[74]

Female orgasm dysfunction

In women, sexual dysfunction has not been thoroughly investigated and the underlying mechanisms are not well understood. Most reported

Table 16.5 Some drugs that may affect female sexual function

Antidepressants (tricyclics, monoamine oxidase inhibitors, selective serotonin reuptake inhibitors)	Gonadorelin analogues
	Methyldopa
	Oestrogens
Antipsychotics	Propranolol
Benzodiazepines	Spironolactone
Cimetidine	Thiazide diuretics
Clonidine	Trazodone
Gabapentin	

problems relate to orgasm dysfunction, reduced vaginal lubrication or loss of libido. Female orgasm involves involuntary rhythmic vaginal and pelvic muscle contractions; it can be assumed that the neurovascular control is similar to that in males.[2] Thioridazine has been known since 1961 to inhibit ejaculation in men, but it was not until 20 years later that the first report of inhibition of female orgasm was published.[65] Failure to achieve orgasm (anorgasmia) is one of the most common sexual adverse effects of psychotropic drugs in women. This problem has been described with SSRIs. Delayed orgasm or anorgasmia has been reported with MAOIs, TCAs, clozapine and risperidone.[65,66] The anti-hypertensives clonidine and methyldopa have also been linked with anorgasmia (Table 16.5).

Multiple spontaneous orgasms have been described in women treated with fluoxetine.[75,76] There have also been occasional case reports of spontaneous orgasm induced by yawning caused by clomipramine and by fluoxetine.[77,78]

Altered libido

Loss of libido or sexual desire is frequently attributed to medication in both men and women. For example, all drugs causing central nervous system depression can potentially decrease libido. In women, loss of libido is the commonest reported form of sexual dysfunction; it is extremely difficult to quantify and manage.[79] Changes in desire may be due to illness (e.g. gynaecological disorders causing pain on intercourse), stress or fatigue, or may be drug induced.[58] In controlled studies women have rarely been questioned about the effect of medication on sexual function, and therefore most reports of altered libido are anecdotal or case reports.

Several antihypertensives, including clonidine and methyldopa, reduce female libido. Studies of both men and women taking methyldopa report an incidence of decreased libido ranging from 7 to 14%.[58] Spironolactone has antiandrogenic effects and is clearly linked with decreased libido. Propranolol, thiazide diuretics and calcium antagonists are believed to have mild effects (if any), and captopril appears to have no effect. Psychotropic drugs affect sexual desire in men and women by several possible mechanisms, including sedation, effects on central or peripheral neurotransmitters, or effects on hormones (e.g. prolactin). Antidepressants have been reported to decrease sexual desire. MAOIs, particularly phenelzine, are frequently implicated.[65] The SSRIs have all been reported to decrease libido, possibly as a consequence of an indirect effect on dopamine; the incidence in men and women may be as high as 40%.[66,80]

In general, rates of sexual dysfunction appear to be greatest with the SSRIs, followed by MAOIs then TCAs. Rates of sexual dysfunction appear to be similar for all the SSRIs, and it is not known whether switching between them will diminish sexual side effects. Case reports of decreased libido with anxiolytics have been published: centrally mediated sedation and muscle relaxation are thought to be responsible.[80]

Cimetidine has been reported to cause loss of libido, possibly because of its antiandrogen activity.[81] This is likely to be dose related. The problem is not seen with ranitidine.[13] The influence of testosterone on libido is well recognised, and any drug that reduces serum testosterone may lead to a loss of sexual desire. In men, this includes drugs such as oestrogens, antiandrogens and gonadorelin analogues.[82] There are preliminary data linking protease inhibitors with loss of libido, and also with erectile dysfunction and problems with ejaculation.[83,84]

Increased sexual desire is a rare adverse effect. Trazodone has been reported to increase libido in both men and women, possibly by decreasing prolactin levels or by increasing dopamine.[85,86] Levodopa has caused hypersexuality in men with Parkinson's disease. The reversible inhibitor of monoamine oxidase A, moclobemide, has been reported to increase sexual desire in some patients.

Management

The management of drug-induced sexual dysfunction can be difficult. Occasionally these problems may remit spontaneously over time. In some situations it may be possible to change therapy to a drug in another class that is less likely to cause problems, e.g. changing from a thiazide to an ACE inhibitor in hypertension. There may not always be an effective or tolerated alternative, however. Other possible options may include dose reduction, delaying dosing until after sexual intercourse, or advocating 'drug holidays'. Pharmacological management of drug-induced sexual dysfunction with agents such as cyproheptadine or sildenafil is seldom indicated.[49,69,87]

Sexual dysfunction due to medication is relatively uncommon and probably not an issue that healthcare professionals will be consulted about very often. If approached by a patient or partner about the possibility that a sexual problem may be drug related, the healthcare professional should be sympathetic. Complex and sensitive issues surround sexual dysfunction, but consideration should be given to possible drug causes. In most cases the individual should be advised to discuss the matter with his or her GP in the first instance.

CASE STUDY 16.1

Mrs S is a 38-year-old woman who was diagnosed with rheumatoid arthritis 4 years ago. She is currently taking diclofenac, co-codamol, omeprazole and ferrous sulphate. She tells you that she and her husband would like another child. They have a 9-year-old son, but she has been unable to conceive despite using no contraception for the last 3 years. She asks you about this, as her community pharmacist, when buying an ovulation predictor test. She has done some internet searching and found some information suggesting that non-steroidal anti-inflammatory drugs might be involved in infertility. She has not yet discussed this with her GP or rheumatologist, but asks whether you think she should stop taking diclofenac.

Could the failure to conceive be related to the diclofenac?

NSAID therapy has been associated with unexplained infertility. NSAIDs act by inhibiting cyclooxygenase, the enzyme responsible for prostaglandin synthesis. Prostaglandins have a wide range of reproductive functions, and NSAIDs may interfere with these physiological processes. COX-2, one of two cyclooxygenase enzymes, is active in the ovaries during follicular development. Its inhibition is thought to cause luteinised unruptured follicle syndrome, an anovulatory condition characterised by clinical signs of ovulation but in the absence of follicular rupture and ovum release. As yet the evidence linking regular NSAID use to unexplained infertility is inconclusive, but published case reports implicate diclofenac, piroxicam, indometacin and naproxen as possible causes. The problem appears to be reversible; in most published cases the woman conceived shortly after NSAID withdrawal.

→

CASE STUDY 16.1 (continued)

Would another NSAID be less likely to affect fertility?

There is no clear basis for advocating a switch to another NSAID, as the effect on fertility is thought to be due to prostaglandin inhibition, a class effect. Prescribing information for selective COX-2 inhibitors (e.g. celecoxib, etoricoxib and rofecoxib) states that their use is not recommended in women attempting to conceive.

What advice do you give Mrs S?

Although women trying to conceive should ideally avoid using any medicines, treatment is frequently necessary in those with inflammatory or connective tissue diseases. However, the possibility that NSAID therapy may be a factor in Mrs S's failure to conceive should be considered. Mrs S should be advised not to stop taking her diclofenac before she has discussed the problem with her rheumatologist and/or GP.

CASE STUDY 16.2

JD is a 35-year-old man who was diagnosed with schizophrenia 10 years ago. He has been taking risperidone for the past 6 months. The dose has been titrated gradually at an outpatient clinic and he is now taking 4 mg daily. The patient has begun to notice difficulties with sexual function, specifically an inability to ejaculate. He has never experienced such problems in the past.

Has risperidone been linked with ejaculatory disorders?

Prescribing information for risperidone indicates that ejaculatory dysfunction has been reported. In retrograde ejaculation, semen passes retrogradely into the bladder during ejaculation. It can occur as a consequence of surgery or may be drug induced. Retrograde ejaculation is a recognised side effect of typical antipsychotics, especially thioridazine, but the problem is thought to be less likely with atypical antipsychotics.

There are a small number of published case reports of retrograde ejaculation with risperidone.[88,89]

→

◗ **CASE STUDY 16.2** (continued)

What is the mechanism of this adverse effect?

To date, all drugs reported to induce this problem have alpha$_1$-adrenergic blocking activity.[88] Risperidone is a potent alpha$_1$-adrenergic receptor antagonist.

How should the problem be managed?

Dose reduction may lead to complete or partial resolution of this problem. In this case, the patient should discuss the problem with the prescriber.

References

1. Tomlinson J. ABC of sexual health. Taking a sexual history. *Br Med J* 1998; 317: 1573–1576.
2. Forman R, Gilmour-White S, Forman N. *Drug-Induced Infertility and Sexual Dysfunction*. Cambridge: Cambridge University Press, 1996.
3. Collaborative Working Group on Clinical Trial Evaluations. Adverse effects of atypical antipsychotics. *J Clin Psychiatry* 1998; 59(Suppl 12): 17–22.
4. Bateman DN. Drug-induced sexual dysfunction and infertility. In: Davies DM, Ferner RE, de Glanville H, eds. *Textbook of Adverse Drug Reactions*, 4th edn. London: Lippincott-Raven, 1998: 875–884.
5. Cooke S. Treatment of infertility: the general approach to the infertile couple. *Prescribers J* 1996; 36: 42–45.
6. Healy DL. Female infertility: causes and treatment. *Lancet* 1994; 343: 1539–1544.
7. Ledger WL. Female infertility. *Medicine* 1997; 25: 48–52.
8. Wu FC-W. Treatment of infertility: infertility in men. *Prescribers J* 1996; 36: 55–61.
9. Nudell DM, Monoski M, Lipshultz L. Common medications and drugs: how they affect male fertility. *Urol Clin North Am* 2002; 29: 965–973.
10. Buchanan JF, Davis LJ. Drug-induced infertility. *Drug Intell Clin Pharm* 1984; 18: 122–132.
11. DeMars LR. The impact of cancer therapy on reproductive function. *Obstet Gynecol Surv* 2001; 56: 251–253.
12. Rogers M, Kristjanson LJ. The impact on sexual functioning of chemotherapy-induced menopause in women with breast cancer. *Cancer Nurs* 2002; 25: 57–65.
13. Beeley L. Drug-induced sexual dysfunction and infertility. *Adv Drug React Acute Poison Rev* 1984; 3: 23–42.

14. Chasle S, How CC. The effect of cytotoxic chemotherapy on female infertility. *Eur J Oncol Nurs* 2003; 2: 91–98.

15. Radford JA, Shalet SM. Fertility after treatment for cancer. *Br Med J* 1999; 319: 935–936.

16. Longhi A, Macchiagodena M, Vitali G, *et al.* Fertility in male patients treated with neoadjuvant chemotherapy for osteosarcoma. *J Pediatr Hematol/Oncol* 2003; 25: 292–296.

17. Lenz KL, Valley AW. Infertility after chemotherapy: A review of the risks and strategies for prevention. *J Oncol Pharm Pract* 1996; 2: 75–100.

18. Tangir J, Zelterman D, Ma W, *et al.* Reproductive function after conservative surgery and chemotherapy for malignant germ cell tumours of the ovary. *Obstet Gynecol* 2003; 101: 251–257.

19. Franchi-Rezgui P, Rousselot P, Espie M, *et al.* Fertility in young women after chemotherapy with alkylating agents for Hodgkin and non-Hodgkin lymphoma. *Haematol J* 2003; 4: 116–120.

20. Sussman A, Leonard JM. Psoriasis, methotrexate and oligospermia. *Arch Dermatol* 1980; 116: 215.

21. Aubier F, Flamant F, Brauner R, *et al.* Male gonadal function after chemotherapy for solid tumours in childhood. *J Clin Oncol* 1989; 7: 304–309.

22. Wallace WHB, Shalet SM, Crowne EC, *et al.* Gonadal dysfunction due to cis-platinum. *Med Pediatr Oncol* 1989; 17: 409.

23. Kaczyk M, Machtens S, Bokemeyer C. Sexual function and fertility after chemotherapy for testicular cancer. *Curr Opin Urol* 2000; 10: 473–477.

24. Drife JO. The effects of drugs on sperm. *Drugs* 1987; 33: 610–622.

25. Korelitz BI. Pregnancy, fertility and inflammatory bowel disease. *Am J Gastroenterol* 1985; 80: 365–370.

26. Birnie GG, McLeod TIF, Watkinson G. Incidence of sulphasalazine-induced male infertility. *Gut* 1981; 22: 425.

27. Riley SA. Lecarpentier J, Mani T, *et al.* Sulphasalazine-induced seminal abnormalities in ulcerative colitis: results of mesalazine substitution. *Gut* 1987; 28: 1008–1012.

28. Cann PA, Holdworth CD. Reversal of male infertility on changing treatment from sulphasalazine to 5-aminosalicylic acid. *Lancet* 1984; 2: 1189.

29. Timble EL. Update on diethylstilbestrol. *Obstet Gynecol Surv* 2001; 56: 187–189.

30. Mitka M. CDC Resource focuses on DES exposure. *JAMA* 2003; 289: 1624.

31. Anon. Late sequelae of DES. *Prescribe Int* 1996; 5: 149.

32. Palmer JR, Hatch EE, Rao RS. Infertility among women exposed prenatally to diethylstilbestrol. *Am J Epidemiol* 2001; 154: 316–321.

33. Røste LS, Taubøll E, Haugen TB. Alterations in semen parameters in men with epilepsy treated with valproate or carbamazepine monotherapy. *Eur J Neurol* 2003; 10: 501–506.

34. Hamilton M. Treatment of infertility: anovulatory infertility in women. *Prescribers J* 1996; 36: 46–53.

35. McIver B, Romanski SA, Nippoldt TB. Concise review for primary-care physicians. Evaluation and management of amenorrhea. *Mayo Clin Proc* 1997; 72: 1161–1169.

36. Dickson RA, Glazer WM. Neuroleptic-induced hyperprolactinaemia. *Schizophrenia Res* 1999; 35: S75–S86.

37. Kim YK, Kim L, Lee MS. Risperidone and associated amenorrhea: a report of 5 cases. *J Clin Psychiatry* 1999; 60: 315–317.
38. Korbonits M, Grossman AB. Drug-induced hyperprolactinaemia. *Prescribers J* 2000; 40: 157–164.
39. Smith S. Effects of antipsychotics on sexual and endocrine function in women: implications for clinical practice. *J Clin Psychopharmacol* 2003; 23(Suppl 1): S27–S32.
40. Guillebaud J. *Contraception. Your Questions Answered*, 2nd edn. Edinburgh: Churchill Livingstone, 1993: 127–128.
41. Potter C, Willis D, Sharp HL, *et al.* Primary and secondary amenorrhoea associated with spironolactone therapy in chronic liver disease. *J Pediatr* 1992; 121: 141–143.
42. Killick S, Elstein M. Pharmacological production of luteinized unruptured follicles by prostaglandin synthetase inhibitors. *Fertil Steril* 1987; 47: 773–777.
43. Kennedy SH, Forman RG, Barlow DH. Non-steroidal anti-inflammatory drugs and infertility. *J Obstet Gynecol* 1991; 11: 151–152.
44. Akil M, Amos S, Stewart P. Infertility may sometimes be associated with NSAID consumption. *Br J Rheumatol* 1996; 35: 76–78.
45. Smith G, Roberts R, Hall C, *et al.* Reversible ovulatory failure associated with the development of luteinized unruptured follicles in women with inflammatory arthritis taking non-steroidal anti-inflammatory drugs. *Br J Rheumatol* 1996; 35: 458–462.
46. Mendonça L, Khamashata MA, Nelson-Piercy C. Non-steroidal anti-inflammatory drugs as a possible cause for reversible infertility. *Rheumatology* 2000; 39: 880–882.
47. Stone S, Khamashata MA, Nelson-Piercy C. Non-steroidal anti-inflammatory drugs and reversible female infertility. Is there a link? *Drug Safety* 2002; 25: 545–551.
48. Norman RJ. Reproductive consequences of COX-2 inhibition. *Lancet* 2001; 358: 1287–1288.
49. Woodrum ST, Brown CS. Management of SSRI-induced sexual dysfunction. *Ann Pharmacother* 1998; 32: 1209–1215.
50. Wagner G, Saenz de Tejada I. Update on male erectile dysfunction. *Br Med J* 1998; 316: 678–682.
51. Ernst E, Pittler MH. Yohimbine for erectile dysfunction: A systematic review and meta-analysis of randomised clinical trials. *J Urol* 1998; 159: 433–436.
52. Feldman HA, Goldstein I, Hatzichristou DG, *et al.* Impotence and its medical and psychosocial correlates: results of the Massachusetts Male Aging Study. *J Urol* 1994; 151: 54–61.
53. Korenman SG. Advances in the understanding and management of erectile dysfunction. *J Clin Endocrinol Metab* 1995; 80: 1985–1988.
54. Anon. Sildenafil for erectile dysfunction. *Drug Ther Bull* 1998; 36: 81.
55. Gregoire A. ABC of sexual health. Male sexual problems. *Br Med J* 1999; 318: 245–247.
56. Rousseau P. Impotence in elderly men. *Postgrad Med* 1988; 83: 212–219.
57. Keene LC, Davies PH. Drug-related erectile dysfunction. *Adv Drug React* 1998; 18: 5–24.
58. Duncan L, Bateman DN. Sexual function in women. Do antihypertensive drugs have an impact? *Drug Safety* 1993; 8: 225–234.

59. Bulpitt CJ, Beevers G, Butler A, *et al*. The effects of anti-hypertensive drugs on sexual function in men and women: a report from the DHSS Hypertension Care Computing Project. *J Hum Hypertens* 1989; 3: 53.

60. Chang SW, Fine R, Siegel D, *et al*. The impact of diuretic therapy on reported sexual function. *Arch Intern Med* 1991; 141: 2402.

61. Lim PO, MacDonald TM. Antianginal and beta-adrenergic blocking drugs. In: Dukes MNG, ed. *Meyler's Side Effects of Drugs*, 13th edn. Amsterdam: Elsevier, 1996: 575–628.

62. Katz IM. Sexual dysfunction and ocular timolol. *JAMA* 1986; 255: 37–38.

63. Grimm RH Jr, Grandits GA, Prineas RJ, *et al*. Long-term effects on sexual function of five antihypertensive drugs and nutritional hygienic treatment in hypertensive men and women. Treatment of Mild Hypertension Study (TOMHS). *Hypertension* 1997; 29: 8–14.

64. Mitchell JE, Popkin MK. Antidepressant drug therapy and sexual dysfunction in men: a review. *J Clin Psychopharmacol* 1983; 3: 76.

65. Clayton Do, Shen WW. Psychotripic drug-induced sexual function disorders. Diagnosis, incidence and management. *Drug Safety* 1998; 19: 299–312.

66. Segraves RT. Antidepressant-induced sexual dysfunction. *J Clin Psychiatry* 1998; 59(Suppl 4): 48–54.

67. Rosen RC, Lane RM, Menza M. Effects of SSRIs on sexual function: a critical review. *J Clin Psychopharmacol* 1999; 19: 67–85.

68. Hirschfeld RMA. Management of sexual side effects of antidepressant therapy. *J Clin Psychiatry* 1999; 60(Suppl 14): 27–30.

69. Gutierrez MA, Stimmel GL. Management of and counselling for psychotropic drug-induced sexual dysfunction. *Pharmacology* 1999; 19: 823–831.

70. Harmon WJ, Nehra A. Priapism: diagnosis and management. *Mayo Clin Proc* 1997; 72: 350–355.

71. Thompson JW, Ware MR, Blashfield RK. Psychotropic medication and priapism: a comprehensive review. *J Clin Psychiatry* 1990; 51: 430–433.

72. Banos JE, Bosch F, Farre M. Drug-induced priapism. Its aetiology, incidence and treatment. *Med Toxicol* 1989; 4: 46–58.

73. Keoghane SR, Sullivan ME, Miller M. The aetiology, pathogenesis and management of priapism. *BJU Int* 2002; 90: 149–154.

74. Burnett AL. Pathophysiology of priapism: dysregulatory erection physiology thesis. *J Urol* 2003; 170: 26–34.

75. Morris PL. Fluoxetine and orgasmic sexual experiences. *Int J Psychiatry Med* 1991; 4: 379–382.

76. Garcia-Campayo J, Sanz-Carillo C, Lobo A. Orgasmic sexual experiences as a side effect of fluoxetine: a case report. *Acta Psychiatr Scand* 1995; 91: 69–70.

77. McLean JD, Forsythe RG, Kapkin IA. Unusual side effects of clomipramine associated with yawning. *Can J Psychiatry* 1983; 28: 569–570.

78. Modell JG. Repeated observations of yawning, clitoral engorgement and orgasm associated with fluoxetine administration. *J Clin Psychopharmacol* 1989; 9: 63–65.

79. Butcher J. Female sexual problems I: Loss of desire – what about the fun? *Br Med J* 1999; 318: 41–43.

80. Gitlin MJ. Psychotropic medications and their effects on sexual function: diagnosis, biology and treatment approaches. *J Clin Psychiatry* 1994; 55: 406–413.

81. Pierce J, Rush JR. Case report. Cimetidine-associated depression and loss of libido in a woman. *Am J Med Sci* 1983; 286: 31–34.

82. Kirschenbaum A. Management of hormonal treatment effects. *Cancer* 1995; 75(Suppl): 1983–1986.

83. Martinez E, Collazos J, Mayo J, *et al.* Sexual dysfunction with protease inhibitors. *Lancet* 1999; 353: 810–811.

84. Colebunders R, Smets E, Verdonck K, *et al.* Sexual dysfunction with protease inhibitors. *Lancet* 1999; 353: 1802.

85. Sullivan G. Increased libido in three men treated with trazodone. *J Clin Psychiatry* 1988; 49: 202–203.

86. Gartrell N. Increased libido in women receiving trazodone. *Am J Psychiatry* 1986; 143: 781–782.

87. Shen WW, Urosevich Z, Clayton DO. Sildenafil in the treatment of female sexual dysfunction induced by selective serotonin reuptake inhibitors. *J Reprod Med* 1999; 44: 535–542.

88. Loh C, Leckband SG, Meyer, *et al.* Risperidone-induced retrograde ejaculation: case report and review of the literature. *Int Clin Psychopharmacol* 2004; 19: 111–112.

89. Shiloh R, Weizman A, Weizer N, *et al.* Risperidone-induced retrograde ejaculation. *Am J Psychiatry* 2001; 158: 650.

Further reading

Forman R, Gilmour-White S, Forman N. Drug-induced infertility and sexual dysfunction. Cambridge: Cambridge University Press, 1996.

Korbonits M, Grossman AB. Drug-induced hyperprolactinaemia. *Prescribers J* 2000; 40: 157–164.

Nudell DM, Monoski M, Lipshultz L. Common medications and drugs: how they affect male fertility. *Urol Clin North Am* 2002; 929: 965–973.

Stone S, Khamashta MA, Nelson-Piercy C. Nonsteroidal anti-inflammatory drugs and reversible female fertility. Is there a link? *Drug Safety* 2002; 25: 545–551.

Index